I Am
On
A Love Diet

Nicole Perry

Copyright © 2020 Nicole Perry

All rights reserved.

ISBN: 9798625088190

Third edition

Disclosure

Before making any changes to your diet or life, please consult your physician. The information contained in this book is for entertainment and inspirational purposes only and does not represent medical advice. Nicole Perry assumes no responsibility for errors or omissions in the contents described herein. Any events, characters, places, businesses, and/or dialogue are drawn solely from the author's experiences and thoughts derived from those experiences and any resemblance or similarity thereof is purely coincidental. The content within this book is not intended, nor should it be construed as medical advice, therefore, in no event shall Nicole Perry be liable for any special, direct, indirect, consequential, or incidental damages, or any damages whatsoever, whether in an action of contract, negligence or other torts, arising out of, or in connection with, the information revealed in her debut book entitled "I am on a Love Diet".

Nicole Perry

Love Power

The love power symbol is placed throughout the book, at the beginning of Nicole's personal love diet as it evolves, and at the beginning of a poem or haiku.

More importantly, the love power symbol is also placed as a signal to the reader that what they are about to read is based on the authors' experiences, and thoughts derived from those experiences, about living with anxiety and depression as well as being a suicide attempt survivor, and may bring out challenging emotions for the reader.

National Suicide Prevention Lifeline

"Reaching out does not define me as a weak person. It only defines a moment in my existence when I needed strength."

<u>*One does not have to be in crisis to call or connect*</u>.

Text CONNECT to:
741741
Massachusetts State-Wide Samaritan's Helpline:
877-870-HOPE (4673)
National Suicide Prevention Line:
800-273-TALK (8255)

Nicole Perry

Dedication

I'd like to dedicate my debut book to my best friend and husband Steve and to my kids with whom in each I have a favorite; Logan, Reece, Greenleigh, and Duke. You are the extension of my world, but also my underlying life purpose.

To my mother Susan, who has become an irreplaceable best friend and confidant. Thank you for placing that small spark of desire into my heart to write a book. To my sister Candy, and my brothers Scott, and Brandon, I thank you for your kindness, (yes kindness) and necessary laughter.

But most of all, I would like to dedicate my book to the people in the world, both old and young alike, who, like me, have struggled with body image, anxiety, and depression. My hope is to inspire you to find a healthier mindset and spirit—that you can live with—through sustainable love.

Table of Contents

1	The Immaculate Conception	1
2	Emotionally Consumed	43
3	Curiosity Killed the Mindset	76
4	But Am I Still A Victim?	101
5	Knowledge IS Power	128
6	To Carb or Not to Carb	159
7	Tell Me Something Good	187
8	Too Little, Too Late	212
9	Taking Back My Power	246
10	I've Only Just Begun	273
11	It's Time to be Free	300
12	Putting My Mouth Where My Mindset Is	331
13	What's in My Gut Could Help My Butt	357
14	Ignorance is Bliss	384
15	What Do I Want?	415
16	Embracing My Why	437
17	The Calm Before the New Norm	459
18	I Love My Diet!	485

Introduction

When the idea came to me to start this journey, I had no idea where it would take me. All I knew was that I needed to change what I was doing. Period. I was not healthy. And I wasn't loving myself nearly as much as I could have.

So, why did I continue to write and stay on this journaling path, even when many times I wasn't placing myself in a good light? Because I was sick. And in order to save my own soul I knew I had to strip away what I had consciously learned over the years as well as what I had subconsciously absorbed through the world and my environment. I knew I had no other choice but to start over.

Albeit there were a few health concerns within my body when my journey began, I was still not feeding myself nearly enough love. Somehow deep in my core I knew by sharing my story and putting my thoughts into the written word would indeed be one of the greatest lessons in my life. But more importantly, it would be the greatest gift I would ever give to myself.

Nicole Perry

*For 365 days,
I am feeding myself love.*

Chapter 1
The Immaculate Conception

"Perhaps there is a secret ingredient that most diets are missing—and perhaps that ingredient is love."

Day 1: 198 lbs. Wednesday, October 4th

I don't know anyone who likes the word diet. The word "diet" itself weighs so much more than the amount of weight I want to lose, and I tried to remove the word from my vocabulary too, but there's no other word to replace it with—we are human, and our diet is what we eat.

I had thought about creating my own diet and tried to once, but I was doing what all the other diets were doing by coming up with a "food" diet. One time I asked the universe to send me someone to tell me what to eat. This will be perfect I thought! Ask a skinny, healthy person to give me a daily menu. Be careful what you wish for: that person arrived, and it sucked.

I don't like to be told what to do, let alone what to eat.

I keep saying "I'm not going to do it," and then I do it—again. I go on diets. I work at eating cleanly and then I salivate when others are eating the types of foods that I wish I could eat. I say screw it—and give in to temptation. Yesterday was the last fad diet that I quit. It lasted five days. The stress of it has me holding onto at least two-three pounds I'm sure.

A sustainable diet is what I want to create for myself and I want my diet to be about mindfully loving myself more. I want to cut out the self-criticism and incorporate more love and positivity. And I want my diet to be realistic and easy for me to remember. I want to create a foundation to fall back on—regardless of where I am, whom I am with, or what stage of life I am at.

My diet is going to be a journey and I'll share the thoughts I have been conditioned to hear and believe, as well as my attempt to turn this undesirable mindset around. The effort that it takes to eat the right foods can be challenging as we get older, but I know that I am perfectly capable of sustainable and long-lasting change. We are all capable of moving in a positive direction—simply by loving ourselves more.

So here we go, taking a few glances in that rearview mirror, but mostly looking ahead, looking inside, and looking into what feeding myself more love will look like.

Just before my love diet idea, I quit another diet and subsequently had eaten two—I'm sure they were not the healthy kind—large muffins, due to a busy day, lack of time, and convenience too. I found myself in that starvation mode—twice. So, I ate what was available—a blueberry muffin for lunch and a chocolate chip one for dinner.

I AM ON A LOVE DIET

When I woke up the next day, I didn't feel that bad from those muffin meals and I wasn't any fatter. I felt a little free—like I could breathe. Still, I really don't want to eat like that or eat like crap every day. I know it's important to love myself and care enough about my own body. What I want is to get to a size that's right for me—a healthy size that I can feel good about and be proud of.

Becoming a size zero isn't my goal, nor is getting back to my birth weight. Currently, I am a size 14/16 and we all know the power in the phrase *I am*. Getting to a size 12 would be good; I have some great clothes in that size! Size 10 would be fantastic. I've got those jeans that give me the cute *Underalls* looking butt from the '70s commercial—ding-ding shrinks each cheek. I wondered if size eight would be too small. Now there's a limiting belief if I ever heard one. Much like my Baby Bear Dachshund, size eight might be just right. So that's it. "I am" on a mission to become a healthy size eight. I wonder what number my scale will show me when I get there, or if at that point, I will even care.

My husband and I laughed about those muffin meals and I said to him, "I'm going to create my own diet. But I need a positive word to balance out the negative word "diet", because eliminating the word altogether isn't realistic." I said, "I've got the perfect positive word, love! I'm going on a Love Diet!" "Genius," my husband said. "Pure genius."

So why hadn't I been able to do this on my own before? And why now? Because I am tired of constantly searching for solutions "out there", that's why. I'm not a victim—anymore. I am powerful. And I am perfectly capable of getting my act together and doing this for me. I can love my body today as it is and I can love it enough to take care of it, even more. There is plenty of room for more love in my life, and I'm guessing there will be plenty of room in my size 14/16 barely breathable jeans by this time next week.

Perhaps diets and even the good ones are just Band-Aids and not really helping me at my core. Perhaps the search for something magical "out there" is not where the magic will come from. *Perhaps there is a secret ingredient that most diets are missing—and perhaps that ingredient is love.*

I am on a mission now for sure. To create a customized diet just for me. And it's not going to be 10 days to a skinnier me, or three months of rigorous training, counting, measuring, adding or eliminating. For 365 days I am on a mission to give myself more of what I've needed for years. I'm feeding myself more love. It might take a little longer to shed these fatso cells, so one year might be the perfect amount of time to get to where I want to be. So, I am going on a Love Diet. And I can't wait to see what I will look like on day 365. More importantly, I can't wait to see how much love I will consume and how I will feel.

We were out of yogurt and I had no time to cut up any fruit. I was in a hurry and had to get out the door fast to a recording, so I needed something sustainable to carry me for a few hours. Toast was fast so I had two slices with butter—and a little peanut butter on top of that. It was delicious buttery goodness and it had protein. I had enough time for that, and I made it with love! Every bite was full of delicious love!

Grabbing a store-bought salad from the fridge to take with me I noticed it had that chemical cocktail dressing in it. But I had to throw something in my bag for lunch, it was only 258 calories, and for crying out loud, it was just a salad. There had to be some love in it. It was not 100 percent clean love, but I had to go. So, I took it with me.

Day 2: Thursday, October 5th

That peanut butter toast was easy and delicious, and I was in a hurry again, done. I remember several years ago when I was about 40 pounds less than I am now, I was talking, I mean complaining, about my weight to my hairstylist, I mean my therapist. And she said smiling, in her skinny voice and body, "I eat an english muffin with peanut butter every day for breakfast." I wanted to punch her. So yeah, I had what she was having.

Rushing home to make an 11:30 a.m. call, I opened the fridge to find a container of leftover broccoli. It was what I call fast and good-enough love, heated up with a little butter, salt and pepper. It was a healthy snack and I was grateful that I didn't overcook it into mush the night before. Al dente vegetables hold more nutrients, which is good for my body. I am loving broccoli! Sing it with me... I am... eat... tin... bro... cah... leigh!!!!!

We had a kid thing to go to, so we had to whip up something fast because by the time we would get home, it would be too late to cook dinner. Shrimp is one of my easy "go-to" meats because I can defrost a couple of bags quickly in the sink. And I enjoyed picking the tails and shells off those little critters. Those crustaceans were providing us with some fast protein love. I think I read somewhere too that women don't eat enough protein with each meal.

I was being very mindful while I stood at the sink and thought about my day prepping my little shrimpies. And cheap shrimp taste so much better wrapped in bacon! There was no time for a starch I thought, just some more broccoli with bread and butter for the kids. Eating starch with each meal used to be an intentional part of dinner, right? In the '50s and '60s, and even into the '70s. Now it seems like necessity we try to remove.

Bacon and shrimp were not allowed on that last diet I was on. But I thought what's the harm in a little extra fat since there was no pasta, no potatoes, and no rice. This was good love and I had three kids with me to share the love—with plenty for my husband when he got home.

When I saw the 10 toothpicks on my plate I thought, did I really eat 10 shrimp wrapped in bacon? We did cut each slice of bacon up into three pieces, so it was technically about three total pieces of bacon that I ate. And I think the average slice of bacon is only about 35-40 calories. I think it was fine.

Day 3: Friday, October 6th

It was almost 11:30 in the morning and I forgot to eat breakfast. The most important meal of the day—so we've heard. And I usually feed myself something at each start. But I forgot. And the only love I had fed myself was two cups of black coffee. Which frankly was love—because it only has one ingredient.

It was not that hard to give up the sugar after receiving that $2,500 bill for some major dental work that I had to have done. "You are coating your teeth with sugar all morning long," my dentist said very matter-of-factly. Fast forward six months and we had no milk in the fridge. I thought maybe that was my cue to go black and to never go back. Lots of people drink black coffee and I know my mom does. Maybe I could too.

I gave it a shot. It took about three weeks of absolutely despising my coffee, but I stuck it through. And one fine day I was finally free from sugar and cream. My coffee was delicious again. Black is the new black! Everywhere I go the coffee is fast, good, and easy, just like carpool karaoke!

Loving myself with two cups of black coffee each day on

my love diet is love! No need to write that down. Back to my immediate need for some breakfast I ate one of the oranges on the counter before the clock turned to lunch. It was full of delicious and juicy natural love. I was beginning to believe that this love diet could totally work for me! I wasn't feeling deprived at all. I didn't even feel like this was a diet. And so far, every day— I was on a fantastic love high.

Our daughter's dance practice was being moved to each Friday, so we decided to squeeze in some quickie date nights. "Yes please, I will have a glass of chardonnay, maybe two!" I said to the barkeep. The Ahi-Tuna is one of my favorites at this restaurant and it was delicious. We were both still hungry after eating our Ahi meals and still had some time together, so I said, "Let's get some stuffed mushrooms—with a side of truffle fries!"

Rationalizing is what I was doing, and I was imagining our food arriving with love. I had worked hard at this love diet for almost three whole days and I was more than halfway through most diets I tried. I certainly deserved a little treat. My eyes were alive and opened wide by the mushrooms and fries when they arrived. I do tend to eat with my eyes. But did those stuffed mushrooms really have that much of a hold on me? I enjoyed a few bites and the puddle of sauce that they sat in, but I realized that it was all "brown" food—so I gave my husband the rest.

Next were the truffle fries, which were yummy and so was the ketchup. But I stopped after eating only a few. A restaurant is the perfect place to ditch any diet, even a brand-new love diet. But tasting a few fries was good enough for me and I was ready to go back to feeding myself more love.

Nicole Perry

Day 4: 194.5 lbs. Saturday, October 7ᵗʰ

Two cups of black coffee were in, and I thought I would have the orange that sat on the counter. The one that clearly no one else was going to eat. I only needed something small. My son was home from college for the weekend and I told him I'd take him out to eat breakfast.

I thought for sure the restaurant would have some love on their menu for me to eat and they did. I was proud of my choice. I usually order and cook myself two eggs. But at my age did I really need two? "One egg over easy please and skip the hash browns," I said proudly. It was just a guess, but I didn't think there would be very much love in that side. Almost immediately I second-guessed myself as she walked away. But sticking to my plan was smart so that less fat would stick to me. I ordered a side of grilled tomato and spinach and I accepted her whole wheat toast and buttery side offer.

Ahhh butter, now that is pure love. We used to say to the kids when they were young; "Yes honey you can have another cookie. Food is love!" Then over the next several days and weeks we would elaborate on our clever inside joke and say, "Yes you can have more cheese. Cheese is love!" "Butter is love!"

Well, butter is love and I'm French, so having to eliminate butter several times throughout the years on my dieting journey was pure torture. Come to think of it, I have a French diet book collecting dust somewhere. I wondered if butter was allowed in there. My love diet will absolutely allow butter. Plenty of real butter—solid and melted.

Interestingly, I didn't feel deprived at all when she placed his giant apple filled waffle slathered in whipped cream on the table about a foot and a half away from my mouth. I was happy for him to be able to enjoy those chemical flavors and empty calories that he will probably burn off by the time he's finished eating it. Good for him!

Sitting outside for that late breakfast with my oldest son home from college was nice. We were both filled with love and left for some power thrift shopping. And we arrived to unload our trash—before going inside to collect someone else's treasures. I do love repurposing and I thrive on finding each treasure—more than the bargain itself.

Back at home, we shared our new thrifty discoveries and I said, "Yes hon, I will have a glass of wine with you." But it went down fast—like water, which was why I had recently switched to mostly red wine. It's full of antioxidants and I tend to sip it much slower. Well, two glasses were in and we moved on to more weekend celebrating with a glass of sherry.

Continuing the discussion about our genius discoveries I wondered, was this love? Was it love sitting with my husband outside on our deck on a beautiful fall day, drinking wine and sherry, laughing and relaxing together? Yes, it was love I decided.

For the evening we planned to visit my mother-in-law for a quick dinner and update on her surgery and recovery. I brought a restaurant salad for myself and two frozen pizzas for an easy dinner for everyone else. I looked forward to eating my Greek salad with feta cheese, black olives, chemical dressing and one of my favorite pleasures—pepperoncini peppers. Most if not all the ingredients were not allowed on the last diet I was on, except for the lettuce.

After stalking them while they ate their delicious pizza, I said to my youngest son Duke, "Are you gonna finish eating that one?" One small half-eaten piece would be okay I thought, and I certainly didn't want it to go to waste. So, I ate it. I love pizza. And I wanted pizza to keep loving me.

It was a very nice dinner and I saw my mother-in-law in a whole new light. She had good color, recovered from the surgery almost 100 percent, and she looked happy. She is more than my husband's mother I had recently learned. She is the grandmother to *my* children. And she gets an A+ for her grandmotherly love.

Shortly after arriving home, everyone wanted to watch a movie. *Popcorn would be involved.* Was that love? It was healthier popcorn, but it was microwavable. And I think I read or heard something about popcorn and microwaves being a dangerous new combination. Would I be loving myself if I ate any of that dangerous popcorn? Yes, I thought. And I had me some of that popcorn love in my new thrifty white ceramic portion control bowl that says popcorn on it. My kids told me afterward that it's the actual bag that's dangerous. And we put it on our to-do list to find a better solution so we could keep the delicious and convenient snack in our future.

Holding the substantial ceramic bowl was better than that of any plastic and I continued consuming my well-deserved popcorn love. Even when my bowl was empty, and I stole a handful of my daughters'. I was still consuming love—topped off with some squealing 12-year-old daughter love. We were all consuming love together. As I took a sneak peek around the room while everyone was glued to the movie screen—it looked like my kids had all struck gold.

Day 5: Sunday, October 8th

"Good Morning!", I said, with a sustained giddy high from this new love diet on day five. My energy was off the charts. Like an out-of-control toddler monkey in a diaper jacked on pop-rocks. "Pipe down, Nicole," my loving friends' voices popped into my head.

Spotting some bananas on the counter that looked so good and ripe to perfection I took one. Really, they were. No hints of brown or green. Bananas were not allowed on that other diet I was on—which was very confusing to me. How can something as natural as a banana possibly prevent me from getting my body to a healthier place or size? Why must we purge whole foods from our diets to shock our bodies? Why is the new trend to "shock" our bodies? What is not shocking to me—is the number of diets I was willing to try with very little success.

Starting each day with a delicious whole food such as a banana, is a great way to lead me to a new healthier size body—*I'm guessing said no diet book ever!* Thank you, God, I will eat your love banana and I will praise you with some lovely gratitude. Oh, this love diet is going to be so good!

A few hours had passed and of course, I was hungry again. My stomach was growling like crazy. Years ago, I learned somewhere that when your stomach growls, your body has no choice but to reach into its reserves, so it's a good thing to wait. Did I mention that the word wait is one of my least favorite words? I do remember telling that new magical reserve diet secret to my mom and sister when my two oldest were very young. What I thought I found was the answer to my prayers. Or the actual fountain of youth. I was not shrinking down as quickly as I thought I should after having two children and a second miscarriage at the ripe old age of 33.

I'm not sure about that reserve thing now. And I'd much rather listen to what my body is telling me, which is that I need to feed it. And I did. With some nuts. Another whole food that was not allowed on that other diet—at least not at the beginning.

It appears I have been conditioned and maybe you have been too: to believe that the only way to achieve a healthier size body is to shock it and remove almost everything—even the good stuff. But no thank you—anymore. I would rather take the slow and sustainable route. So, I put those love nuts into a lovely tiny dish that traveled from the lovely country of Bermuda and continued on my own lovely road, to my new—it may take me a little longer to get there—lovely size.

After listening to my radio show, we cooked an early family dinner and it was delicious. My husband made pork chops dipped in egg then cornmeal and grilled them with a baked potato side. We grilled some brussels sprouts too, adding shredded parmesan cheese toward the end and topped off everyone's plate with a bright red quartered tomato. Bright whole food—full of color—is definitely love.

"Make sure someone grabs the butter and sour cream, please!" I said, also reminding the kids to wrap up a meal for their Grandmother when they cleared the table. It was something I had thought about the night before—after our visit. And bringing her some occasional leftover meals filled with love solved so many things on so many levels.

There I was on day five of my new love diet without a single sign of guilt or deprivation in sight. I even ate that piece of pizza my son didn't finish.

Day 6: Monday, October 9th

I started my day with another banana, and then a pre-packaged strawberry Greek yogurt. You know the one with the paragraph of ingredients we can't pronounce. I do prefer to eat clean yogurt and add my own fresh fruit and cinnamon, but I needed something fast. I am not looking for perfection on my love diet, just progress.

The kids were home from school for the holiday and I had to remind them to eat lunch. I needed another portion of quick and good enough love for myself too. So, my son Duke and I had peanut butter and jelly sandwiches together. His eyes are big and full of pure fun love! The sandwich was one of the simplest things to make. I toasted some bread to make mine a little more grown up and devoured my childhood fun love sandwich with my lovable one son.

The clock said 5:30 pm and I realized that I had forgotten to take something out for dinner again. Planning and preparing healthy meals can surely help me stay on track. But it was too late for that. We each grabbed ourselves some leftovers and I popped a bag of frozen chicken tenders into the oven to seal the meal. I was very aware that it was an unhealthy packaged food with a paragraph of ingredients, but I was choosing not to read it.

A lot of ingredients are not good for me or my kids. When my oldest son was little one of his first teachers sort of between the lines suggested neurological testing. In our minds what we heard was, "please medicate your child." And what we knew about medication scared us.

About one year before that we did have a couple of evaluations at the suggestion of his preschool teachers and those tests went nowhere. They all said our son was quite normal and adorable. They would say he was so cute and looked like a little miniature Harry Potter. Long story short, we ignored his teachers almost retired advice and decided to keep on providing a loving environment for our child.

The food we feed our kids is part of our environment, so

we made several healthier, kid-friendly changes right away to our pantry and learned quite a bit through the process. I even typed up a list of the healthier choices we found that easily replaced the unhealthy packaged foods using the simple rule of fewer ingredients—and I shared that list with a few other moms.

Making a mental note about the chicken tenders that I had just served and eaten was good because we are all aware that jar food, canned food, box food, and frozen bag food is not the best food to feed ourselves with. One diet wanted me to write everything down into a journal or type what I ate into an app. The quantities, the ounces, the calories, and points. I even had to count the glasses and calories of wine!

Adding something else to my already very long daily to-do list would make things more complicated. Been there done that! I couldn't help but resist the very thought of having to do that again. What I wanted to do was to keep my love diet simple with one thing to remember—feed myself love. I don't want to track portions, ounces, calories, or servings, because in my opinion it all leads to more negativity. And it's time-consuming. It's also placing the focus on everything "out there."

Sharing bite-size pieces of what I am doing and what I want to do is as specific as I want to get. I could simply acknowledge that I ate a small amount of packaged chicken tenders on a small plate, with a small amount of yellow mustard to dip it. I was mindfully loving myself with food to live—and with what we had on hand.

Day 7: Tuesday, October 10th

My day began with a pre-packaged blueberry yogurt for some fast, easy breakfast love to accommodate the appointment I had

I AM ON A LOVE DIET

sandwiched between two meetings.

Ahh sandwiches. I sure do love them. Juicy ones too like the French Dip or Au jus. It really sucked that every diet I was on made me give up sandwiches or swap out the bread for an obviously even trade of lettuce. Eliminating bread was the sucky part. I think I'll keep an occasional sandwich on my love diet thank you.

On the way to my meeting, I ate a banana in the car for some quick stamina love. While it was not ideal to eat while driving, and I prefer to floss and drive, I needed to feed myself something to sustain my body for a few hours. It was day seven of my love diet and I was still high as a kite in love with feeding myself more love. As I got closer to the meeting location though, I noticed the drive-thru restaurant that I had visited many times in my recent past.

After the meeting, I could just get a small fry before eating my apple I thought. I was getting sick of apples. And I was eager and ready for a little treat. After that meeting, I drove toward that drive thru because I deserved it.

Pulling up to the stomach-candy menu I imagined how I would feel after eating those fast food french fries. Would I feel guilty? Would I feel like I had betrayed myself on my own love diet? Then I asked myself a better question. What will my body feel like after eating it? But I did really want those fries. It was almost my turn at the window, so I asked myself one more question. What do I really want? Do I want bloated, fat, greasy, french fry regret? Olivia Newton John is there something else on the menu that has a little more love?

I said to the voice box lady, "Oh hi, Yes, I'll take the chili please, and make it a large, thank you." I needed a little more love I thought. "Did you remember the saltines? Ok, thanks." Just a little more love would make my chili right. Halfway through the chili I popped the lid back on to save it. I was finished adding drive-thru burnt tongue to my day—and to my body.

My final meeting rounded off with an enormous unsweetened cold tea cut with half water. While watching one of my favorite reality shows with my kids, I enjoyed a few slices of swiss cheese and a couple of glasses of wine. Week one in my eyes—a complete success.

Day 8: Wednesday, October 11th

After working and plugging along for a couple of hours I wasn't really drinking my coffee. Had I only had a half a cup? Was I acquiring more energy organically on my love diet?

I needed to eat breakfast, so I made another fresh cup of coffee while frying up an egg and grilling up an asparagus bunch. A double pleasure was waiting for me with a scrambled egg leftover asparagus lunch. Yum. Double mint gum. It's chemical fun, said my tiny Forrest Gump voice. I topped off my open-faced lunch omelet with some salsa and then sour cream. Low-fat must have low love and I was glad to have full love sour cream on hand.

For dinner, I made pasta with mussels in a tomato sauce because mussels are easy to defrost. For myself, instead of pasta I shredded a raw zucchini that looked like green spaghetti on my plate. It was a great trick a friend had taught me, and I liked the idea. It was tasty and easy enough to do. I couldn't imagine living a completely raw diet, but one raw zucchini every now and again was close enough for me. I certainly didn't need to start another trend and fail before it ends. I liked my love plan.

We all rushed out to one of my kids' activities and when we came back home there were lots of dishes and pasta leftovers lying around. I started to pack up a nice meal for my mother-in-law and moved on to putting the rest away while catching up with everyone and found myself shoveling in several mouthfuls of the delicious, too bad it was cold, spaghetti. Was that a five-minute pasta binge? Five heaping bites were already in. I hoped it was a temporary love loss on my way to getting thin.

Day 9: 194 lbs. Thursday, October 12th

After the tiny pasta binge, I looked to see what crazy number my crystal scale had to show me—hoping it wouldn't make my hazel eyes blue. What the heck? I was down a half pound! Then I stepped on and off the scale a few more times to be sure. I stripped down and went pee too. Yes! My crystal scale was true. My body was changing. Loving myself more was working.

Giving up weighing myself once or twice over these past few years didn't really work for me. I tried to let go of that control. I thought it would be a great idea because it occurred to me that "watching" my number might actually be "keeping" me at that number. Did I finally have the answer I wondered? Was it that simple to just stop weighing in?

Long story short. It was simple, not that easy, and not the answer. Not stepping on my scale was a green light to eat whatever I wanted and to not care. It quickly became crystal clear to me after gaining about five pounds that I wanted to go back to watching and maintaining my number. Then I said that again in my head with my tiny Forrest Gump voice, "After gaining about five pounds, I went back to watching and maintaining my number." Cue the bus.

After getting my kids on the bus and before checking emails, I had breakfast. I wanted to be sure I ate enough to sustain myself for well into the late morning. I cut up an apple with my new paring knife my husband had bought me. Thank you, Ste-Bay. And since I was not in a rush, I topped off my apple with some clean yogurt, cinnamon, and some granola in my lovely bowla. What a great concept—put the real fruit in first before adding the cereal. And easy to remember.

A bad hair day was in full force and it was going to be a windy day—not a good combination. But I dry shampooed my hair to get through my morning meeting and then went to the salon. As I pulled into the parking lot, I thought about how ready I was for a change, even though it was my regular, I can't believe it has only been four weeks, gray cover-up visit.

The chatter filled the air about calories, carbohydrates, and grocery bills. Everything you could possibly think about was being shared and debated. To shake or not to shake was one question. What to eat, when and why, and some portion control exactamundo's. My mind racing over to Leather Tuscadero, Suzie Quatro's alter ego and how I missed my calling in a backup singer trio. I could have rocked those little outfits with Joanie on Happy Days and oh what I would give to have that cute little body of mine back. Even an older crepey, but wiser version would be better—smaller is better.

Sitting in the salon chair, I wondered who it was looking back at me in the mirror. Or where did that person come from? When I was in my 30's, in my mirror was a woman who wasn't younger or skinnier anymore. It was hard to see since I was coined "the youngest and skinniest" for so many years. And I stopped looking into that mirror for a long time, pointing my nose into a book before I got up the courage to love my hair salon reflection again. Which really wasn't love at all. But merely acceptance in disguise.

With all the conversations flying around I could hardly catch a point or concern. They were each feeding off one another. Then I smiled to myself and thought, all that noise was music to my ears. My love diet could solve all that intense exact portion control. Which brought me right back to my frustration.

We are all focusing on what and when and how much and how little and do this and do that. Some people are finding themselves in their own success stories which is great. But most women like me, have struggled—and are still struggling. What we need is more love. All we need is love.

What we need is to stop listening to all the chatter and stop contributing to the chatter. We need to slow down, get curious and think about what we are feeding our bodies. Are we feeding ourselves enough love? Is love even on the menu? Is love on our plates, in our bowls and in our cups? In some cases, is there too much love? We need to stop talking and do things differently. We need to stop falling prey and victim to every latest and greatest thing that comes along. Some outward things can give anyone a jump start for sure. But are those jump starts where we need to start? Is love even playing a part?

I think my love diet is going to help me tremendously. On my love diet I will not be eliminating good, nutritious, whole foods, nor will my love diet be a quick fix. It will be about incorporating more love and introducing long-lasting love that's sustainable. It is a beginning, rather than a means to an end, or a path to just another trend. I won't be counting or writing down any quantities or exact measurements. I won't be eliminating, introducing or combining anything—unless it stems from love.

The unknown can be scary, and I don't know what I will look like on day 365. The thought had also occurred to me that I may not lose much weight at all. But I only have one me and I only get one life. At the very least, I will love myself so much more on day 365 than I do now.

I want to face this challenge wholeheartedly because nothing else has really worked for me. Not in the last six years anyway. I am a little scared that I might fail. But my desire to make a change is strong. I am done pushing myself into panic mode just because I need to fit into a tight dress for an event. I am through with coming down hard on myself for not sticking with the latest fads and trends. My intentions are clear. And I am choosing to start with love.

I am sure that there will be plenty of moments moving forward for the rest of my life, that my brain will want to resort back to old ways and tired habits. But loving myself more will no doubt help me to avoid those old ways and lead me down a better positive road. I would rather focus my mind on loving myself more and as I am today. I would rather pour my thoughts and heart into love. It's kind a funny how all I seem to hear since I started writing the book are love songs. Love is clearly in the air everywhere I look around.

My hair was done and looked fabulous. Confidently walking out into the wind I remembered the little café upstairs and lucky for me I was starving. Although their foods are all prepared with love, I hopped into my car and went home to eat instead. I had one more event to attend and I needed to get some work done first.

Driving home with my great new look some things that I don't like about my body found their way into my thoughts. I quickly switched gears and focused on what I love, which filled up a little bit more of my love cup.

"Thank you this looks delicious," I said. Hors d'oeuvre number one was in. I was at a networking event and just as the second gal with a tray started to walk away, I said, "Come back, come back!" like Rose said as the boat started to leave right before she jumped in the water to get the whistle. Appetizer number two was beef somethington and went down the hatch with a small glass of red juice. It's not real wine when it's cheap my husband taught me.

Standing in a triangle discussion one woman shared her exact weight out loud enough for many other people to overhear. She went on to say that nothing comes off because she loves her body, that's her problem. I thought to myself, she might slim down if she read my book because if she does love herself a lot already, there's always room for more love. Just like Jell-O. I said, "Yeah I was 198 when I started my new diet," loud enough for the two people I was with to hear, and of course they didn't.

We have all seen and heard many success stories every day and everywhere, more than ever before. This person went on this diet and lost 110 pounds. That person lost 35 pounds by doing this or that. This person started eating this and lost 53 pounds. That other person lost 72 pounds and has kept it off just by doing this one thing. Most of these people are people we don't even know. Their stories come to us in the form of postcards that come into our homes or in commercials or on television. And some of them are real people in our real lives—which can be frustrating to those of us who continue to try, but I wondered—are those people succeeding because they are secretly adding the ingredient of love?

Trying something new does stick for some beyond the jump start. But for me, nothing has stuck. Except for more fat to my thighs and more jelly to my belly. I want to be that person that figures this out and has a success story—an awesome success story. I want a love story!

As I lovingly unloaded more positive energy from the evening onto my husband's plate, I watched him generously knife a wad of extra frosting onto one of the cupcakes that my daughter had made. Those cupcakes didn't even tempt me I thought to myself—several days later.

Day 10: 192 lbs. Friday, October 13th

I was finally over the hump! You know that hump where you lose a few pounds and you linger, and then one day magic happens to your crystal scale, and a new number takes the stage. The attention to love had paid off and my love diet was working! I was feeding myself more love and I was living my own amazing love success story *in real time.*

Waking up I immediately thought about the book and how I would most likely self-publish and enlist a friend to help with editing. This is my first book and I see it as a practice book, just like my first marriage. Not worrying about how I will publish, will undoubtedly help me to focus on writing what I am passionate about. I could figure out the editing and publishing part out later. I have a lot of lovely friends. And just by letting that go I already felt like a huge weight had been lifted from my shoulders. Which might be part of my problem. Pouring unnecessary pressure onto myself was senseless. And part of what I might have is stressed up pressure weight!

I got dressed into a cute outfit, styled up my new hair, painted on some makeup, and was off to my wellness doctor appointment. I was still on a love high from the networking event the night before and was almost uncontrollably giddy. I could feel the people in the waiting room stealing curious looks at the smile I couldn't wipe from my face.

After checking my blood pressure three to four times with no luck the nurse and I laughed it off. We agreed that I should come back another day or stop at a pharmacy and call in my numbers. I told her that I had never had high blood pressure before, not even with any of my four, full-term pregnancies. And we both assumed that her reading must have been wrong. Then I wondered if I was so pumped about this love diet, maybe that was the reason, we couldn't get a good reading. I shared some bits and pieces with my doctor about my book and suggested maybe that was why my pressure was high. I couldn't help but try to read her mind.

I was laughing and giggling throughout the entire appointment and she looked like she was trying to figure out if I had just smoked some pot in the parking lot. Then I saw that she couldn't hold back her smile any longer. My love high was officially contagious. It's legal and it's free. It's needed and it's healthy.

I am sure many of her patients would love to learn about my new love diet theory. And by the end of the appointment, they both said they would love to read my book and agreed with my husband's original assessment—that it was pure genius.

Driving home I recalled telling a few friends that I had been so excited about writing the book and creating my own diet that I felt like I might explode. After sharing what I had learned, my husband said to me, "Yep. You might just do that Nicole. You might literally explode."

It was scary to think that my reading may have been spot on. And I started to think about the things I could do to lower my pressure. A glass of red wine was a good thing to keep on my internal calming list as well as a cup of "decaf" chamomile tea and some meditation. Breathing, yes, I could add breathing to my love pressure list too.

YouTube informed me that there are many ways to help bring blood pressure down including mineral water with lemon, eliminating ketchup, and removing canned food. I could work in some of those little pressure tricks right away too, then get back to the doctor's office on a calmer day. I had that routine blood work to do anyway.

Day 11: 192.5 lbs. Saturday, October 14th

Sometimes I type, and sometimes I write, and on occasion, I utilize the weekends to get caught up with my daily revelations.

I was invited to a yoga class though and said goodbye to my keyboard for a few hours. It had been quite a while since I had loved my body with some exercise, and I was happy to get it in gear. I ate an apple in the car on the way and remembered to take my water. Apples are great—especially when it's the only food on hand if I'm starving. It's auto-magic whole love, even if you get sick of them.

I arrived at the yoga studio on time and we took to our positions. It can be awkward and uncomfortable trying something new, going to a new place, or doing something we haven't done for a long time. And I was not entirely thrilled when we were asked to face each other at the start of the class.

Really? Could this get any weirder? Am I the only one who feels awkward? Don't look, don't look, I thought to myself. Just pay attention to the stain on the ceiling that looks like Plankton from SpongeBob. I didn't want to look at anyone else's body and I certainly didn't want them looking at mine. At least not with any judgment or social elitism. I might fall prey to negative thoughts rather than stand in positive positions.

I wondered how ridiculous my body looked from the window to any passersby during that last pose I tried. My current size can barely maneuver, and my butt needed to keep kissing the mat. I wasn't sure if falling would have been funny or just plain embarrassing. But I sure did laugh a little bit, inside and out, during that yoga session. I was cracking myself up about how great my comedy yoga idea would be.

On my imaginary stage, I would place my yoga mat right next to the real yogi person. They would do the real poses as I attempt my, out of shape older lady ones. I think it would be helpful to a lot of women who may be holding on to that "what's the use" mentality and not want to go. And I think it could be fun!

It could help some women break through those barriers that make us cancel that session or not join in the first place. Frankly, it would help myself since I have the same fears and anxieties. The good clown deed of mine would still give everyone the benefits of the yoga session and make it more fun and entertaining. Turning any potential judgment into laughter is healthy. I certainly don't mind being laughed at especially if I am the butt of my own joke. And I believe people would be laughing, you know, "with" me.

My tree pose would turn into weeping willow in the wind. My down dog would become an injured dog, then lazy dog, and eventually sleeping puppy. My cat/cow would become peeing pig as I lift my leg and really work those outer thigh muscles that cramp up during sex. I'm not sure if pigs lift their leg or not to pee, but it does make me laugh. It would take Laughter Yoga to another level! So yes, I think my comedy yoga is a fantastic idea.

On the drive home, I turned my car around to see if a nice lady wanted a lift out of the sudden down pour of rain that she was walking in. I don't stop for every stranger, but some strangers are kind and need help. She was clearly grateful for the offer but appeared to be more grateful for the all-natural cleansing from mother nature. I could use a great cleansing like that!

Shortly after arriving home, the kids told me our dog was doing yoga too. I assumed she was doing the down dog obviously since she is a dog, but they both said, "No her legs are bent and spread out to the side." I said, "Aww she's doing down frog!"

After the yoga session, I was happy to find some celery in the fridge and... oh yes cream cheese! Cream cheese is a lost love of mine that I was thrilled to have back. It was not allowed on any of the diets I had been on for at least the last few years anyway. No bagels either—but I agreed with that. I looked for green olives to add and we had none. That last diet I was on didn't allow jar food and I had dumped it all. But mostly into meals for my husband.

I had no idea how a tiny toy knife got into our real-world silverware drawer, but I used it to spread some cream cheese moderately onto a celery stick. I ate two of them, standing in the kitchen with my eyes closed, savoring each bite with delight. Yum. I decorated three more sticks with the cream cheese and then some walnuts, my back-up idea to the salty green pimento stuffed olives. It certainly was after yoga love. And I had three more, satisfied with my cream cheese celery nut love lunch.

My husband and I whipped up an early family spaghetti Bolognese dinner. It was about three o'clock in the afternoon and I chose to eat the pasta with everyone. I loved myself with a smaller plate of course. We were eating and talking, and I noticed I was eating slower, which was a huge good sign for me.

Growing up I learned to eat fast, real fast, as well as to eat the good food first, before we got stuck eating the rest. To clarify, the "good" food consisted of things like english muffins, individually processed cheese, sugary cereals, and canned beef stew, just to name a few.

English muffin pizza with premade jar marinara sauce was another one of the good ones and the rest of the "stuck" food was having to make anything from scratch. Like homemade french fries from an actual potato vs. the yummy, already done for you crinkle-cut kind that toast up perfectly in the oven. The "stuck" food was basically what we had to prepare. Obviously, I know now as an adult, that preparing food from scratch is the best way to eat and to live. But as a kid, I worked in quite a few habits that I am now working out.

Our meal was finished and my husband and I each poured ourselves another glass of box wine before moving into the living room to watch a free movie. Earlier in the day we discovered we were bleeding money from our budget. We pulled the reins back hard and I was grateful we weren't bleeding love.

The movie was great. Especially that nap I had during the second half and woke up in just enough time to see the ending. I treated myself with a small ramekin of the kids' school snack pretzels. And then I went back for seconds. I knew it had salt, which was not good for the newer and higher than usual blood pressure. And they had a lot of salt. Had I suddenly stopped loving myself? Was I slowly going back to unlovable ways? Or did I just get sidetracked by letting an old habit momentarily creep back in?

Nicole Perry

Day 12: 192.5 lbs. Sunday, October 15th

I couldn't sleep and neither could my husband and I wondered how many calories we just burned. I wondered too if God would bless me with one more cycle for old time's sake.

Before anyone got up, I went into the kitchen and sliced a few ginormous tomatoes in half, popping them in the oven with a little olive oil, garlic and sea salt, a recipe from one of the many dieting books I had collected over the years. Pfft, salt.

It was too late for those tomatoes, but I knew I would get the hang of it. Adjusting to any diet takes time. Even my love diet. They baked for about 2 hours on low at 275 which gave me plenty of time to do some writing. After they were done, I made myself two slices of white toast with butter and topped each off with two of the roasted tomatoes. I loved myself a little more with a few on the side too. This was what I called yummy fresh oven love!

During some editing I cleverly changed the font of my love diet title to "frosting for breakfast" in my laptop document. I know—it's the perfect font. But the weird thing was, my computer wouldn't let me change it back or even change the text. It wouldn't let me backspace a single letter. Interesting. I am one of those people who are somewhat software challenged, so I immediately moved my manuscript to a safer location. It must have been a sign that the title was meant to be mine.

Once when I was helping a client with my top ten to-do sales tip guides, I reached over to get the list out of the printer and number six and seven were missing. It was very freaky Friday. I looked back at the computer—and numbers one through ten were all clearly right there on the screen. I thought how ironic. The universe just helped me to see where my client needed the most help! Later that day she confirmed it. Not being able to change my font was so similar and probably mercury retrograde rising love!

When the idea about my love diet came to me the title came first, and frankly, I told my husband that I didn't want to look online to see if there were any other diet books out there even remotely similar. I was sure it would just crush my lovely ideas. He agreed. There is no one like me and there are no two people alike. However, my love diet might just be the very one size that fits all.

There was a game on tv, and we were not having our usual family meal together. So, I whipped up a comfort food leftover spaghetti and meat sauce sandwich on white bread with butter. My family had given up on wheat bread, and whole grain bread too. They do the grocery shopping and as of late, they had only been buying locally made white bread, which I do love.

My favorite comfort food sandwich from childhood is a Spaghetti-O's sandwich—which I had the pleasure of having a few times when my kids were little. It's not a meal suitable for company as there is no graceful way to eat it and reminds me of its delicious sloppy joe brother. I ate my comfort food sandwich with the white bread and shortly thereafter felt like little miss fatty pants. Three times must have been enough pasta charm.

Day 13: Monday, October 16th

My day began again with another banana for breakfast and two cups of black coffee. When I realized my hand was stuck in the position of my mouse, I took a break and toasted up some more white bread with a leftover roasted tomato inside. I needed some crunchy fast love.

Fast forward a few hours and I wolfed down half granola

bar that I saw on the counter opened and left for dead. The kids got home from school and I was still typing away without a single thought about dinner. Quickly, we chucked some more chicken tenders into the oven since my husband was about to be home any minute.

While our delicious dinner was cooking, I printed the first few pages of my book and folded it to give it that look of a real book. I turned the pages as though it was already in print and then handed it to my daughter. Pouring myself a glass of chardonnay I eagerly watched her smiling eyes absorbing my witty words and very vulnerable thoughts.

Day 14: 194.5 lbs. Tuesday, October 17th

Early to rise for a presentation I happily hopped on the scale since I didn't eat very much food the day before and I couldn't believe that I was up to two pounds. This certainly couldn't have been anything I ate—or didn't eat.

Then I let the number consume me. Maybe I don't want to succeed? Or maybe God wanted me to come down off my happy go-lovy-high so I wouldn't have a heart attack. My husband told me it's not a heart attack I needed to worry about, it's a stroke. Well isn't that special. But he's right.

Obviously, it could have easily been the quantity of pasta I had been eating, along with the white bread. Was I thinking about love each time I was eating? I wasn't really loving myself, was I? Pasta and white bread were both full of empty calories and have practically no nutritional value whatsoever. I was doing a lot of rationalizing—more than I was loving.

Bringing my focus back on feeding myself more love is what I needed to keep doing. I had not loved myself enough throughout the years and I know I'm not alone. But was it possible that I loved myself too much at the beginning of my love diet? Or worse, was I crashing down from my love high already?

For the moment I wanted to get back into the swing of love, so I started by loving my hair into a fabulous look. Do I love my skin? It wasn't looking as good as it did the day before. I must have forgotten to swipe with my acne pads. Swiper no swiping! It's amazing how sayings from cartoons have stuck into my brain files from umpteen years ago. I hoped my dirty face girl habits wouldn't stick around like those catchy cartoon shenanigans did. Immediately, I fed myself some clean face love.

Since fasting would be involved for the blood work I needed to have done and I had early meetings on my schedule for the week—I kicked that needle down the road. I had a presentation to give and I was extremely mindful that I needed to stay calm with this new blood pressure thing. And staying calm was far from easy for me. I get so excited that I just can't hide it. And it sucked to have to stifle my energy. But I sniffed some lavender and drank some chamomile tea before my presentation and then after to keep my pressure in check.

Would I ever have to go on medication I wondered? And would it accidentally make me—I mean help me to lose weight? I was still doing it. Looking for something "out there" to fix my "in here." Becoming a healthier size is important, not focusing on weight. But just as the words landed on the page, I could see that I was doing it again. I was still focusing on size and weight, rather than love. What I needed was to focus on loving myself all day, and every day. And then my outward appearance would automagically fall into place. It just had to.

Was the banana that I ate for breakfast going to take me there? Tangled up in this web that I had weaved I couldn't help but let the number on my scale continue to consume me. Then I found something positive to cling to. My body may be adjusting and re-adjusting. My love diet isn't really a diet anyway. It's just a means or path to loving myself more. And so far, keeping it simple was the key.

<u>*My Love Diet*</u>:

1) *Feed Myself Love*
2) *Minimize Sodium*

With a little extra time on my hands, I popped into a pharmacy to get a pressure check. It was so convenient to be able to take my own blood pressure.

A quick internet search told me about 75 million, or 29 percent, or 1 in every 3 Americans in fact, have high blood pressure. OMG, there were six Americans in my household alone! I wondered about the rest of my family—and my friends too. My pressure was higher than it used to be. It was not dangerous, but it was higher. So now—I was not just on a new mission to feeding myself more love with a byproduct of fitting into a size eight—I was on a mission to getting my blood pressure straight.

A banana for breakfast and only one cup of coffee chased down with that granola bar followed by a chamomile tea, another banana, and another tea was a good start to focusing back on loving myself again. And instead of going out to eat for lunch I went home. Lord knows how much salt was out there. A spinach omelet topped with salsa seemed nice and simple enough and I hoped the salsa low in salt since I had already dumped it onto my plate.

The pharmacist had said my numbers were not that high and not that alarming. But it was alarming to me. I was proud of my normal numbers during all those pregnancy years. I didn't even have preeclampsia or gestational diabetes. I just had bigger than average baby bumps.

Since the blood pressure diagnosis, I could barely think about anything else. It was pressure just thinking about my blood pressure! It was what it was though—and at least I was in the know.

Peanut butter on a slice of bread would be enough of a snack before my next meeting to keep the hunger curves and my pressure levels at bay.

Day 15: 193.5 lbs. Wednesday, October 18th

Yoga and meditation are great ways to bring the blood pressure down. But for some reason, I had not made it a priority, yet. *I had not made me a priority.*

For a while, I had created a great daily meditation and yoga routine. But then I started to blow it off, again. I did have that pattern—do have patterns. We all have and create patterns. And I was still placing other things ahead of my own health, which I know, was not feeding myself love.

Pre-meditation yoga was a good idea. I started out slowly and introduced a few minutes of stretching then settled myself in to meditate. Each day I introduced a few more minutes of yoga to build up my stamina and desire. It was working but then the pattern kicked in again.

No longer did I have time for 28 minutes of yoga *and* 20 minutes of meditation. So as any smart savvy person would do I shifted and recalculated. I cut back the yoga to 18 minutes followed by 20 minutes of meditation. It was a perfect solution. I could do that!

Once again, it began to consume almost an hour of my morning that eventually, you guessed it, I didn't have time for. I began doing little things first like checking a few emails and tidying up my desk. And I kept doing just a few more things before getting to that workout. It didn't take long before I lost momentum and was blowing it off again completely—into three weeks or more of doing nothing. Not even the meditation—which clearly wasn't the answer.

Yet, I had another brilliant idea. Alternate each day with yoga or meditation! It was the best solution yet! So why hadn't I found the time for that? What was I waiting for? I didn't know. But I certainly made the time to spell out my day and accomplish some writing. I made some more time for breakfast with a yogurt and fresh fruit. And I noticed that the kitchen looked like an explosion, so I squeezed in even more time to clean that.

I had a lunch date to go to with my sister and my financial advisor was arriving at the house. Part of loving myself more was spending time with my family and planning my future. Exercise is important. I just needed to figure out what would work for me long-term.

Sitting with my sister Candy, I shared some of my book ideas with her. I thought it might be good to have someone to do this with, after a friend told me that she had people read her book before publishing it for the testimonials. What a fantastic idea! My sister was on the fence about the invitation though. She had a lot going on and wasn't sure she would be able to commit, especially without knowing any real details and all I could tell her was that I was feeding myself more love and that my love diet was a work in progress.

On my way home I spotted a different pharmacy and ran in to get a quick pressure check. They were old school though and the pharmacist had to search for a form. She looked past me with annoying eyes as she handed me the piece of paper and pen. Pointing to the chair in the corner she told me to sit, fill out the form, rest and then she would be right over. What I heard was "Sit and wait, and I'll get to you when it's convenient for me."

What I wanted was fast and easy and what I had was no patience. That seat in the corner looked like a tiny stage of punishment like an elementary school dunce chair from the early '70s. It looked like a shameful place to sit in this twenty-first century and it looked like a place for someone other than me. I rolled my eyes in the air at the sight of the unfair chair and I left. I know, two rudes don't make it right.

Later my son Reece dropped me off at a networking event conveniently across the street. I took the opportunity to entice two more friends to see if they would like to try this new diet of love with me. Not because I think they needed to lose weight, but for the testimonials. And accountability for myself.

Regardless of whether I have anyone on board my love diet train I still wanted to do it for me. I was not afraid of failing, because I knew that even if I did fail, with failure would come discovery. And I was more afraid of what my future would look like if I didn't pour more love into myself now. I wanted to succeed at simply loving myself—more than ever before.

Day 16: 192.5 lbs. Thursday, October 19th

My day was beginning ever so blissfully. I didn't know how it was possible, but I managed to eat a clean yogurt, print all that I needed to print, be still in meditation, get my hair and makeup done and have a few minutes to spare to stop and get gas. The universe was somehow in alignment with me.

After my meeting, I popped into a nearby pharmacy to find a wicked cool blood pressure machine this time. Nice technology! This machine was smart enough to email me the results or something—but I still took a couple of old-fashioned iPhone photos just in case. My pressure was better. I was no longer in the "high" range. Now I was just "at risk!" Whoo-hoo! Changing my diet was working by watching my sodium. Loving myself more was working and it looks like my future may just be—medication free.

I stopped to meet a colleague right quick before rushing off to a lunch 'n' learn and handed off some paperwork for an event that evening. I said I would not be attending, and a look of shock spread across her face. I kindly said with a smile, "Look, I shouldn't have to apologize for my absence. I have already been out one night this week and have another event tomorrow night. Tonight—I am choosing to stay home to be with my family." She mirrored my smile and nodded in agreement. And it felt really good to stand up for myself with love.

Day 17: 192.5 lbs. Friday, October 20th

My days had been filled with pure bliss. Every moment felt like love magnified. Even when driving down the highway all I could see was pure clarity and unlimited potential in my beautiful mysterious future.

Starting my day with me I got still in meditation. I drove to a coffee meeting and ordered oatmeal with fresh fruit, raisins, cinnamon and a touch of honey. Mindfully, I was being fully aware and present in each moment.

Rushing home for an eleven o'clock call, I found my package had arrived. The uncut tarot cards that I created had been overnighted. They looked beautiful. I poured so much love into every single card—all 80 of them. I wrote the copy keeping in mind everything that I needed and that most businesswomen needed. Everything I could think of that most women entrepreneurs deserved. I read each one slowly to find almost no errors. Excitement poured through my soul at the thought of the book being next.

My husband and I were sitting outside on our deck while I devoured the card proofs. We both had a home office day and I had an event to attend later that night, so we enjoyed lunch together outside under the warm sun sipping our wine grateful for the peaceful easy breezy clever swirl. My evening event was just as fantastic. And I remembered some of the cha-cha steps from my recent dance routine debut. Life is good. Living with Love.

Day 18: 191 lbs. Saturday, October 21st

On the weekends it can be challenging to meditate with all the noise and controlled chaos that fills our house, so I took advantage of my time by writing. And as I typed the word "yoga" onto the page, I realized it had been too long.

Letting go of the keyboard I hopped onto the mat, and worked in 18-minutes without hesitation, wearing my regular street clothes. I wondered how it would be received to show up to a yoga class in my boyfriend jeans with a cute pullover sweater. If I can do yoga like that at home, then why wouldn't it be acceptable in public? Obviously, I'd take my heels off.

Who created that yoga pants rule anyway? This could be part of my genius yoga idea, wearing jeans or even better, a dress. People could do their yoga and then go right to work. Good-bye pre-natal and hello pre-office!

After my 18-minute private casual comedy yoga session, I got in a little more writing and then met my mom for lunch. I had shared with her the beginning of Chapter 1 and hoped that she would want to love herself with me.

After lunch, we met at the jewelers. She had many years of experience in this department and I wanted her input on what to do with some tired and broken pieces. I hadn't been to the jewelers for a few years and we were both eager to transform our good, bad, and not too ugly, into beautiful brilliant creations.

I was so grateful for the decent dirty diamond earrings that would soon be mounted into a beautiful ring with a Peridot added to the center from my mother's bag of jewelry tricks. Peridot, Periwinkle, and yes even Perimenopause are some of my Perry loves. My husband thinks my love for the Periwinkle crayon as a child was me getting a glimpse into my Perry future. He's so cute. I can't wait to read his book.

Some cool jewelry made this birthday extra special and I continued to live my life high on cloud nine. My mom spent a pretty penny on me at this milestone and I was feeling pretty good about my age. I was turning 50. Mid-life crisis, pfft. My mid-life was more like a circus and the next act was sure to be the greatest.

I am enough, she whispered on stage behind the curtain I heard through the social media grapevine. I am enough too I knew, but I hadn't always felt that way. I recently shared on air, and in print, that I am a suicide attempt survivor. I was only 16 at the time and I only attempted once.

What I didn't know at that age was the amazing life lessons and experiences that I would have missed. From the excitement of receiving little raises and praises for jobs well done, to the feeling of accomplishment at my High School graduation. Then becoming a woman and experiencing marriage to becoming a mother while holding the memory of a miscarriage.

I would not have felt the heartache of having a newborn baby hospitalized, nor the fear of doubt sending a young child into surgery for his two eyes. How could I have known what my future had in store for me, or how those experiences would make me the woman I have come to be? How could I possibly have known that I would be happy turning 50, with those experiences behind me, and still so much more that I have yet to see?

When I was 16, I had no idea that I would experience so much love, heartache, happiness, and dismay. I had no idea that I would become strong and live through a lot with grace, struggle or even ease. For every experience, I am grateful. Even the not-so-great experiences, I am very grateful. Even this experience of learning what to feed my body, and how to love myself more, I am still grateful.

My husband came downstairs clean from his shower and asked if I wanted to go out for a quick bite. I jumped out of my chair and shouted "Yes! I will go grab an appetizer and a glass of wine with you!" My daughter laughed because of the recent budget lock-down. College seemed so far in the distance when our kids were first born, but it had finally arrived in our lives.

Everyone lives through it—or so we've heard. She knew I

was excited for the tiny break from the tight cuffs. Our budget lock-down had only been in place for about six days, but it was still nice to have a conjugal restaurant visit.

We ordered two appetizers, but I was still a little full, from the half turkey Reuben sandwich I had at lunch with my mom that had the extra thousand island sauce for dipping, that took a thousand times too long to arrive. I was surprisingly satisfied. I had a few bites of the first appetizer and let my husband eat the rest.

Watching a movie later I finally had room for a little bowl of popcorn. I mindfully enjoyed eating one pop at a time, albeit still the microwavable kind.

Day 19: 191.5 lbs. Sunday, October 22nd

Coffee was brewing and my kitchen was tidy enough. So, I snuck into my office to get some writing in. I grabbed a banana and settled into my document for several hours taking only a short break to say goodbye to the kids. They were off to secure Halloween costumes and asked if I wanted anything. I said, "I'm all set. Every outfit in my closet is already a costume."

Listening to my show we snacked on some crackers, cream cheese, and some tomato jam we picked up from the Cape, Yum. I went down to the basement while dinner was being prepped and tackled the dreadful room. Our son needed a studio apartment—stat. He was coming home from college every couple of weeks and the couch was not serving any of us long term.

The pork chop family dinner was another hit and I thought about how everyone would have their own separate space in our home, which hadn't happened for about ten years since our last child was born. People would ask me all the time,

"Where will you put the baby? You only have four bedrooms." All I could think about was how my Grandma Baker used a dresser drawer for one of her newborn babies. "It will all work out." I would say confidently. And it did. We turned my walk-in wardrobe into a nursery—and a few months later our baby came out of the closet.

Day 20: Monday, October 23rd

Hardly a sip of coffee in my system I noticed what I notice almost every Monday morning, that my house was a wreck. Even though I washed dishes the night before it was still a disaster. We had lived without a dishwasher for about three years, probably longer, which some think is crazy for a family of six. But a dishwasher doesn't collect the dishes nor does it load, or unload is what I say—mostly to the people who live here. I continued to kick that expensive can down the road, waiting for the day of fewer kids to create the mess and more importantly, fewer kids to help clean up.

Each day I aimed to start with me, so I chose to spend a little time cleaning up quietly by myself. I moved some plants, swept, and rearranged some furniture. I folded some laundry and put a few things away. It was as though every move I made was happening easily, efficiently, and quickly but in slow motion too.

I was being fully present. I had accomplished more in an hour and a half than I had all week it seemed. With a whole banana under my belt, I was ready to organize my desk. It is a great life, the life of an entrepreneur. Every day is mine to be there for my children and pursue my dreams.

For dinner, I made chicken marsala—minus the marsala. It was pretty good, and the kids easily picked out the mushrooms.

Nicole Perry

A glass of wine and a few crackers with swiss cheese closed out my evening and I quietly thought to myself, this love diet must be too good to be true.

Chapter 2
Emotionally Consumed

"From emotions—to eating—to emotional eating—at my age, I am still learning how to choose to rise above—from within."

Day 21: 193 lbs. Tuesday, October 24th

Sometimes I let outside energy influence the choices that I make. And I'm pretty sure I'm not alone here. I'm talking about emotional eating. It's so apparent in the aftermath but by then—it's usually too late. I know everything is a choice and everything I do is my choice. But still, on occasion I find myself consumed in emotions or wrapped up in unnecessary frustrations.

Ultimately, I end up shifting my own original intentions and sometimes pretty darn quickly too. It's like someone flipped a light switch that I wish I could flip back just as quickly. And it may seem weird to say—that it's my choice whether I let other people get me down or even heated—but it's true. Otherwise, I would be admitting that everyone "out there" has total control over my "in here."

I am still learning how not to let outside energy affect me. Unless it's good energy of course. And I am still learning how to look away and more importantly when to walk away. Regardless of whether the trigger is large or small I have to own every choice I make. *From emotions—to eating—to emotionally eating—at my age, I am still learning how to choose to rise above—from within.*

So here I was in a conversation with a person who was leaning toward the negative while I was developing a positive bigger picture. As I watched their sky virtually falling, I tried to catch it and cleverly spin it back toward the light. In the end, they stood even stronger in their dark room.

In what seemed like no time at all I had betrayed my own soul. And as most of us know—all energy has to go somewhere. I just needed to keep it from entering my atmosphere. But I let their energy take over me and my glass felt just as empty as theirs actually was. By the end of the conversation the energy that I attempted to help change—I allowed to change me. In no time at all I was all out of love.

Had my cup runneth over? I didn't want to be out of love. I wanted to be full of love and I want to effortlessly hold the power of love. What I needed was a protective layer of love. My current layer was so thin it was practically transparent—and evidently it had a few holes in it.

It comes easily to some to hold their invisible force fields high, but not for me. Not yet anyway. I wished I could be like Glinda the Good Witch who was quick to dismiss her wicked sister with a simple wave of her wand by saying, "You have no power here! Now begone with you."

Empathy had me visibly spent, so I said to a friend at breakfast, "What can a person do?" She looked at me and smiled knowing exactly what I was feeling. Waving her magic wand, she shared with me that black tourmaline stones can absorb bad energy. Ask and thy shall receive!

Did a potential solution just magically appear? Could black actually be the new black? "You can put it in your pocket," she smiled optimistically. I don't even wear black, I thought. But I smiled. Maybe I could slip them into other people's pockets... "It works in a windowsill too." She sold me. "You should try it!" Well, I don't like to "should" upon myself, but I was in desperate need of something fast and easy. Those magical stones might help turn my lacey layer of love into skin thick like leather. Naturally, I ordered a bunch.

Throughout the years, there have been many times when I've had more stones than two good men put together. But there have also been just as many times when my so-called stones had retracted back into their ovary positions. And retracted they were. I couldn't wait to get those new stones into my hands and give them a try. Even though it would take a while for them to appear. Snail mail on a slow boat from China is how they would get here.

Overall, breakfast was lovely, and I felt like my spirits had already started to lift. I had an egg sandwich with sliced tomato— on what I believe to have been whole-made-grain-bread. It was big enough to save half and trick my breakfast into lunch. I am totally loving this diet!

Later at home, while enjoying some leftover broccoli and rice for a snack with my hot saucy friend Louisiana, I noticed a plant had been moved. I took his plant and raised him two more.

My husband and I were having our yearly pissing plant match. He moves a plant to where the sun will hit it most perfectly and I move it to a place that is perfectly good enough. It's one of the ways I like to get in some exercise—and sneak in a hint of equality.

Day 22: 192.5 lbs. Wednesday, October 25th

It was about seven o'clock in the morning when I walked toward my car in the driveway and stopped short surprised by the sight of a deer. She was ginormous and beautiful.

She froze. I froze. And our eyes locked. Bambi placed enough trust in me momentarily to hear my whisper, "Awww, hi honey, hello." I was grateful to see her, and she appeared to be grateful for our pear and apple tree breakfast—full of organic residential love.

Shortly after that amazing deer sighting, I arrived at a place where gratitude was nowhere to be found. The lab. And I could feel the no cream, no sugar, and no breakfast irritability squeeze me as I entered the room. Keeping my lacy love layer held high I consciously let go of the brief empathy surge.

It was a simple routine visit for me so when they called my name it was no big deal to give in to the empty vile or the idle chit-chat. Aside from some extra weight that was no longer serving me I was confident my blood would come back free from any unwanted disease.

Leaving the cotton bandage on throughout the day like a decorative wound I waited for the perfect moment to rip it off with reckless abandon. Next on my list to loving myself more— a colonoscopy. And I hoped to manifest a lovely and gentle woman.

It might actually take the entire year for me to slim down naturally, to where I want to be. I had only lost a few pounds so far, which felt like it took forever. But paying closer attention to what I had been feeding myself was still a good thing to do.

Ideally, it would be great to shed about 40-50 pounds. And just a few short years ago—it was only 20. Deep inside my heart, mind, and soul, I knew I had what it would take to let it all go though. To rid the weight that clung to me—the weight that had a hold on me.

To have and to hold, for better, or for worse, in sickness and in health, one can pledge their faith to oneself. I was committed to looking closer at what I had done to what I wanted undone. After all these years, looking for solutions "out there" was literally the heaviest price to pay. And we all know there is usually a price to be paid—for anything and everything.

We had another plan to "talk" about our budget, which for my husband and I had become a code word for "argue." Our current budget wasn't working. Whether for richer or for poorer it's easier for anyone to embrace a fat wallet, than it is to face any skinny account. And boy we were stuck in a crept-up web of financial frustration. What we were doing was not supporting our relationship—nor our future.

My husband has always been good at the planning and I have always been good at the bill paying. Except for that time when I was pregnant and sent our mortgage payment to the cable company. But regardless of our pros, neither of us had been on the same page about saving. And I know saving and paying attention is love. Don't they say money is what makes the world go around? Money definitely makes our conversations go round and round—and yeah, back around.

Nicole Perry

Day 23: 192.5 lbs. Thursday, October 26th

Just before my daughter pulled away from our quick little get on the bus kiss—my silent afterthought was to say I love you. Did I say it enough?

At that moment I didn't dare say it to her, because then I would have had to shout it out to the other two. And they were even further away—which would have been devastating to their "she's not my mother" spirit. Sharing more love beyond myself was something I needed to do too though, and I made a mental note to say it when they got home—and more often.

Later that morning, the downpour of rain brought a little gloom to our meeting room. So, I played some fun music to lift the energy. And it immediately shifted as I clicked through some of my favorite oldies, disco, pop, and current hip-hop music playlists. Rolling my eyes at their eye rolls I said, "What? I'm just an average person."

As a teenager, I specifically recall thinking to myself how truly average I was. But in a good way. I was the average height and size and my grades were average too. I had average looks and even had average hair. Not too curly and not too straight. My family was not rich by any means, and there were definitely more that were poorer than we were.

I am still average in many ways and have probably gained the average amount of weight over the years for a woman with my experiences. Collectively, I suppose one could coin me as slightly above average. To this day though, I feel like I am just like the average person. I didn't graduate from Haarrrvid and I'm no dummy either. I've got street smarts and street cred!

What I wished I had was healthy body image cred. This world of diets and dieting is getting scarier by the minute moving at flying speeds inside the internet. I read somewhere that only two percent of dieters keep the weight off, which seems crazy. And the average person like myself is constantly doing whatever it takes—or whatever we are told it will take—to do better and live healthier. And those many short attempts at thinking I was doing right for my body had spilled into several years. God only knows how that translated into dollars.

How much money does the average person spend on weight loss is what I searched and evidently, it's a $60 billion business annually—just from us Americans. In fact, we are engaging in the diets that we think are most ideal for us and for our lifestyles. We are doing what we think will work for us and we are most definitely willing to try new things at whatever the cost. But aren't we all just lost and getting sucked into fads that may or may not produce sustainable results?

I don't think anyone who starts a new diet believes that they are at the starting line of their next failure. And anyone can see that a lot of people are not successful. All we have to do is take a simple look around. And in my case—into a mirror. If we were succeeding, we would stop at the finish line and more than two percent of us would stay there. We would drop down to the size of our dreams and move on with living our lives. Clearly, that's not what's happening.

Nicole Perry

It's not just me.

But like many I have looked inward often.

Self-criticism. It must be me.

But I am clever. I'll be better.

Self-sabotage. I hate my size.

I ate my size bigger.

We think we just need to stay motivated,

or it's our metabolism that's out of whack.

And we keep looking deeper—

for what we think we lack.

We hold our heads high on the outside—

in hopes that one day it will click.

And someday,

we'll find our own magical trick.

Back to real life I headed to my home office for the day. And the kids were home from school for at least an hour before I managed to peel myself away from the computer. Finally letting go, I let them know, that I was heading to the store to pick up dinner and a spota box of wine. (It's spota be in a bottle.)

Driving right past the store and straight toward the pizza restaurant I was proud of my takeaway surprise—for them of course. It was not in our skinny account, nor was the glass of chardonnay I ordered while waiting followed by the small salad with grilled chicken since I wouldn't be eating the pizza. Nonetheless, it was just another small price to pay, right?

Reality set in when I got home with the pizza. I caved within seconds by the delicious and oh so familiar smell. The uncontrollable salivating that was happening inside my mouth wasn't helping either, but I sliced a small piece into a clever, skinny little half and felt a great sense of pride. Then I wolfed it down like Dr. Jekyll ate Mr. Hyde. Did I even chew it? I picked up the unclever half and ate that too, shoveling it in so fast, that there was literally no time to stop myself. More importantly—no witnesses. *Awareness is the key to everything I remembered.*

Standing in my kitchen talking with my kids I realized one of *their* pizza crusts was in *my* hand. I stopped, looked at the crust, then back at my kids, then back to the crust. *Ahhh, the lust I had for crust.* Begrudgingly, I rolled my eyes as I put it back in the box letting out a tired and familiar sigh. Will I ever get the hang of mindful love? Am I addicted to pizza? Which also made me wonder. Am I addicted to bread?

Bread. Could I eliminate it, and would I even want to? Would it be realistic? There was that time when I thought about getting tested for celiac disease. It's the thing to do these days since a lot of people have it. But it was just that. A passing thought at what I could do. Our bodies do crave what we feed it, but is there such a thing as mindfully and moderately eating bread? And was that too much bread I had just eaten?

My husband sat with me unknowingly, as I contemplated all of those questions in my head—about bread.

Day 24: 192.5 lbs. Friday, October 27th

Was my love diet concept sustainable? I had only dropped down five and a half pounds in 24 days, but I had dropped. I wasn't losing weight as quickly as I wanted to, but it was happening. And equally important, my mind was shifting in a positive direction. I knew that I still had to be careful though. In the past, whenever I saw positive results like my crystal scale numbers shrinking or my clothes fitting better—it was usually an invisible green light. And you know what they say, history is the greatest predictor.

Prior to starting my love diet, I had dropped down a few pounds, a few times. Of course, I gained it right back. At one point, I had even lost up to 13 pounds. I remember feeling so great and strutting my stuff in my skinny size 12 very tight pair of grey dress slacks. But once again—I put that weight right back on. While I was sitting there watching my kids scurry to the bus, I half whispered out loud, "I love you guys." and wondered if this little five and a half pounds was really gone for good this time.

Most days, I plan to start with a quick meditation or a few minutes of yoga and have a clean yogurt with fresh fruit. But I've added writer to my gifts in titles. And on many occasions, I have skipped over the healthier choices—like exercising or meditating and reached for foods that take little to no effort—like eating a packaged granola bar. And that's exactly what I did. The granola bar was only 200 calories and it was effortless. Could it be possible I was spending most of my days—and years—making little to no effort?

On my way out the door, I saw my doctor's name flash up on my phone and the nurse informed me that my cholesterol was high, and they wanted me to come in to discuss it. Really? First high blood pressure and now high cholesterol? Doctor—my eyes have seen enough fears.

Ironically, the morning meeting I attended was a presentation about our health and the crisis our country is in—if we don't do something about it. Individually and collectively. It can be a challenging subject and provoke a lot of emotions, but the meeting was full of good energy and positive forward thinking. Even though I had just earned another strike against my own health—I am doing something about it. I am loving myself more than ever before. And after the meeting, a friend confirmed what I was already thinking. It all boils down to our diet, and exercise.

My theory was simply to stick with this love diet of mine and all my numbers would come down in time. I was sure my doctor would agree that they would get to where they needed to be—to where they used to be. And I was eager to prove my unwavering determination to get healthier and live healthily. My health is important to me and I was willing to avoid medication by changing what I was doing—significantly.

I'm not saying all medication is bad. I for one have been extremely grateful for the many times that I have needed it and my family has needed it. But immediately fixing either of these two new discoveries with medication from the get-go—in my opinion would be like taking a Band-Aid approach. And if I put that Band-Aid on right from the start—it might never come off.

Over the hill was not quite me yet. And I figured I could afford to take some time to change some things. The blood pressure and cholesterol were both brand new discoveries for me, and they were both still within fixing range. I am smart, so obviously if my numbers don't change after I change my diet a homeopathic approach was next. And only then would I introduce a synthetic one. Ideally though if I could simply change what I put into my body—my body would adapt.

I couldn't wait for my doctor to feed my non-medical mind and help me turn my numbers back into normal ones—with a little more time. I'm pretty sure my cholesterol was higher simply because of my age, but it's quite possible it had to do with all those diets I was on. I was eating a lot of eggs and yogurt. And my historic love for real butter may sadly have something to do with it. So yeah, I was pretty sure I could turn this around with some effort and attention—simply by making a few shifts to my existing diet.

We both sighed as we watched our two oldest cautiously drive away ahead of us. They were going out to eat as we were. It was an equally proud and scary moment like many other parents have experienced before us. And we both wondered if our kids were doing most of the learning—or if we were.

At our restaurant, I struggled a bit with the menu after sharing with my husband the recent cholesterol news. And it occurred to both of us that since we ate most of our meals together, he might be in for a rude awakening himself.

Day 25: 192 lbs. Saturday, October 28th

I did it. I loved myself on purpose. And if I were to give it a number, I'd say it was around 80 percent. I ordered fish and chips for dinner—a long overdue green light—but I only ate a little bit. Albeit there is evidently quite the debate online about whether an occasional fish and chip meal was, in fact unhealthy, it was still fried food. I enjoyed a few savory bites knowing full well that perhaps it would be my last before getting serious for real. The love I have for myself was growing much stronger and I felt super confident that I was going to keep off the six pounds I had lost.

My sister-in-law was visiting from Paris, and my mother-in-law planned a family dinner. I knew she would make it with love, but how much cholesterol was the question. And of course—she served steak. I couldn't remember the last time I had even enjoyed a steak dinner or a bunless beef burger for that matter. But surely, eating one last cholesterol filled meal would be fine—for my now pressure sensitive and cholesterol-filled body. Then I would get serious for realsies.

Day 26: 192.5 lbs. Sunday, October 29th

Each summer we take a mini-church vacation—confident that God forgives us each time we go back. This year we were off to a late start, but we finally fed ourselves a little church love. Neither one of us was raised with any kind of religious routines, but when we had our first baby, we knew we wanted to gift our children with some type of religious background. At least a loose foundation they could build upon. Unusually, the day we decided to go, there was no gospel, peace, or communion.

Ahhh, communion. That tiny thin round wafer that helps minimize hunger for a fast minute when you're starving. My mind wandered to the aroma that was filling up our kitchen at home. It was a delicious chicken, rice, zucchini, tomato, and celery stew. We all couldn't wait to taste it. And on the ride back home after the service we prayed out loud that our church would bring back the three essential ingredients that would bring us back.

Day 27: 192.5 lbs. Monday, October 30th

Our day began with a power outage followed by no school. I continued to sleep a little longer to make up for the several hours that I couldn't during the loud storm. Still, I planned to keep my doctor's appointment.

I was beginning to feel blessed for the new information I was receiving, but I was just not entirely sure why it was happening to me now. I had always been a healthy person and I started to assume this was just normal with aging.

It seemed like just yesterday when my husband had his blood work checked for that Life Insurance policy that we had opened several years back. He was so healthy that they informed us that he had been bumped up to athlete status. It was shockingly great news and certainly made me happy since I'm the one who feeds him. I must have been right there with him at athlete status too. Back then we were athletes—or at least amateur runners. We started running in 2010 and even ran together in our neighborhood on occasion—until I got sick of the spitting.

Tears welled up in my eyes as I struggled to see my family cheering me on when I crossed my very first 5k finish line. It took me less than 30 minutes back in the spring of 2012 after a few months of training. But somewhere along the line we both got tired—and just like Forrest Gump—we just stopped running.

Hanging in there a little longer than my husband did, I stopped shortly after I ran a half marathon in the late summer of

2014. I finished tenth… to last—but I finished. The crew had all but packed up and gone home, but hey, I ran a half marathon! I must have subconsciously decided to spend the next chapter of my life getting back to something a little softer—like yoga.

Shortly after complimenting me on how lovely my outfit was, the nurse took note of my weight and said, "Huh, I never would have guessed." She continued with, "You look more like 160." I thought, "Why was I even self-conscious about being up a half pound for the last two days?" Whether this was a true compliment or a left-handed one—it fed my doubt.

The fact that she didn't think I "looked" my size made me wonder if I should reveal my actual weight in the book at all. But who was I kidding? I had never had the desire to lie. Not even about my age—unless I lied higher. Lying about my weight seemed pointless, until that moment. Except for my driver's license of course. Oh, and that CORI form I had just filled out.

Receiving any bad news is just the first hard blow to one's ego. On top of the weird high blood pressure and my now unusually higher cholesterol my doctor asked me if I had something called Graves' disease. I said, "What? I don't have that. What is that? My last primary care physician said I had a very small thyroid issue. He said on a scale of one to a hundred, my issue was so small that it was in the five percent range, so I didn't do anything about it. And he was more hung up on the eight-pound weight gain back then, which annoyed me since he was obviously clueless about what menopause can do to a woman's body. Even though that was several years ago, if he said I had a 'disease', I would've remembered. Especially something called Graves."

She skipped over my resistance to the other issues at hand with her "don't kill the messenger" aura. Animal fats and sodium are what she said I needed to pay attention to and pretty much keep them down to a minimum in order to bring my numbers back to where they needed to be. I was happily willing to reduce and even eliminate just about anything to love my body back. So, I asked her how long it would take to see any changes and she said about three months.

I flashed my doctor a lovely smile of confidence, because for the first time in years—I had real information about my health and realistic goals to set and pay attention to. I had an important mission now—that I could stick to—unlike the fad diets that never stuck with me. I let her know that it wouldn't be a big deal since all of those other diets I was doing had me eating tons of yogurt and eggs and sometimes I was eating two to three a day of each thinking I was eating my way to healthy. I also shared with her that we didn't really eat red meat in our family. and preferred healthier options like chicken, fish, and pork.

Her expression told me she hardly seemed convinced. She must be a poker player. Then she clued me in about pork not being as healthy as we think and that an occasional tenderloin was ok because it was less fatty. "But I thought that pork was the other white meat?" I smarted her. And then I dug myself deeper and said, "And we eat healthy things every week like shrimp. I can definitely stop wrapping them in bacon."

As I was checking out, I said to the staff, "Really? The day before Halloween I'm told I have something called Graves' disease?" I wondered if receiving this information was what it was gonna take for me to get healthier. Any autoimmune disease is enough to give a person a good kick in the fat pants. In the car, I texted my husband, "OMG, do I have one foot in the grave?" "No, Nicole," he grounded me, "Graves is just the name of the person who discovered the disease."

I did nothing about the Graves and didn't want to—until I met with a specialist. Well, I did nothing except worry. But the anger I pointed at the messenger slowly dissipated from resentment into gratitude. And my eyes were opened wider than ever before. With that knowledge I felt powerful and helpless at the same time.

Focusing on the two things I could change—I thought about what else we could educate ourselves on, reduce or even eliminate. And I was already turning my "me" into "we" for the sake of my family. When I started this journey, I wasn't planning to introduce or eliminate anything—unless it came from love. And it appeared that everyone I love may just receive a few fringe benefits.

Pork chops, bacon, and sausage are some of the things my husband loves and my kids too. And I do like to cook and feed them what they love, but we had to shift. And my husband was dragging his feet to this new starting line. He had agreed with me that what I was doing was better for all of us, but he came home from the food shopping and "forgot" to buy the tenderloin. They must have been out.

My life was turning into an emotional health roller coaster. Was this just the beginning and was there more to come? I sighed when I opened the fridge to find something to eat when I got home from the doctor's office. It appeared that all the food in it might kill me. So, I walked over to the pantry. Nothing in there was going to keep me alive either. With my head hung low—I wobbled to and fro. Back at the fridge I finally decided on white bread toasted. It was the only thing I could wrap my brain around and added only a hint of butter then peanut butter.

Since the kids were homebound and I couldn't really focus on work I said, "Hey let's start making our little bags of tricks. I need to get out of my head and at least get something accomplished." After that, my daughter and I looked in the pantry to read some labels and see what we could come up with for dinner. "How much sodium is in that?" I asked. "A lot!" she said. I surrendered, "It looks like I won't be able to eat soup in a can anymore—or probably at a restaurant either."

Managing a deli in my late twenties I learned something very important about the bottom line. Salt and sugar sell. My daughter and I were both horrified at the sodium levels we found in our own home until we looked at the large can of crushed tomatoes. And then I asked her, "What does the pasta package say?" Done. My doctor said that hard cheese was better than soft. So, I said, "Chicken parmesan it is!" Pasta obviously wasn't a healthy choice—but it was the devil we knew.

My husband plunked into his TV chair and I sunk even more into my head. "You're not dying Nicole." he said and continued, "We're just getting older and we need to pay closer attention to our health." Right then a commercial appeared with healthy vivacious skinny white-haired people happily enjoying life, riding bicycles and climbing mountains at ages 20+ years beyond ours. They were selling medication though. And they climbed their commercial mountain in less than three minutes.

Was it all an illusion? Are there really people in the world that are healthy, happy and medicated? Could I be healthy, happy and medicated? More importantly, would I be able to get off the medication ride—if I ever had to get on it?

Day 28: 193.5 lbs. Tuesday, October 31st

Of course, my weight was up even more. "My weight." Placing the word "my" in front of the word "weight" was taking ownership of something I didn't even want. Was I the one making myself fat? Or was it beyond my control? And was I stuck at denial by continuing to feed myself useless worry? With too much work to do I researched nothing about Graves' disease, the thyroid or autoimmune disorders. I can only imagine what it feels like to receive even graver news.

When my previous doctor talked about my thyroid, he made it seem like my issue was nothing compared to his other patients. But I should have gotten a second opinion. I could have cared more about my own body. Instead, I complained about his bedside manner or lack thereof and wasted a bunch of precious time, years in fact, before finally replacing him.

Being blissfully ignorant is who I was and ignoring the signs my body was giving me was what I had done. When did it start? Age 40, 45? Which issue came first, and did it matter? Thank God I was learning about all of this at an age I could turn it around. I hoped I could turn it around. Had I taken a deep breath since the Grave news? Everything I was learning was feeding my emotions with additional stress.

At first, I practically laughed off the high blood pressure confident I was capable of fixing it myself. I knew I was using too much salt. And changing that bad habit was easy-peasy almost. The second issue about cholesterol added a bit of a challenging layer and knocked my confidence down a peg or two until I plummeted at the third news into the Graves.

I didn't know what to do about my thyroid issue—the real

health issue that I needed to deal with. "Deal with." I prayed that the Graves' disease would somehow be reversible and in time would be something I could look back at vs. become a serious obstacle in my near future. All that was ahead of me was still sinking in. And it was better to wait and seek professional advice from a thyroid specialist—before I scared myself straight on-line. I made the appointment and a colonoscopy too. To love myself more from the inside out.

Sodium and cholesterol both affect the heart… so I did a tiny quick search on that. I found that one in every three women die each year from cardiovascular disease and stroke. Those numbers were not new to the internet—just news to me. I really did think I was smart. I knew too much salt was bad. We all know that. But I never realized how much salt I was consuming beyond the table though—and beyond my own cooking control. I didn't think I would ever have high blood pressure or have high anything. I had no idea that my cholesterol levels were in danger. And it never occurred to me that it was possible to eat too much clean yogurt, pork or shrimp.

The short list of things I needed to avoid was simple. It's easy enough to remember without having to count or write anything down. And I was already minimizing the no brainer items right away. An actual list of don'ts was hardly necessary. It's silly to write down what I couldn't or shouldn't eat. And what would I write? No bacon. No yogurt. No soup for you!

Day 29: 193.5 lbs. Wednesday, November 1st

Stepping off my pity-pot I stepped into my big girl panties. After waking up, I found a little pep in my step and even caught myself singing out loud.

Was I accepting the Graves as a gift? A 'Wake the hell up—what's it gonna take Nicole gift? Halloween was over. I didn't die from nibbling on a few Doritos, eating three small slices of cheap frozen pizza, or drinking that extra very necessary glass of wine. It was sort of the last hurrah.

My journey began with the intention of focusing on feeding myself more love. And I kicked that off by feeding myself a few wellness visits. In turn, the truth was revealed about the love I was lacking on the inside. And it all made me wonder. Had my love diet become a medical intervention—turned confession?

Still, I needed to get back to my original intention. Which was to adjust my diet in a way that was easy and sustainable—for me to adhere to—for the rest of my entire life. The least I could do would be to avoid the foods and ingredients that were no longer serving me. And that simple step to loving myself more would help me realistically shift my mindset over the next few months until my follow up appointments—and beyond.

I can create something simple that I can live with—and something that I want to live with. And yeah, I want to live! I want to live a life filled with love and mindfully love myself more by paying closer attention to this one body that I have—in this one life that I get to live. My body and mind needed to be simply fed. So, cheers to the start of my love diet. And here's a second glimpse at the beginning of a beautiful relationship with food—that will lead me to a healthy new body filled with love.

Nicole Perry

<u>My Love Diet</u>:

1) Feed Myself Love
2) Minimize Sodium
3) Reduce Animal Fats

For breakfast I had a whole banana and two cups of black coffee. Following a meeting I had a bowl of granola with almond milk, a sliced banana, some cinnamon and honey. At lunch I made a simple tuna fish sandwich with a little mayonnaise on white toast. It was too dry, but I could work on that.

Dinner was at a networking event which was not very healthy, but not too unhealthy either. I ate moderately to make it just right. And since this was all new to me, I decided not to be too hard on myself if sodium or animal fats accidentally make their way past my lips, into my blood, and onto my hips.

Day 30: 193.5 lbs. Thursday, November 2nd

What I have are hopefully modest health concerns. And I wasn't quite sure what to say when it was my turn to speak at my morning meeting. I didn't really know enough to articulate what was going on with me. I fumbled through my one minute. And said next to nothing. After the meeting I was so tempted to cancel the rest of my day. I could have easily gone home and crawled under a warm blanket to love myself with a little thing called compassion wrapped inside a good old-fashioned nap. But I didn't.

There was a pretty big event that I wanted to attend and continued with my day by having lunch in the car. Another still too dry tuna fish sandwich was what I packed along with an apple and granola bar. Next on my agenda was a sales seminar, which was followed by the infamous happy hour.

At dinner I could almost see the sodium in the lumpy pile of gravy on my plate. I scraped it off to the side, avoided the mystery meat, and devoured the veggies and mashed potatoes. A few bites of the apple pie too. There was a slim-to-none chance I would win the award for my specialty show entry—but I remained full of hope. Just like that time I thought I could actually be the one crowned prom queen—at someone else's prom.

I didn't win first place that night or the merit award, but it was okay. I was already a winner at the suggestion to enter—and there would always be a next time.

Day 31: 193.5 lbs. Friday, November 3rd

I stuck to simple foods all day until it was time for our date night. And I thought it would be nice to order the baked fish topped with tomatoes.

The fish was delicious, but it appeared they thought I asked for a side of salt with spinach. I couldn't even bear to eat it. Interestingly, after just a few short weeks of being mindful and reducing my sodium I was already beginning to taste the salt in everything. Really, that side of spinach was so awful I wasn't sure why I bothered to bring it home because it ended up in the trash.

Day 32: 193 lbs. Saturday, November 4th

I made a delicious egg sandwich with a slice of tomato and added a little hot sauce while we all discussed the grocery shopping list. The kids were really starting to get involved—I'm guessing so we would keep purchasing some of their junk food requests. "Ok no more buying shrimp, bacon, or pork please and we need plenty of different types of chicken." I begged, "And please," I continued, "For the love of God, bring home an abundance of fresh and frozen vegetables for me to work with."

Later that night we celebrated one of our traditional "day of your actual birthday" dinners for my husband. And since pizza is always the most economical choice for a family of six—we landed at one of our regular go-to pizza restaurants.

One roll slid into my thoughts. I could eat just one roll. I had been so mindful and doing so well that one little dinner roll, house salad and a single slice of pizza would not be a big deal. I could continue the journey of loving myself more right after this special dinner. Heck, I still want to have fun! But what I ate were two rolls and three slices of pizza. Yup. I fell two rolls forward—and three slices back.

Day 33: 194.5 lbs. Sunday, November 5th

My crystal scale was beyond blue. I had changed some things, but some things remained the same. As in eating too much pizza. It's ridiculous to think that after eating a bunch of pizza and rolls that I would somehow magically be lighter. What's that saying about the definition of insanity?

Nonetheless, I moved onward and upward to cereal. I hadn't had cereal for at least a year after a good friend clued me in to how dairy could be the cause of my acne. Rosacea is what I have though, which is a tad bit more extreme than acne. If I were convinced that dairy was feeding the issues in my tissues, I would have eliminated all of it. What made more sense to me though was that my rosacea was instigated by hormones and stress.

I wasn't sure if I was consuming too much dairy, or that dairy was the reason for the acne that appeared in my 20's, came back in my 30's with each pregnancy, and showed up for the final tour of menopause in my 40's. But I am open-minded and removing cow's milk from my diet seemed like a good idea. It might have done nothing—but it could make all the difference in the world too. Replacing cow's milk with almond or any other non-dairy milk for my protein shakes was the least I could do, and I said good morning to my long-lost love cereal! I added some granola, cinnamon, a few yellow raisins and a couple of walnuts and I was in cereal heaven.

After approaching our bills like one would approach a wild animal running loose in the house—we started to cook an early dinner. Evidently, a little earlier than usual since the clocks had turned back without us. And dinner seriously sucked. Salmon, white rice and broccoli, oh why? Why can't I cook fish like a normal person? It sucks to be salmon challenged. And we all agreed to look for a few good salmon recipes to make it better the next time. I basically begged my family for help and wrapped my evening up with another bowl of delicious cereal to make up for it.

Day 34: 193.5 lbs. Monday, November 6th

I was having a good solid home office day, but I couldn't help but wonder if I was gonna be okay. I knew I wasn't dying and just needed to take the information in one bite at a time—but still, in my mind I worried.

Dinner sort of sucked again. We fought over some

chicken tenders, had plain broccoli and picked at the brown rice on our plates that was sticky and weirdly gritty. Uggh. I desperately needed to fall in love with healthy recipe cooking again.

Day 35: 194.5 lbs. Tuesday, November 7th

Some days the scale is what it is. And yet I still keep stepping on it. I pretty much weigh myself every day first thing in the morning and even before going to bed. It's automatic for me. Except for that brief time when I stopped looking and gained that five pounds.

My obsessive compulsiveness to see my number magically change is not good I know, but I still don't think weighing in is a horrible thing to do. To be aware is not horrible. I am, however, fully aware that my mind is still conditioned to look outward. I was still looking for a magic number to appear that would change the current me—into who I wanted to be.

The subconscious mind game I was playing with myself was not love. I knew it. I don't even want to play it. And I am working so hard to keep shifting my focus back to love and toward love. Perhaps someday, when my body settles into my ideal size, I may be able to auto-magically let go of my crystal scale. For now, I want to keep my numbers in check because it's the simplest way for me to measure—whether I get stuck or I progress.

It was early afternoon and I decided to unpack the crock pot. It's such a great assistant in the kitchen when I need to run errands. I threw some frozen cod into it along with two diced zucchinis, a can of tomatoes, some minced garlic and onion powder. There were not a lot of ingredients, but I knew it would make a delicious meal over pasta for dinner, because the flavors that were there would slowly meld together over several hours. And I wanted to make up for the last two embarrassing meals hardly worth mentioning.

While our dinner was cooking all by itself, I dropped my daughter off at her dance studio and popped into the pharmacy to get a few things. I saw a blood pressure machine and decided to sit down for a quick check to see what my numbers looked like. And they looked good! My OCD got the better of me and I decided to do a quick comparison.

October 17th results: Take 1~ 136 over 96 with a pulse rate of 73. Then I did a simple double check since no one was waiting. Take 2~ 133 over 98 with a pulse rate of 75. My heart rate was okay and within the normal range of 60-100, but I still had some work to do—to get to the normal pressure range of 120 over 80.

October 19th results: Take 1~ 131 over 91 with a pulse rate of 76. Then I cleverly tested out a calming technique. You know—to get a fake reading. Take 2~ 125 over 87 with a pulse rate of 69. *Interesting.*

November 7th current results: Take 1~ 113 over 83 with a pulse rate of 56. Wow! What I'm doing is working! I should have taken my candy and left the party, but I got a little excited. Take 2~ 124 over 81 with a pulse rate of 56. Then I got a little pissed… Take 3~ 134 over 89 with a pulse rate of 55. *Dammit!*

All-in-all it's just like stepping on and off the scale a few times or taking the kids' temperatures. I kept the one I liked the best. From simply being mindfully aware and making a few tweaks—I had dropped 20+ blood pressure points. It was so uplifting and was just the thing that I needed to lift my own spirits.

It was a huge sign of progress for me. My love diet was working, and I was healing my body from the inside out.

Shortly after tossing some mussels into the stew I realized that they may be full of cholesterol just like their cousin shrimpie and possibly high in sodium too. So, I asked myself a simple question. Could I let go of the delicious foods that I had grown to love over the years—if they no longer served me? Interestingly, not a sign of resistance appeared. So, yes. I was totally willing to let those mussels go next—if I really had to.

Day 36: 192.5 lbs. Wednesday, November 8th

Thank you, crystal scale!

Immediately upon waking up I thought about changing my 18-minute yoga idea to eight minutes and follow that with a meditation. But I didn't do either and fell right back into my computer.

Using my work as a crutch was an easy way to skip exercising and meditation altogether. There was so much work I had to do and there's always more. Interestingly, the good number on my scale gave me even more permission to skip the workout. But what I had really done was skip over loving my body.

Cereal had to be healthy and good for my body, right? Each item in my bowl was individually healthy and whole. Some things in it were common sense healthy like the oats, nuts, and berries. Yet there is so much information out there that contradict my instincts. Carbs are good. No wait, carbs are bad. Fat is bad. No, wait, fat is good. Sugar is bad. Yes, sugar is bad. And carbs turn into sugar. Wait, our bodies need some sugar. It's enough to make any amateur nutritional head spin.

Lying in bed at the end of the day, I realized that each day my intention had been to start with me, but each day began with dogs, kids, and emails. My office is where I was meditating so moving the location from where I meditate as well as when may just do the trick.

Day 37: 191.5 lbs. Thursday, November 9th

A few weeks ago, my son Duke said very matter-of-factly, "Mom you're just putting the word love in front of everything you say and eat." To which I replied, "Yes I am!" And then I realized that I hadn't done that in quite a while. I hadn't been talking about love—out loud.

Reconditioning my brain is what I was working at, which had not been the easiest thing to do. I had to sift through years of limiting beliefs as well as bad habits. And as slowly as it was happening, I was still doing it. My crystal scale was reflecting some positive change too and what I needed to do was simply get back to talking more about the love I wanted to keep feeding myself. Loud and proud. But it was already eight o'clock in the morning—and I was doing it again. I was putting myself last. So, I put money where my mouth was and dropped everything to meditate—before I betrayed myself yet another day.

On our date night, we decided to share a pizza. And settling on a topping took quite a bit of convincing. There was no way I was having sausage or bacon. And if my husband really wanted it, I suggested we order individually. But we finally settled on a large BBQ chicken. And after all of that back and forth, I wondered how many times did I really need to order and eat pizza as a meal each week?

When we got home, I asked each of my kids, "If you were stuck on a deserted island, and you had that one wish to order whatever you wanted to eat, what would you order?" One said ice cream, another said steak and mashed potatoes, and the other said calamari. Huh, interesting—each of their wish food meals were high in cholesterol. I thought my dream meal would be sushi, but who was I kidding? It was pizza! I was beginning to believe my love for pizza was slightly beyond normal—perhaps even qualified as OCD or OCPD.

Day 38: 193.5 lbs. Friday, November 10th

Fun fact: In my early 20's I was at a bar, (that's not the fun fact) and noticed a few started singing the lyrics to the Righteous Brothers You've Lost That Lovin' Feelin' song. I quietly enjoyed humming along on the side lines while my date was in the bathroom.

Standing there alone and waiting so long I must have actually looked like I had lost that loving feeling, because a few more people started to chime in and before I knew it—I was being serenaded. My boyfriend missed the whole thing. Turns out—he was in the bathroom doing drugs. So, I dumped him and quickly lost his "I can't believe you're a dealer," number.

Getting that lovin' feeling back is what I wanted to do so I dropped everything and headed upstairs to my serene bedroom to meditate again. And later that night I took my phone with me to bed. That way I could start my day with a meditation—before I even got coffee—to keep that loving feeling for myself alive and strong.

Day 39: 192.5 lbs. Saturday, November 11th

My daughter Greenleigh and I had quite a day ahead of us with a photo shoot and I made myself a simple egg sandwich before the long ride. Eating a good solid breakfast was obviously a good thing to do but I wasn't sure what the traffic would be like on our way there or on the way back. I brought two apples and a few granola bars too—just in case.

My mother had to take all four of us kids to a pediatrician in Boston once when we were little, and the waiting room may as well have been called "the torture chamber for children." It seemed to have taken forever and a day to be called next—which meant when the appointment was finally over, we were all tired and hungry. And I'm sure we were not easy to control and grumpy. In my memory, when we got back to the car, we all turned into something like vultures over an innocent sleeve of Ritz crackers. I don't even remember if it was a full sleeve or not. Who knows how accurate my recollection was, but nonetheless—perception may as well be the reality.

When I became a mother myself, I was very mindful of such potential circumstances. And I made it a point to always be prepared. But my kids are no longer newborns or even toddlers though. And it was probably not necessary to have food so handy in my car anymore. My daughter didn't even eat anything I brought. I was the one who ate one of the apples and a granola bar. Both unnecessarily on the way there.

We were exhausted from the day and my daughter convinced us to go out to dinner. Shockingly, we decided on pizza. I was smart this time though by filling up with salad first before eating my one proper ladylike slice. In hindsight it was hardly worth the calories or time spent chewing it because it was cold by the time I did eat it.

Day 40: 193 lbs. Sunday, November 12th

After another egg stamina breakfast, I made my grandmother's bread pudding recipe for an event the next day. It was not the healthiest recipe when baked, but each ingredient was simple and there had to be something to be said for baking a recipe at home.

Grandma Baker's Bread Pudding:

One large casserole baked @ 375 for one hour
6-8 slices of bread broken into pieces
3 eggs beaten
1 c. sugar (or ½ regular and ½ light brown)
2 c. milk
⅛ tsp. cinnamon
⅛ tsp. salt (#pinch)
¼ tsp. vanilla extract
½ stick oleo, aka butter pads, placed on top

I usually double up on the recipe too because every time I make it, everyone devours it—inside my home and out. Sometimes I add grape nut cereal, walnuts, oatmeal or raisins. And I have always skipped over the pinch of salt, not really understanding the point of it.

Spraying each casserole dish first, I sprinkled cinnamon sugar into the sticky pan. I hate it when I forget that part. Then I fill up the pan with the broken pieces of bread. Stale bread works as I'm assuming the recipe was born from the depression era.

The liquid goes in next drenching the broken bread pieces and I top it off with several pads of butter—and sprinkle more cinnamon sugar on top. It's home cooked, it's traditional, and it is one of my grandmother's love's.

Climbing the scale creeps up slowly.

A few pounds I climb higher.

Then I inch back down.

Nothing to panic about.

The next time it's higher.

It lingers there.

Then comes back down.

But not all the way.

At the beginning of my journey I had so much hope that introducing more love was the answer to my skinny prayers. But beyond the thoughts that have occurred to me—learning how to love myself all day and everyday—has not been as easy as I thought it would be.

Nicole Perry

Chapter 3
Curiosity Killed the Mindset

"She was the friend I kept close—but was quickly becoming the enemy I kept closer."

Day 41: Monday, November 13th

Over a couple of decades, I had a history of overindulging. Dating back into my 20's even, which has led me on the path to engaging in a variety of diets. And in doing so it became instinctual for me to always, yes always, do my best to stay away from any foods remotely appearing to be fun. Especially in public.

We can't hide our size. And if I dared to venture off the healthy eaten path—I felt like I had to stake an intentional white flag into thy plate. Yup, look at me, I'm overweight and I'm

I AM ON A LOVE DIET

cheating again!

Eating fun food was the obvious visual that meant I wasn't trying. Fun equaled bad. I was used to settling nearly every time we ate out choosing meals that I thought I had to eat, or I "should" eat. After all, I had no business eating anything but greens. Especially as I got older and especially with all the excess weight I had to lose.

Unless of course, it was pizza! Pizza had become the one indulgence that almost anyone could overlook—and seemingly without judgment. Pizza felt like the one exception that easily brought people together with plenty of smiles and forgiveness. Pizza also made me feel like I was choosing the "healthier" fun option. Don't we all play that internal rationalization game? All in all, reading menus had become a game of diminishing and hiding my cravings—to seeking anything more interesting than salad. Who was I becoming?

On this occasion we went to a restaurant downtown outside of our typical go-to pizza locations. It was one of our family's traditional "day of" birthday dinner celebrations and of course everyone at my table was eating the menu with their eyes the minute we sat down. They were all ready to indulge.

My desire to love myself more was quickly tossed aside with those salads by that good ole' American phrase we have all come to love called screw it. But why? And what was my intention? The Ahi-Tuna could have been a fun and healthier choice for me and at least it wouldn't have been salad. But I felt alone. And I was tired of being the only one who was trying. I was so tired of being the only one who cared. Caring was exhausting.

So, I ordered the Buenos nachos! There was some salad-ey stuff on it and at least it wasn't pizza or pasta. I wanted to work some nachos into my love diet anyway. Again, I rationalized. It was research.

I gave in to the temptation and ate into those nachos like there was no tomorrow. While I was chowing down, I imagined refining that 1970's meal into something better suited for this 21st Century. It would be more than a task, but I could help shift this meal to keep it in my future. Especially if it aligned with my personal and current needs as well as my family's not-so-great-at compromising ola-resist-once. And then I realized—this was quite possibly energy not well spent.

But I headed straight for that border anyway and began designing a healthier version in my mind. Perhaps I could create something even a little more ladylike too. Like introducing turkey in lieu of beef as well as finding organic corn chips. Every little bit helps. I could swap out the cheese for a lower in fat version and switch to light sour cream too. Both of those were easy no brainers. So yeah. If I made a few tweaks and introduced some portion-control this Mexican fiesta could be filled with lots of love—for everyone, not just me. But who was I kidding?

No one was judging me. But I sat there afterward and judged myself. Not just for my own weakness, but more for the stupidity about gaining the weight I shouldn't have gained in the first place. I had made my own bed—and it sucked that all I wanted to do was go lie in it.

Despite our happy occasion what I was doing was still eating emotionally. And I felt bad that I barely tried to muster up a hint of will power. We hadn't even paid the check and the choice that I had made was settling in and I was feeling sick to my stomach. *Having no will power was one thing—but having no love power was weakening.*

Day 42: Tuesday, November 14th

My dinner carried with me into the morning sticking to my ribs like a ton of bricks. I was slipping back into old ways and tired habits again—and fast.

Someone's leftover fries were in the fridge, so I tossed them into the oven without a second thought, placing them onto a baking sheet right next to a piece of pizza—and a large piece of leftover squash I already had no intention of eating. I was losing my desire to love myself more and sat alone in my kitchen blatantly eating junk foods. Almost proud of it. I knew I had to muster up some curiosity—to kill this old and tired lingering mindset.

Day 43: Wednesday, November 15th

Every now and again it shows up for me and usually when I least expect it.

When it comes to anxiety and depression, I do my best to work my life around it. It is what it is and living with it is what I've learned to do. It's part of who I am. What is refreshing to know is that nothing lasts forever. And the good news is—I always come out of it.

Yes. I used and use the word "always" here very specifically. It's a strong word and it's the worst word to use in any argument just like its counterpart "never". But in this context, it's true. The word "always" fits, because literally nothing ever stays the same. In that moment of melancholy, I felt solace knowing that my emotions would change.

And change is good.

Day 44: Thursday, November 16th

My son had a low-grade fever and a cough, so my energy shifted towards my motherly instinct—which was compassion. See, change happens!

Very appreciative of my entrepreneurial freedom I shuffled a few things around to stay home. Still, I didn't dare show how concerned I was because kids can smell fear like a good watch dog. And I think most mothers could probably become good enough actresses after a few short child-raising years. I got him settled in and then I felt a sense of stability, so I snuck in a brief meditation for myself. *My kids all need me to be healthy.*

Later that morning my thyroid specialist called and suggested I come in sometime mid-January. I asked her, "Are you sure that's a smart thing for me to do? You know, wait two whole months?" I was really looking for some more insight, so I emphasized the words "smart and wait." The look on my face must have been priceless when she told me that my file was stamped "not urgent". I was so tempted to hold her hostage with more questioning, but she sounded busy, so I booked the two-month appointment and settled for their waitlist.

Hanging up the phone I let out a huge sigh. It was less about relief and more about the amount of time I spent worrying and wasting my energy pouring "what if's" into my thoughts. My issues had all but taken over my mind. Regardless of how serious this disease was for me, having a health issue no matter how large—or evidently in my case how small—can introduce a lot of unnecessary stress.

Day 45: Friday, November 17th

One sick kid had turned into two which introduced more underlying stress. But we looked on the bright side. At least it was viral and not bacterial. And thankfully my husband took a home office day to help so I wouldn't have to cancel my entire schedule. Scratching off a couple of morning meetings I was grateful to be able to keep the one at lunch.

When I arrived, I was tempted to take one of my favorite Greek salads from the cooler but noticed the excess feta cheese on it. Making a slight shift I made a better decision by ordering a chicken salad wrap with craisins and pecans with a hot black tea instead. Great choices I thought to myself—and delicious! I was really getting the hang of this love diet.

Our kids were feeling much better too which helped me to feel more like myself again. The worrying weight on my shoulders lifted just a little and I took a deep breath. We kept our brief parent-teacher conference in the late afternoon and grabbed a quick bite afterward.

The wrap I had for lunch was surprisingly still with me, and we both agreed to order something on the light side. Beginning with a healthy egg roll appetizer to share, the greasy brown food wrap that arrived looked nothing like the photo. But I ate my half anyway and then searched the menu for a cleaner dinner item to make up for the egg roll disappointment.

A vegetable option on the menu looked good to add chicken to, but when it arrived my husband commented about how weird the chicken looked and his power of suggestion hovered over my plate while I picked at it. Finally, I asked for a side of simple white rice to disguise my funky white chicken.

Considering my meal was not very good, and I wasn't very hungry to begin with—I certainly did order and eat a lot of food.

Day 46: Saturday, November 18th

If we have free will—it will do its thing is what I learned. My only Reiki experience was just a few minutes and a few years ago so I was really looking forward to my one-hour session. I was such a believer and I was thinking of taking a class or two and getting certified myself. It was something I had sort of seriously thought about. Reading energy and then having the ability to clear it seemed like the gift that would keep on giving!

When I got home, I made myself a cereal snack with fresh diced apples and craisins before we tackled the bills. And oh my God, for the first time in ages we discussed everything calmly like a happy and proactive married couple! Afterward, we enjoyed a simple family dinner with salmon, risotto, and peas, followed by a movie. The Reiki must have spilled into my family—free will, once removed.

Day 47: 196 lbs. Sunday, November 19th

We put off—putting out the Christmas decorations again.

Looking for something to eat, it seemed like I had opened the fridge at least three to four times to grab a prepared yogurt—only to put it back. Not because of the chemicals—but because of the animal fat. It kills me now to think of all those days I would eat two or even three yogurts per day—convinced that I was eating smart. It was scary to think about what was going on inside my blood—leading up to my heart.

Day 48: Monday, November 20th

It never ends. The twists and turns our lives take when we become parents. The coughing began around three o'clock in the morning and the kids were homebound again.

We had experienced much worse with newborns and I thanked God this turned out to be a typical viral cold. I was grateful too—that their doctor patronized my plea and was supporting me. She helped convince my son that actually wearing a winter coat is important—not just having one. Insisting he start to wear socks was next. Walking back to the car I felt relieved that neither one of them had pneumonia.

We each had some leftovers for lunch, and I ran out to get their meds while they watched some good ole' fashioned cartoons and rested up. And while I was out, I bumped into a friend. The conversation began with kids and sicknesses but then shifted to our own health. And I shamefully admitted to eating some Halloween candy myself. Guilt evidently had more of a hold on me than love.

Day 49: 194 lbs. Tuesday, November 21st

Receiving some unconstructive criticism, a bit of rejection, along with a hint of abandonment was what finally led me to reach for more Halloween candy.

Yeah, I caved. The road I was on was a little bumpy, but I hoped it would be short, because blatantly I dove headfirst into emotionally eating cheap chocolate—again. In that moment of weakness, I was still mindful as I slowly exposed each sweet little treat. I searched the calories in a mini Butterfinger—only 33. So, I ate another, and another. Eventually, I sat there staring at all six wrappers on the counter in full view. The evidence was clear. But I looked past the negative and saw two positives. Ha! The candy was low in sodium and fat. I sat there and made a mental note of the quantity and calories but more about the emotions I was feeling before, during, and after. And what did I feel? Frustration, satisfaction, and guilt. And two out of three is kind of bad.

For years I thought I had an eating disorder. I knew I didn't have Anorexia or Bulimia, but I was sure I had a problem. Of course, I had a problem. Why wouldn't I have a problem? Don't most women have a problem? I know that I sometimes eat emotionally, but was there more to it than that?

When I was about 27, I purchased a women's size eight business suit. And while I was trying it on in the dressing room, I remembered thinking I was fat. The kind of fat that made me too embarrassed to come out and show everyone kind of fat. That type of fat that shamed me into thinking I "should" be a smaller size.

Most women have experienced the very same thoughts that I did and still do, and those negative thoughts of mine continued. Why wasn't I fitting into a smaller size six? It's what I kept thinking back then; that it was more of a respectable size. I knew I should have been skinnier even when I was—and I was positive something had to be wrong with me.

At an even younger age I had a barely-there one-piece bathing suit that still stands out vividly in my memory. Shifting my body in the mirror into the sexiest position possible I looked desperately for the positive. But the negative thoughts programmed in my mind were too strong. In that mirror all I could see was the not as good as, the bad, and the definitely ugly.

I never actually wore that bathing suit in public and eventually let go of it. Even in my 20's I felt better about myself covering up with clothes. At such a young age I was already finding more confidence—by hiding.

Day 50: Wednesday, November 22nd

Thankfully, my husband went to our last parent-teacher conference because I was not in the mindset of going out in public.

Getting out and about usually helps pull me out of any slump. And having human to human contact is such a great way to lift my own spirits. I don't even have to talk to people that I know. A simple grocery store line conversation can help bring out the smile in me. But I wanted to hide a little bit longer—to get myself emotionally stronger.

My spirits were a bit crushed and I wondered why was I allowing outside energy to consume me? Why was I giving my power away? I sat in my office and thought—what was it about me—that made me think I needed to stay in such a place of stuckness? This time I reached for some resources to help raise my own vibrations. No, not cheap Halloween chocolate. Essential oils, mists, and my new protective stones.

Beginning with cereal for breakfast I went through the motions of the day doing my best. I had turkey chili with a baguette for lunch, and a healthy piece of white fish topped with homemade breadcrumbs and a side of grilled brussels sprouts for dinner. It would have been a good enough ending to my day had it not been for the seasonal eggnog cake I had taken a few bites of just before heading up to bed. The good news was that I was almost back on track.

Day 51: *195 lbs. Thursday, November 23rd*

When I went to bed, I could feel my grey skies sort of lifting and when I woke up—they actually did. Ironically, an older song entered my head. "Grey skies are gonna clear up, put on a happy face..." Humming the lyrics as I made my way over to the coffee machine, I sang a little bit out loud and naturally had to YouTube it. Dick Van Dyke and the lovely Janet Leigh.

Thanksgiving had arrived and I was thankful. I was also very aware of what can potentially be consumed during a typical holiday and I was grateful to have created a protective love diet for myself.

Because I tend to eat emotionally, I paid remarkably close attention to everything I ate and drank and more importantly to how I felt each step of the way. Was emotional eating my problem? And was I a binge eater too? I wondered if emotional binge eating was an actual eating disorder. A quick search told me that Anorexia, Bulimia and Binge Eating are in fact, the three eating disorders. Interesting.

After all these years of assuming I had an eating disorder, had I finally acquired one? I'm not sure that eating six mini Halloween candies in one sitting qualified as "binge-eating" or nibbling on some cake without getting a plate. But merely getting curious was important. Awareness is the key to everything, and we all know that acceptance is the first step. Or is it?

I was very proud of myself for eating really well on one of the easiest days of the year to say screw it. I was mindfully aware all day. I sipped on a couple of glasses of wine and I was very reasonable with my portion controls. Especially since I had a plate full of six sides, gravy, and a hanging off the edge roll.

My Thanksgiving rounded off with some shopping in my

mother's closet and the additional necessary room of hers. And I also I learned from my brothers during dinner that mussels and clams are actually superfoods.

Everyone was in good spirits throughout the day and I have to admit, it was one of the best family holiday dinners ever.

Day 52: Friday, November 24th

Decorating is one of the ways I like to sneak in some exercise. When I get on a roll, I just go, go, go, and it seems like I can practically move mountains.

When I was about 36, I actually moved a large love seat up a short flight of stairs—alone. It was a mini-mountain and I sure did move it! Never underestimate the power of a willful woman right? I'd love to have that ambition again and I tried to manifest it by spending a good portion of my Black Friday cleaning my beloved built-in living room bookshelves. They needed a good fall cleaning and I thought I might as well move my body. It's also a great way to love my house again.

When I get on a roll cleaning like that, I can get so consumed with the task at hand I can forget to eat. Sometimes I can work my body into such a state of hunger—that I have to force myself to stop what I am doing just to eat something, just so I won't pass out. It's such a beautiful feeling. To not have my mind consumed and controlled by food.

Day 53: Saturday, November 25th

No surprise. I was the last to get sick and woke up with the kids' cold. But I refused to stay in bed.

It was my birthday and a big one. But 50 really is the new

40 and might even be considered the new 30. I felt a lot younger than I was anyway. Except for the cold that was kicking my butt. And except for when I got on the floor to organize my living room bookshelves and got stuck in the sitting position. Other than that—I felt pretty young!

For my 50th birthday breakfast my husband and the kids made me an egg on toast with some delicious leftover roasted veggies on the side from Thanksgiving. I felt so happy and blessed. But come to think of it—I felt happy and blessed most days. And it didn't even feel like my birthday, which could be part of my problem. Maybe I was treating each day like it was a holiday. A reason to cheat when I eat holiday.

Meeting a friend for lunch, I made a good enough choice and ordered the squash soup, a baguette with butter and a hot green tea—completely forgetting about my built-in no soup love diet rule but I let it go because I was sick.

When I got up from our booth to leave, I noticed that it felt like I had pulled something in my back. Of course, I dismissed it. I spent the next few hours thrift shopping with my daughter and when I was loading the car, I felt my knee pop. Of course, with so much to do—I dismissed that too.

We all went out for my "day of" traditional birthday family dinner. And what I really needed was love in the form of comfort food. I ordered the chicken alfredo with broccoli. It had only been about a month into my new cholesterol regime and I was still trying to let go of foods that were no longer serving me. The chicken alfredo was not part of my love diet with all of that salt and fat, but I was sick. So, I mindfully ate it slowly and packed up half to go.

Day 54: Sunday, November 26th

The kids all helped string the lights outside and as sick as I was, I had to run out there and give them some guidance.

Running in from the cold I warmed myself up with another egg over easy nestled in the roasted veggies. Throughout the day we continued with our Christmas decorating and pulled out the last of the pork chops from the freezer for dinner. I wasn't exactly sure if my husband was somehow sneaking pork chops into the house, so point blank, I asked if he was hoarding pork. He assured me that he was not and genuinely said he was appreciative of all that I had learned and was sharing with him about pork not really being the other white meat.

He is all about taking preventative measures when it comes to his health and said he was completely on board and following my lead. We paired the last of the fatty proteins with one of my favorites—some leftover mashed carrots and turnips from Thanksgiving. A traditional family holiday recipe from my French side—naturally traditious.

When we pulled into the driveway a few days later, the lights that decorated our home looked like they were completed by underpaid and underqualified children.

Day 55: Monday, November 27th

The meds I took did not seem to work at all because basically I slept like crap. I tossed and turned all night while being nudged a bunch of times for snoring. I wished I could have stayed in bed for several more hours, but everyone's alarm clocks were going off—one by one. Five in total and to the point I didn't even need one.

I got up and showered immediately to feel better. I wanted to get in a crystal scale check anyway before I consumed even a drop of coffee. Most people drop down in weight when they get sick, but not me. I'm apparently one of those people that has a body designed to hold onto *every last bit of fat* at every chance it gets. I was under the weather and it was just Thanksgiving, but I was really bummed by the number revealed by crystal. *She was the friend I kept close—but was quickly becoming the enemy I kept closer.*

Thinking positively, I moved on and started my day with a clean slate—a small bowl of cereal. The thought crept up on me again that I may regret sharing my actual weight in this book—let alone all of these vulnerable thoughts and feelings. What if I hardly lose any weight on my made-up love diet? What if it doesn't work? What if love isn't the answer?

Day 56: Tuesday, November 28th

Getting back on track with breakfast I grabbed my Vitamin D's and multivitamin. It's another great way to love myself and I had been forgetting.

I get nauseous if I don't eat vitamins with a meal, which does take a little effort to coordinate. Not that much effort but some. And I mostly forget. Each day they sit in their pretty little pill-popping dish and I somehow get side-tracked. Before I know it, the next day appears. It's one of my fears—the medication thing—I can't even remember to take a vitamin!

Just then the phone rang, and my attention was diverted again. A thyroid appointment had opened up and I wished I could have gone. But there was no way I would have been able to run out the door in less than 10 minutes—even if I wasn't sick. I chose to love my body and stay inside my nice warm home and rest. I did, however, drop everything to meditate for the first time in about a week.

It appears that when I remove carbs from my diet, my body seems to go into some kind of starvation mode thing and holds on to *every last bit of carb storing fat*. On the flip side, when I eat carbs, my body seems to go into some kind of packing it on mode thing and *welcomes even more carb storing fat*. Am I damned if I do, or damned if I don't? I think I read somewhere that eating carbs before noon or two o'clock is best. Maybe this could be something to test.

<u>My Love Diet</u>:

1) Feed Myself Love
2) Minimize Sodium
3) Reduce Animal Fats
4) Reduce/Remove Carbs After 12 or 2pm

Just before heading out to a board meeting, I stuck a sticky note to the fridge with my four-item love diet list directly under my sign that says; *Having no plan, is the same as planning to fail.*

Day 57: Wednesday, November 29th

It probably would have been a better idea to stay home and miss that board meeting. I woke up feeling sicker on day five than any other previous day.

I came down to the kitchen in the morning and lost all

patience at the sight of the mess and the lack of chore support. Especially when I needed it most. Snapping at my children I barked out a few ridiculous new rules then guiltily sent them on their way to the bus.

Leftover white cod with stuffing and brussels sprouts was a great quick lunch on a small plate. My healthy lunch choice was immediately followed by three—I feel like crap and want something sweet—Halloween chocolates. Of course, they were minis. But they were not on my love diet list. That list that was on the fridge and nowhere near the bowl of candy.

On day 57 I had not loved myself all day every day, yet. I was under the weather so it wouldn't have been fair to beat myself up too much. I made myself a lovely green tea flavored with pomegranate to get back to loving myself more. There were 308 days left of my love diet to go. I had a really great start followed by a rough couple of weeks. So, I loved myself with a little more compassion.

Day 58: 196.5 lbs. Thursday, November 30th

I woke up even sicker sneezing and coughing. I was a giant mess all morning. And it was the ideal time to make myself an early lunch with some good old-fashioned chicken noodle soup.

In my pantry was a tiny can that was ridiculously high in sodium. And then I thought about going out and picking up some fresh ingredients to make a really healthy soup almost from scratch. Could I get away with crawling into the store looking like death warmed over though? I spent all the energy I had taking myself there in my mind but lazily, I opened the can.

Then my brain woke up. It was condensed. The label said

37 percent of the recommended allotted sodium per serving *for the day.* And there were two and a half servings in the can, which almost equaled one full days' worth. After doing the math, I did the smart thing and quadrupled the amount of water even more to stretch my soup into the evening to be sodium safe. Damn I'm smart!

Day 59: Friday, December 1st

Working through any sickness just plain sucks but I managed to get ready in time and still squeeze in a quick bowl of cereal before leaving the house. I gave myself permission to eat a granola bar too, for some extra stamina. It's exhausting to keep my energy up on this hell of a sick road. Equipment, texting, and recordings oh my!

During a session with one of my therapists several years ago I was educated on a thing called chaining and was figuratively slapped for doing it. Chaining is when you list a bunch of issues one after the other and together, the several small challenges can make for a strong and powerful chain. Which of course makes it harder to break free from and on occasion I still find myself chaining. I knew it was keeping me stuck in my own little victim mode, but I had reached my threshold.

It appeared I could tolerate no more. So, to help you gain some perspective—here's my chain gang: I had been diagnosed with higher than usual blood pressure, high cholesterol levels too, and a thyroid condition called Graves' disease. Underneath all that, I was at the height of menopause and had been spotting for well over 40 days. I had a cold that was kicking my butt, a strange pain that erupted in my back and a weird knee popping thing that was also happening. I had a husband that was not thrilled about planning my "surprise" 50th birthday party, or at least not happy about paying for it, and my kids were avoiding chores like the plague. Oh, and I had just turned 50.

Something had to give—which was code for—the people in my home needed to give. And they weren't. So, I snapped. I screamed at everyone into listening. Which they finally did. And I demanded that everyone pitch in. And they did. But it wasn't pretty.

It was what it was. So, was my outburst menopause or thyroid based? Or did it matter? It's really not a huge mystery that I blew a fuse with all that I had accumulated onto my plate. Contrary to what the people I live with may believe; I am not a superwoman. *I am human and I am imperfect.* I make mistakes and sometimes I need help. I say and exude behavior that I am not proud of that I wish I could take back too. I am woman. And boy did I roar.

Day 60: 196.5 lbs. Saturday, December 2nd

I had tucked two whole months under my belt and was down a whopping one and a half pounds. I was so embarrassed to be revealing it. But I continued on.

Cereal was my go-to as of late and I hoped it was a smart choice in the long run. I put my love diet angst aside and began my day with a small bowl. Thank God everyone in my home was chipping in—finally. And I was sort of regretting insisting on having a "surprise" 50th birthday party to begin with. It might behoove me to plan my next self-surprising party somewhere else.

We arrived across the street for a drink while our guests arrived at our home. I had built up so much stress onto myself up to that moment and I was finally able to stop, relax and take a deep breath. Of course, now that I was mindfully in the present moment, the pain in my back was in full force.

I could barely shift without feeling the sharp stabbing pain when my husband boasted, "And that's what scotch is for Nicole!" But I yucked his yummy solution and opted for a girlier Cognac. I was not entirely sure how many calories were in it, so we searched and found a reputable source that stated 96 calories for one and a half ounces. Obviously, I had two.

Magically after a few sips I was able to move and breathe deeper. I had a delicious tortellini-like appetizer that I guessed was about 800 calories—maybe more. I let it carry me throughout the evening that was filled with laughter and love as I climbed over the final mountain of my milestone.

Day 61: 198 lbs. Sunday, December 3rd

There's got to be a morning after. And there was plenty of leftover gourmet restaurant food for me to try. I didn't give myself permission to eat very much at the party due to the calorie filled drinks and appetizers I arrived with. So, I started my morning out by making up for it.

Beginning with three crab Rangoon's and three reasonably sized stuffed mushrooms I moved on to dipping into the broccoli, chicken and pasta alfredo. I was choosing small portions and small plates which was easy enough to do. And my day continued with some delicious baked ziti in the afternoon.

Later in the evening I remembered that my colonoscopy was coming up in just a few days. I thought about what the fasting process would be like while grabbing another glass of wine and enjoying a piece of my birthday cake. Several bowls of chips followed that for a little precautionary—pre-prep—prep.

Day 62: 198 lbs. Monday, December 4th

The small amount of weight I had put on in what appeared to be the beginning of menopause for me started to show up about six years ago. I was only 44. And each year I slowly packed on more. Finally, I reached my personal heaviest at about 203 pounds—just a few months prior to starting my love diet journey. And it was very shocking to see that number since I was not nine months pregnant.

On one side of my shoulder sits a caring angel who whispers sweet everything's into my ear like: "You are making a lot of positive shifts from tired old ways of thinking and eating. Give yourself some credit and compassion. A little understanding goes a long way. You're doing a great job, keep it up Nicole!" Then there's the other side of my shoulder. The mean-spirited side that knocks me down and kicks me back to the ground adding in the infamous mantra voice: "What's the use. Just eat whatever you want. You only live once."

And then there's the real side. The inside—the side that throws real questions at me like: "When will you realize that the choices you've been making over the years are no longer serving you—or this now 50-year-old body of yours?" Thankfully, I did lose nearly six pounds over the past two months because on Day 62 I was right back to where I started from, which made the idea of ordering some take out strong. My original plan was to make a salad and I followed through with the angel right by my inside.

Honey mustard was one of the best choices for low sodium dressing, and since I didn't have any Dijon or honey on hand, I squeezed some yellow mustard onto my salad with olive oil and a skinny drizzle of maple syrup. It was a good enough substitute and I topped off my salad with some oats and a side of beets, which wasn't as full of sodium as I thought. For dinner, we all ate leftover pasta from the party around the island together. Mine on a small plate of course. I couldn't erase the past, but what I could do was keep penciling in my future.

The colonoscopy was fast approaching, and I snuggled up to my television with a bag of potato chips from the party after the kids went to bed. I really wanted to make better choices—even when or if there are still junk foods lying around. But was it realistic to remove all junk foods from my home with a family full of kids? Or the better question; Were the excuses just strings puppeteering my fingers?

I do want to make better choices *on my own*, period. And I want it to come easily without doubt or frustration. Perhaps it isn't ideal to have these junk foods lying around at least until it does come easier. One certainly would not have cocaine lying around if an addict was trying desperately to kick their crack habit.

Day 63: 197 lbs. Tuesday, December 5th

Phase one of the fast had begun. I was limited to chicken, fish, pasta, white bread, dairy, and dessert. No fruit or vegetables were allowed for the next three days. No nuts and no whole grain bread either and nothing with red dye. Okay, I could do this I thought. Cookies for breakfast, lunch, and dinner! Just kidding.

But I did eat two cookies for dessert at each meal, only because it was practically required.

Day 64: 195 lbs. Wednesday, December 6th

The kids were curious why more and more unhealthy foods like white toast, pasta and desserts were on *my* menu. They were the very unhealthy foods I had been preaching about and avoiding. And boy did their eyes bug out wide when I explained that the reason pasta, dairy, white bread, and desserts were all foods accepted during this colonoscopy cleanse was because they have little to no nutritional value whatsoever to the human body, and since there are not too many nutrients for the body to actually absorb, they go right through you. The look they both gave me was priceless.

With four events on my agenda for the day I still followed the hospital rules. My final networking meeting had lots of vegetables that I couldn't eat, so I took one scallop wrapped in bacon, and the procedure-experienced gals I was with gave me two thumbs up on the brown food stuffed mushrooms.

Day 65: 194 lbs. Thursday, December 7th

The no solid food day had arrived, and I was already well passed pissed-miserable. I got through my first meeting and then was off to my hair appointment where I sipped on green tea. Then I picked up "the drink" at the store with lots of other drinks that were allowed along with some mints. Three days of preparing had been okay, but it was the one-day liquid-fast that made me the grumpiest.

No solid food screamed the guidelines in my head. Why

must I be a stick to the rules and not seek loopholes goodie-two-shoes kind of girl? I was beyond starving when I realized *chicken soup broth was, in fact, not solid food.* And I couldn't get the damn can opened fast enough. The kids came home from school and of course the first thing they wanted to know was what was for dinner. I growled at each of them and said, "I am having chicken soup broth because remember, *I can't eat any FOOD today.*" My daughter looked at my noodle-free bowl and the pan on the stove and said, "Oooooh can I eat your noodles?" Pfffft. Wine is liquid. So, I prescribed myself a glass, alternating sips of the broth and the chardonnay.

Ready for the final step I headed upstairs early to get it over with. I sat in my puddle of pissed-off-ed-ness—too frustrated to troubleshoot the TV and surrendered to watching YouTube on my phone. The time finally arrived to begin the drink thing and I managed to get it down okay. The phone rang and I answered it, hoping I would not have to make an urgent escape.

The final 30-ounce Citrate of Magnesium consumption was not as bad as I thought it would be. The straw was a good idea. It did not even hit me until after midnight and as it turned out, the entire ordeal was not nearly as horrible as everyone had painted the picture for me.

Day 66: Friday, December 8th

The morning went by fairly quickly and before I knew it, I was eating my giant unhealthy but satisfying blueberry muffin on the ride home.

The doctor's orders were not to work and to have *a couch potato* day. It's so crazy how many unhealthy things we must do to be healthy. I surrendered though. It had been a long time since

I had watched day-time television and I found plenty of great shows that I could zone out to. My husband made me an egg with toast and I slowly come back to life from my colonosco-peezia haze to check a few emails.

We wrapped up our evening with a quick date night that I insisted on going to. I wanted food. I ordered some mozzarella sticks and marinara sauce for dipping. And he ordered some stuffed mushrooms. We brought home a pizza for the kids. And in the end, I was really proud that I had loved myself from the inside out.

Chapter 4
But Am I Still A Victim?

"A common phrase popped up into my head, you know, the one about how we create our own reality."

Day 67: Saturday, December 9th

No matter how much I tried to focus on my website, my mind wandered. Do I want to be skinny, or do I want to be healthy? Is my desire strong enough? Is setting visual goals a good thing like writing a number on my crystal scale, or hanging up that smaller dress size on my closet door? What will it take to change my mindset? And does it really matter how I change it as long as it changes? Is it my mindset what really needs to change? Am I struggling, or am I resisting? Am I still a victim?

Day 68: Sunday, December 10th

Sharing my colonoscopy experience with my kids was an interesting opportunity and I was glad I was able to do it. I considered myself blessed to hopefully have had a hand in helping them mentally prepare for their own procedures someday. But mostly I hoped I inspired them to be proactive when it comes to their own overall health and wellbeing.

I spent the day writing down my thoughts and getting back to thinking healthier, pre-colonoscopy. I do want to eat wholesome foods that are good for me, like fruits and vegetables, proteins that are lean, nuts, and whole grains. I do want to love my body in a positive way. *I want to be smarter by eating healthier.*

Cooking some chicken for dinner I gave it our "shake and bake" style recipe. It's easy and yummy. After placing the skin-on thighs into a large casserole dish, I drizzled olive oil generously over the chicken. I added parsley flakes, onion powder, garlic, salt and black pepper baking it at 375 for about an hour. And I served it with a side of roasted veggies.

I was proud of myself for taking the lead, straight out of the 50-year-old gate. And I finally received some good news for once. Benign—be nothing. Yay me!

Day 69: 195.5 lbs. Monday, December 11th

Originally, I thought it would be a great idea to have some friends and family do this love diet with me, you know, for the support and accountability. The testimonials would have been great too. But this is no ordinary diet. This is me learning about my health naturally and making the necessary changes I need to make. This is me, standing deep inside vulnerability.

There are only four items on my love diet list and God only knows what my list will look like on Day 365. And revealing all of these health discoveries is way more than I had originally bargained for. Which is why I let go of the initial invitations to a few people to do my love diet with me. I want to experience each and every profound discovery of self-acceptance, unconditional love, and transformation privately—for myself first.

Additionally, I stopped sharing what I was learning about Graves. The door was flung way too wide open for tons of questions and too many suggestions. And a lot of "you should do this, and you should do that's" came flying in too. What I needed was to breathe. I needed to mentally let this process wash over me. Taking on everyone else's thoughts was weighing too heavily on my shoulders and my brain was running on full advice capacity overload.

I am smart. And I had plenty of appointments on top of appointments scheduled to get myself educated. I was taking it all in. And in the midst of everything—I kept moving forward by having my first colonoscopy procedure a week and a half after I turned 50. In and of itself, having that procedure had prompted my husband to schedule his. In essence, I was already doing everything that I could to love myself more—and it was rubbing off on the ones I love.

Day 70: 194.5 lbs. Tuesday, December 12th

Peanut butter on toast was some good enough love for my drive, along with two cups of black coffee. I was giving a Reflection card reading, followed by a quick lunch before my recording.

The eager gal in the sub shop was forced to wait while I studied the menu. And then I made what I thought to be a high-maintenance decision. I ordered their chicken Caesar salad wrap but asked to swap out the dressing for my new favorite honey mustard. The happy-go-lucky gal tackled my order like it was nothing just as eagerly as she originally welcomed me.

A quick search told me that the chicken Caesar salad at this particular place was 770 calories and the sodium alone was a whopping 2,044 milligrams! I was so glad I traded it for the honey mustard, which was 500 calories less, and only 250 milligrams of sodium. I searched some more and found that a traditional Caesar salad has approximately 470 calories, 40 grams of fat (9 grams of which are saturated) and 1,070 milligrams of sodium. I guess this particular restaurant was twice as traditional.

There was no need to study the variety of Caesar brands in any restaurant or dressing aisle going forward. This was a no brainer. I simply, and quickly, removed Caesar from my personal love diet menu. Quite possibly forever. My love diet remained the same from Day 56, with one small adjustment.

My Love Diet:

1) *Feed Myself Love*
2) *Minimize Sodium*
    a. *Remove High Sodium Caesar Salad*
3) *Reduce Animal Fats*
4) *Reduce/Remove Carbs After 12 or 2pm*

Spending over two hours in the car doing activity drop-offs in traffic we finally got home around six o'clock. Quickly, I julienned some carrots, sliced some red peppers and grilled some white cod on the stove, pairing our fish with a side of white and brown rice mixed. So far, lowering my carbs after twelve or two o'clock in the afternoon was something I kept forgetting about.

Day 71: 194 lbs. Wednesday, December 13th

Black coffee and white paper. It was the new alliance in my life that was standing the test of time. I typed in the next few days and dates into my book to stay on track and wondered, could I type in my desired weight? The power of suggestion can be strong, so I put down 193—just to see.

Cooking dinner first thing in the morning is not what I typically do but I pulled some leftovers together and made chicken soup. Tossing the chicken into the pot I added some of the fat and rice, then fresh carrots and celery, water, two teaspoons of chicken base, some white pepper, and a little sea salt. It made about six decent sized servings—after I ate some. I had more for a late breakfast, and then had some again for an early lunch. It was really that good!

At each sitting I enjoyed a small handful of oyster crackers too. The salt content was not nearly as high as I thought it would be. And my day ended with a friend, a delicious tortellini appetizer, and two glasses of chardonnay. Again, completely forgetting about the low-to-no carb rule after two o'clock.

Nicole Perry

Day 72: 193 lbs.! Thursday, December 14th

Would I have hit 193 had I not written it down? Or did I subconsciously nibble my way toward my new number? To hit the number was a good feeling, but I still had a long way to go.

It was snowing outside when I guiltily left my two youngest standing at the bus stop as I drove away. And I felt a sigh of relief just as I pulled out of the neighborhood when I saw their bus entering. Popping open my banana and sipping on my coffee I was grateful for how understanding my kids truly are.

When I arrived at the breakfast meeting, I took a modest amount of fresh fruit, a small scoop of scrambled eggs and two tiny slices of bacon from the buffet. The meeting was a great success and just before I left, I took a good long look around the room admiring all that my team and I had accomplished and what was yet to come.

Next on my agenda for the day was my new love tattoo. My first *word* tattoo. I hadn't been to the parlor in about four years and this would mark my 16th time under the voluntary needle. Body art is painful, but in my opinion art worth having. You just can't be afraid of commitment—or regret.

People often joke about how tattoos will eventually sag and get wrinkly but so will a blank canvas. My colorful body art will have great stories to tell someday and my wrinkles are pretty. Tattoos are subjective like anything else. They can be tasteful or tasteless. Regardless—I choose to see people first.

A luncheon was next and helped to take my mind off the residual pain. Luckily for me the bar was open. But my greater need was to find the bathroom. It was day 12 of this crazy cycle, which had followed over 40 days of spotting. And quite literally, I had a spot on my skirt that I had to hide. I did my best to pretend it wasn't there, even when one of my friends held my hand and was encouraging me to give her a twirl to show off my outfit.

I knew I wasn't bleeding to death. But still, I had what I thought to be normal concerns. Losing that much blood couldn't be good. Obviously, I would have to do some more internet searching. About 1 cup is what the average woman loses in a regular cycle is what I found. *Good Lord, the things I had been searching!* I made an appointment with my OB-GYN anyway just in case I was freakishly hemorrhaging.

Making my way to the buffet, I was moderate again with my portions, but realized afterward that the soup and gravy were probably loaded with sodium. Damn! I was almost there—being mindfully aware.

Day 73: 193.5 lbs. Friday, December 15th

Early to rise I had some simple toast with peanut butter for breakfast, followed by a single baked potato lunch around twelve o'clock in the afternoon. And just before heading out to the post office, I called the doctor to cancel my appointment. I was sure my cycle would end soon. At least by Sunday, bloody Sunday!

After dropping my son off at the Mall, I dashed over to a boutique for a last-minute desperate search for an outfit. We had a party to attend and luckily, I found a sweater with plenty of bling that conveniently hid almost everything.

When I got home, I tried on the sweater with a skirt. The sweater fit, but the skirt looked like shit. Swapping out the skirt for another one I started to regret buying the sweater. Ripping off the fabulous-for-a-minute sweater, I put on one of my typical go-to tops. It looked ok but wasn't long enough to cover my butt.

So, I took off the crap-ass skirt and put on a pair of jeans. Frankly, this was a typical day in the life of my closet.

Almost ready to give up I stood there fingering through my dresses and found a red sleeveless ball gown that I completely forgot about. And as luck would have it, it was stretchy. *Thank God.* And I had only worn it twice. *Perfect.* The only acceptable pantyhose I found had two massive runs in them, but they were hidden by endless amounts of fabric. *Phew.* I was just happy I didn't give myself a hernia shoving myself into them. *Bonus.* I was sucked in, tucked in, and I could easily breathe. It looked like my dress of choice was a well-thought-out plan. *Excellent.*

I did not eat much food throughout the day, so as we were prepping the youngest two on long overdue, repetitive safety tips, I started to feel a little light-headed. It would not be a good thing to pass out at the party, or on the way there, so I nibbled on one of my kids' used pieces of pizza to hold me over. Moving on to eating a slice of my own was smart, but it was early, and the dinner would likely be served late. For good measure I took a few more bites of my son's piece just before walking out the door.

Feeling light-headed was not a good sign, which made me regret that I had just canceled my appointment. But my recent theory was that my friend Flo had just overextended her welcome and she would soon leave. I was done thinking about doctor appointments. I just wanted to enjoy myself for one night. Even if momentarily. Or at least from the waist up. Trying not to think about my uterus falling out wasn't easy. On the flipside, worst-case scenario—my dress was blood red.

I AM ON A LOVE DIET

Day 74: 196 lbs. Saturday, December 16th

I did eat a modest amount of food while my husband loaded up his buffet plate and I only regretted eating a few very small desserts. Not while I was enjoying them of course, but only after I stepped onto crystal. And she was starting to turn into a coal piece of shit.

My breakfast was a simple sandwich. One egg over easy with a little hot sauce. Then for a light snack, I had a small amount of cream cheese on celery decorated with a few walnuts. We had a dance thing for my daughter to attend and while I was getting dressed, I sat in my closet and sort of fell apart. I had been pushing so much deep down inside trying to take everything in stride. And out of nowhere I broke down and cried.

My journey began by taking care of my heart and thyroid. In the midst of it all I took a little side-hustle to work on my colon, which appeared to be the only happy organ in my body. My uterus was bloody freaking angry. And my closet was quickly becoming a place of worship. I tear-begged God for it to stop.

After dropping our daughter off at her dance call time, we headed over to pick out a Christmas tree and I noticed I was feeling light-headed again. Two days in a row was not good at all. I was anemic years ago without hardly having a symptom and with that—I knew something more had to be going on.

Working through an illness is one thing but I had layers of issues going on. We didn't have much time in between getting our Christmas tree and when her holiday showcase started, but I needed food. After securing the tree to the roof, which seemed like it took forever and a day, my husband pulled into a convenient store for me to grab something. I made a b-line for the sandwich cooler and took a chicken salad on a bulky roll to the register without skipping a beat. No one else was hungry but I grabbed a few small bags of chips to share just in case.

When I get sick with a cold, I just take day-meds, drink more tea, stock up on tissues—the usual stuff. Stomach bug, same thing. There's almost always way too much on my plate to even consider taking an entire sick day. And the same goes for whenever I have gotten a period throughout my life. I just go with Flo. I do the best I can, which is hardly less than usual. I can generally plow through any sickness, like any other mother, and only once in a blue moon, do I need a little extra, early-to-bed rest.

Fast forward to my humble request. I had been asking my husband and our kids for suggestions and in-sight on what to do, but no one had a clue. By the look on their faces they didn't even know how to respond. After all, I'm the one who usually gives them advice. I am the one who eases their pain and puts everything into perspective for them. And here I was clearly struggling with what to do about my own health. They were speechless.

Over the past few days, my husband did respond with his quick wit and silly remarks, implying that I may even be a borderline hypochondriac. But I wasn't laughing anymore. I pleaded, "I just want to love myself and care about myself. Please don't make me feel bad about sharing my concerns with you or asking for help. Do you think I made the right decision by canceling my appointment? Should I reschedule? What would you do? Should I go to the ER and suck-up the stupid co-pay? I don't go to the doctor for every little hangnail, bump or sneeze. You know that. This cycle has lasted over 14 days and that has never happened to me before—outside of giving birth. Could I be hemorrhaging? What if I need a hysterectomy? What I need from you is your strength, insight and compassion." Of course, he was even more supportive.

We win from within is a famous saying. I began with wanting to change my size, which led me to focus on healing my heart. It all began because I wanted to shrink my body, and my uterus was the newest concern, cutting ahead in line of my thyroid. I looked for my book, "You Can Heal Your Body", by Louise Hay, but I had no luck finding it and immediately ordered a new one. My family were listening and said they would sit with me in the ER for several hours if need be.

Day 75: 197.5 lbs. Sunday, December 17th

A few months ago, when I first came out about being a suicide attempt survivor, someone had asked me, "Who saved you?" Which caught me by surprise. No one had ever asked me that before. And I told them in a way I guess I had saved myself, because I called a few people.

When I made that attempt all those years ago though, I didn't really want to die, but my mind was in an altered state. During school, our teacher was fast asleep, sitting upright and snoring at his desk. So, I bummed a cigarette from a friend and easily snuck out of class to the bathroom to smoke it. I was flippant and didn't even try to hide.

What I felt was next to nothing. No pain, or guilt. I got caught, of course, and was informed that I would be suspended—again. I don't remember my response, nor the bus ride or the walk home. But I do remember that I did still care about myself. And it showed by making those phone calls.

At the emergency room I remember feeling judged. And I could feel a strong *shame-on-you-vibe* shooting at me through thin air. Like, how could you do something like this *to your family*. Maybe it was just pity. But when I was moved to a semi-permanent hospital, I was in the company of several people who were much older than me. Some were just angry, unhappy, or depressed. But others seemed to be psychotic and delusional. They were ill beyond anything I could have ever imagined as a 16-year-old girl. And I knew I was *the one thing not like the others*. In that room I was the one thing that just didn't belong. Why was *I* here, I wondered to myself?

What I had was a lot of compassion for them. Struggling and smoking their cigarette butts consuming ridiculous amounts of coffee. Desperately searching for answers at the bottom of each cup after eight-ounce foam cup. I realized very quickly, even at age 16, that my problems were *petty*-normal. I knew at that first meeting I attended that I didn't *need* to be there. I didn't want to struggle like they were struggling. I wanted to go home.

What I wanted was to be loved. I certainly didn't want to die. All I needed was a little extra love. Regardless of what I had done, I wanted to be forgiven and trusted. I needed attention. And I wanted someone to take the time to ask me questions, listen, and care about my answers. I was a teenager struggling normally just like most teenagers do. The people in my life loved me. But my soul needed more. That's all.

"Oh, they just want attention," is a phrase I've often heard people say. Like what? Shame on people who *crave attention*. Shame on that kid for *wanting so much attention*. Shame on anyone who *needs more attention*. Since when did the word *attention* become a negative word? *Since when did the need to be loved, evolve into a shameful desire?*

We all know there's a stigma or stereotypical angst that comes with the word suicide. Perhaps it will forever be a curse to talk about it, like it's contagious or something. But we have evolved tremendously as a society. And we are able to brave, talk about and fight disease—like cancer. *We need to be able to talk about and be more compassionate about the mental health of others—with suicide prevention.*

Suicide prevention. Two words much stronger when placed together and softened at the same time. And if we really think about it the two words simply mean to care about and support people. The very people that may need a little extra love or attention.

If a person is struggling, we all know it shows up in many different ways. And we could be more compassionate and understanding as a society. We can let go of fear and ask the question. Any question will do. Like, "Are you okay?", or "You do love yourself, right?", and a great one would be, "You wouldn't do anything to hurt yourself would you?" I like to say, "I'm glad you're here." The point is, we could care just a little more. We can slow down and take notice. And that little extra love and kindness can go a long way. *Suicide is permanent. Anxiety and depression are temporary. Love and compassion are everlasting.*

It is my personal mission, to be sure and ask a question. If there ever is a question. I wonder how the statistics of attempts and suicide would subside if more people asked questions and cared out loud. *A person that attempts to take their own life does not deserve to be judged, they simply need to be loved.*

Day 76: 197 lbs. Monday, December 18th

Something miraculous had happened. And I was free. After 15 days, my uterus was finally empty!

I grabbed a cup of coffee and started my day playfully searching one thing on the internet, then another, then several others. I tried to find a video with Dr. Wayne Dyer's philosophy around the number eight, which led me to the Schoolhouse Rock video Figure Eight. From there I clicked over to the old-fashioned Blue Christmas cartoon.

I wasn't blue anymore. Twas' the week before Christmas and all through my house—it was quiet, and I was grateful. Sitting in my kitchen watching a few childhood cartoons and fun videos. I clicked through some more and brought myself up to speed and back to the current world with a little Lady Gaga and Amy Schumer.

Day 77: 196.5 lbs. Tuesday, December 19th

I had a small bowl of cereal again for breakfast and followed that with some leftovers from dinner for lunch.

Everyone loved my turkey meatloaf, and scallop potato side dish. I thought it could have used a little more salt, but they were all happy to add it at the table. They were all being very supportive and coming along on my low-sodium sleigh ride.

Dinner this time was fresh white cod, seasoned and baked with a bag of onion crunchies that are usually meant for the green bean casserole dish. A simple side of grilled brussels sprouts made this dinner a success.

Day 78: 196 lbs. Wednesday, December 20th

This isn't an easy button. And my road may prove to be much longer than the average. But paying attention, looking within, shifting, tweaking, and making better choices would eventually pay off.

Shuffling only the health and wellness cards from my tarot card deck I picked one—and then read the rest anyway. My health is the most important thing to me and it's what I needed the most coaching on.

I kicked off my day with a black coffee and a banana, then headed out to an early meeting. My husband was home office too so when I got back, we made egg sandwiches together for lunch. One egg a day was okay. Before I left for the station, we had a quick snack together with some swiss cheese and crackers.

Later we ordered pizza for delivery. I insisted on no meats or extra cheese and we settled on one small with garlic, spinach and mushrooms and one large cheese for the kids. It was a good enough compromise for all.

Day 79: 196 lbs. Thursday, December 21st

My morning meeting was so great, and I topped it off with some little treats to share. We were almost at the start of the new year, but I gave myself permission to have one.

Resolutions were not my thing. Every time I created them with each passing year as I got older, my self-esteem would get a little more crushed. It was a waste of my time to set unrealistic goals. And it was easier to give up on quitting and failing. And by accident, one of those precious little fluffy chocolate bites I ate turned into three.

I ordered soup again forgetting about the sodium content. It was something I kept doing and not realizing until after I ordered or took the first sip. But I knew it was bound to eventually click. And sitting with a friend at lunch, I sipped on my soup during a very thought-provoking discussion.

She reminded me of the tactic called mirroring. When we see a specific quality in someone else, whether it's positive or negative, it's the perfect opportunity to look within. And we can see ourselves in a whole new light. If we choose to see it.

Afterward I picked up a few kids from school to do some Christmas shopping and while I was waiting, I picked and ate a few more of those treats that were still in my car. Three kids came with me on our Christmas shopping spree, which turned out to be a bad idea. I could only buy things for me.

Against her wishes, I handed our cashier a pile of coupons I had been saving for months and put the single one she wanted, back into my purse. In the car I mentioned the mirroring tactic to my kids and again at home to my husband after telling him about the grumpy cashier and he said sometimes the other person is just who they are, and the quality we see has nothing to do with us. Which makes the mirror more like that of a window.

Day 80: 197 lbs. Friday, December 22nd

Betraying my own new rule, I shared my Graves news with another friend. She wondered and asked me—if my thyroid issue was the over-active kind, then why wasn't I *losing* weight. The good news she gave me was that her medication was keeping her thyroid in check.

It was the first time I had heard anyone say anything positive about their medication. I had been afraid to search for anything before going to my appointment in January and was additionally worried that I may have to get more than one opinion. Terrified might be a better word, but I worked up the courage to search and click the best foods that promote a healthy thyroid. As it turned out, some foods that we know are typically good for us still are, but what I read was, *unless your thyroid isn't functioning properly.*

Quickly printing up a list of the top seven foods that can potentially slump energy, tears of hope welled up in my eyes. I was elated and shared everything immediately with my husband. It was easy to understand, I felt relieved, and I thought I might actually have some control over my body again, and my future. Like I had taken a Thyroid 101 class or had read the latest Thyroid for Dummies.

After sharing the positive information, my husband crushed my hope effortlessly in a matter of seconds. It must be another window. I said to him with slightly gritted teeth, "By all means. If you discover that purple polka-dotted pistachios dipped in raw garlic are the best things for me to eat on Mondays and Wednesdays, between six and one will fix my thyroid issue—then I am all over it like white on rice. Until then, I'll use my new list."

My husband is very savvy when it comes to overall good health and preventative measures and was questioning why I was willing to remove something as healthy as brussels sprouts from my diet. But after our brief discussion, it turned out he was more freaked out about the fact that I was willing to remove pizza.

Pizza is a type of fatty food, which is not good for a *not functioning properly thyroid.* I froze and thought, *maybe he's the one who's addicted to pizza?* I said to him supportably, "Hon, *I* will be avoiding what's on the list, it doesn't mean you have to."

Before decorating our Christmas tree, we gave it several good shoves in the stand. We've had too many trees tip over in the past. So, once it passed our test, I strung the lights, ribbons, and ornaments. "Hey, the tree looks beautiful!" my husband said, both of us knowing time would tell.

Day 81: Saturday, December 23rd

We woke up to find our tree all over the floor. It brought me immediately back to when our tree fell like I don't know, maybe six or seven times in one season. How did we ever survive that? Every year since that year, the stress and anxiety arrive. Should we tie it to the door? Should we get a fake tree? Should we buy a new stand or Charlie Brown it this year? Having our tree fall over multiple times was not funny. What was funny though was the year I drove into the garage with the tree still on the roof. Ooof.

This year, we got a reasonably sized tree, a new tree stand, and gave it several good test shoves before decorating it. It still fell over in the unwanted traditional fashion. There must be a few spirits living in our house having a good chucky chuckle.

Before heading to the market, I made some toast with peanut butter and left. I couldn't even look at that tree, or the mess still all over the floor. We all avoided the entire room. After dropping off the groceries, again without looking into my living room, I headed back out for some final Christmas shopping.

Unable to avoid my home permanently, I went back, made myself a small leftover rice snack, and then faced the music. I ripped off all of the tangled lights and ribbons and collected the ornaments like the sad spirit that I was. And then it hit me. Since it was in the corner of the room this year, I only decorated the front and a little of the sides. Shit! That's why it fell. *A common phrase popped up into my head, you know, the one about how we create our own reality.*

We left to get dinner and I ordered the house salad with grilled chicken and honey mustard, adding some marinara sauce to dip my one roll on the side and my husband ordered the ho-ho-oh-so unhealthy fried calamari platter.

Later that night watching TV I finally worked up the courage to at least get the lights and ribbons back on the tree before heading up to bed. I gave it another good shove and decided to finish the damn thing in the morning.

Day 82: 197 lbs. Sunday, December 24th

Nothing was crystal clear anymore. I had always been pretty healthy and proud of it. But I kept looking at my face in the mirror, and the number on my scale to no avail. Braving my computer again, I read about Graves' disease and wondered if everything I was reading was Google-true. And why my doctor would use the term *Graves.* A term I had never heard before. I was hit with something that was not too hard, but at the same time, in slow motion. It wasn't cancer. But how bad was it? My husband's previous rational supporting text popped back into my head. *"You're not dying Nicole."*

My previous primary doctor had mentioned that the issue I had with my thyroid was so small all those years ago, I didn't think very much of it. At the time I chalked it up to simply being perimenopause.

My primary care physician had a perplexing look on his face that day about my theory that was matched by the look of *you are so clueless* on mine. Sitting there was torture. The room was too tiny for the two of us. And I had to work at mustering up every ounce of patience that I could while he struggled with his own technology. He gave new meaning to the term bedside manner and lack thereof. I wanted to take over his computer and fix whatever he was trying to do just so I could escape and get on with my distorted aging life. I never went back after that appointment and didn't need to look back. Not until my newest wellness visit opened up that very old can of worms.

My current file with the thyroid specialist had said, "not urgent," on it. But searching on my own was on my mind. I cooked one egg over easy with two slices of gluten-free toast right quick. What I found was it appeared that I had many Graves' symptoms. Eight out of twelve from one particular list. I searched and found more. One of the unanimous symptoms was weight loss. Why couldn't I have gotten that one? At least six symptoms were in alignment with menopause. The more I read, the more confused I was.

The list of ailments I was compiling was quite long and had crept up into my life over the last several months and years. What popped into my head were the couple of times I was standing in my kitchen eating a hard-boiled egg and I could feel my throat closing up like I was having a spasm or an allergic reaction. It happened with peanut butter a few times too.

Looking back, I wondered if it was my thyroid all along, cluing me in with a few wake-up calls. Each time I thought I probably ate too fast or didn't chew my food long enough. I did pay attention, and on some occasions, I would eat the same things, and nothing would happen.

The strange soreness in my hips had raised a little pink flag. It was happening more often than not, and it started a few months ago. Usually when I sat in the car or in a chair for long periods. I thought it might be just another sign of aging.

There was, of course, that thing called menopause I was carrying around. The constant state of insomnia had to be from menopause since it was hot flash based. And one of the symptoms of Graves was thick skin, and I had that too. It had shown up on two of my fingers, which I originally attributed initially as one of the signs of arthritis. The list goes on and I would worry.

What if I have something more serious like Lyme disease? The heart palpitations have been happening for a few years. I had assumed nearly everything was because of menopause, and some of it simply signs of aging. Why would I go to the doctor for all of those teeny tiny, almost insignificant little issues? Of course I would self-diagnose. And one of my final searches stated that a person diagnosed with Graves' disease might start to think they are a hypochondriac.

Day 83: Monday, December 25th

The somewhat materialistic holiday with family and food had arrived. I had a small serving of the fatty duck I prepared and stayed clear of the salt-infused ham. I took very small portions of everything; the mashed potatoes; mashed carrots and turnips; brussels sprouts; asparagus; and one candied tomato. And I passed on the gravy this time. For dessert, there were many to choose from, so I took a few small slivers of each just like I usually do at each holiday. Same as it ever was.

My mom took some photos. And I thought I looked really tired in every single picture. I was tired. I was clearly exhausted. Not from shopping or food prepping, but probably from all of the worrying and resisting. To acknowledge everything would be admitting I was not healthy too.

Day 84: Tuesday, December 26th

It may be better for me to break everything down into smaller, more digestible and lovable chunks. My thyroid needed the most love. I was reading mainstream and a little at a time to help me keep processing. Too much information could cause mental and emotional stress, not to mention anxiety.

Stimulants are not good for the thyroid, but one cup of coffee was acceptable. Maybe even two. I had already dropped down to one to two cups of black coffee each day for a few years now anyway. Maybe I could let go of the second cup. Or maybe it wasn't even necessary.

Learning that pizza and fatty foods are not good for the thyroid was very good to know. Basically, foods like burgers, fries, and tacos. I had no idea pizza *was in fact a fatty food.* There's a little cheese yeah, but in my mind, having a slice, or few, was the healthiest option of fast food. Red tomato sauce is supposed to be so good for you, and most of us turn a blind eye to the carb. It never occurred to me that *pizza* was lumped in with other "fatty foods." Fat is good. But evidently "fatty" is bad.

Since reading this particular article about foods that can slump energy, I found it to be extremely helpful. For almost three months I had eaten countless amounts of pizza. Sometimes two to three times per week. After reading about pizza being a fatty food, I decided to let go of that for a while. It helped me to view pizza as the poison that it might actually be for me.

Mentally, I was surrendering to the fact that I might have to take medication someday for something. I was warming up to it and reprogramming my brain, reconditioning my body, and getting healthier. My main goal was far more important to me now than losing weight was, fitting into skinnier jeans, or eating a stupid slice of pizza.

Day 85: Wednesday, December 27th

Letting go of fear again, I searched and found an article that said to eat broccoli and another one that specifically said not to eat cruciferous vegetables. One article said to eat fish and another that said don't eat seafood. Get plenty of calcium from yogurt and milk. Don't eat dairy. Stay away from strawberries. Eat plenty of berries. Everything that I was finding was more and more contradictory "should" and "should not's". All I wanted was to gain some insight and do a little homework prior to my appointment. And I was more confused and frustrated than ever.

Iodine. I did discover that my body may have too much iodine and quite possibly be overproducing it. Our bodies need vitamins and minerals, we all know this, but too much metal was not good. I read the label on my multi-vitamin and it had 100 percent of the daily recommended allowance. For me it might be too much. Thank God I hadn't taken those vitamins for six months!

Day 86: 198.5 lbs. Thursday, December 28th

Seek and ye shall find. But I wasn't sure if I should keep seeking or finding. How many cans of worms would I open? I looked on the bright side. At least I didn't have worms.

Day 87: Friday, December 29th

Somewhere on the net I read that people who find out they have Graves' often discover they actually have Lyme. Oh, my freaking

God! My hips had been bothering me and that was a huge sign of Lyme.

On the path to better self-love I darted out the driveway to get to a minute clinic. But they couldn't check me in without a proper photo ID. *Shit where the hell was my license?!* Frantically I cleaned out my purse and car before I finally drove back home to get my passport, finding my license in a pair of jeans on the floor. I ran back out to the clinic, but the wait had grown to over an hour. So, I took my phone next door for a checkup instead. I knew the urgency when it came to Lyme, but I put myself on the shelf one more time.

Several weeks earlier we planned to take all the kids to the movies because they would all be home together. Lunch needed to be something light and I opted for one egg over easy, broccoli and cauliflower on the side with some whole grain toast and butter.

Our two eldest met us there and we took our two youngest and entered the food court first. In my mind it was like I was entering a land mine. Was there anything I could eat in there? I looked at each menu slowly, so as not to make any sudden choices. My daughter pointed to the deli with enthusiasm. God only knew if the chicken was real or rubber, but I nodded yes, and I added every vegetable that I could into the tomato wrap. I treated myself with a few favorites I had missed like pickles and yellow banana peppers. He topped my wrap off with a little honey mustard and I opted for bottled water.

My meal was actually delicious, and I hardly cared about the pizza everyone else was eating right next to me. It looked good, but something in me was different. There was no way that pizza was getting past go into this pie hole.

I enjoyed plenty of movie popcorn, without butter of course, and several red Twizzlers. I was proud of being determined to eat a healthy meal prior to the movie. And all of my choices were sure to amount to success.

Day 88: Saturday, December 30th

Could I have caught the Lyme in time? Sitting in the express clinic line, I remembered all of the symptoms of Lyme that I had found. The joint pain, dizziness, fatigue, and lower back pain.

Several people have had Lyme in my home over a span of several years and so far, we were lucky enough to catch it early each time. The thought of potentially having Lyme was extremely nerve-wracking though and I didn't know which was worse, the Lyme or the Graves.

Loving myself on this love diet had brought me to an unbelievable place of extreme awareness though. And moving forward I decided that Web MD might be the better and more reputable place to continue doing any of my touch the surface research. I did my best to not think about the Lyme test and hoped the results would come back sooner rather than later.

Eating protein with every meal is something I learned that we're supposed to do a long time ago and additionally, most women don't follow that protocol.

Lunch and dinner seemed easy enough but what would I add to my cereal? Perhaps a side of cottage cheese? With cottage cheese on my brain I found some saltines and red pepper jelly. It was a good enough snack and might even carry me to dinner. Pulling the box of saltines back out of the cabinet I read the label for calories and realized that I didn't even care. Not because I don't love myself, but the calories don't really seem to matter anymore. What is important is what I eat, and if it will help my thyroid.

The dogs were swarming all around me as I spread the cottage cheese on each square and topped them off with the delicious hot pepper jelly. My dogs may have bad manners, but they definitely smell the importance of protein.

Interestingly, exercising was not a good thing to do especially with the heart palpitations that I had been having. At this point I was afraid to get my heart rate up at all. Yoga was a better choice. But rather than to do the smart thing, I did the dishes instead and put away my china.

But why avoid breathing and stretching? What was it about me that made me believe that I didn't need to breathe, stretch, or move my body? Barely stretching my body, I bent over the front stoop to pick up my new thyroid book that arrived.

Day 89: 198 lbs. Sunday, December 31st

Starting out the last day of the year I had one cup of black coffee with a banana. Cleaning my kitchen was on my to-do list and I gave my office a bit of a U-Haul. It was exactly how I envisioned wrapping up my year.

My daughter and I were going to the movies again, this time just the two of us. And we would be eating popcorn again and possibly a few Twizzlers. But first I got some good nutritious food into my body with one egg over easy and a side of zucchini. It was perfect.

After the movie, we looked for something fancy for each of us to wear to dinner. I spotted a beautiful sharp business-like off-white dress with a built-in gold choker. On the hanger it was gorgeous and perfectly my style. But trying on clothes after a movie was almost as bad as trying on a bathing suit in the winter. Who was that roly-poly woman in my mirror I thought to myself? With not one, but two spare tires.

It was the first time I hadn't spent New Year's Eve with my husband in over 25 years. He had purchased Celtics tickets, which was a long overdue promise to our boys and didn't realize the date. He continued to not think about the date when we made New Year's Eve plans together and booked a dinner reservation at one of our favorite fancy restaurants. We continued to plan the entire evening out together, so it was a bit of a shock as the information about the date and time of the game slowly unfolded.

What choice did I have really? I took my daughter and a friend to our couples, date night. There weren't a whole lot of singles or children in the restaurant. Well, there were, they were just all at my table. I ordered the pan seared scallop dinner but asked to trade out my side dish since it had cranberries, one of the foods on my list of "unsure abouts".

The scallops were teeny tiny, and the substitution didn't fit. My meal was not the greatest, but my daughter and friend enjoyed theirs and I was with two people I loved. And when the clock struck nine-thirty, my husband humbly surprised me and crashed our singles party.

Chapter 5
Knowledge IS Power

"And I thought to myself; don't mess with a woman who's on a mission to care for herself as though she were her own child."

Day 90: 198.5 lbs. Monday, January 1st

Knowledge is Power. It's the last thing I say at the end of my radio show. I'm not sure when I first heard the saying, but it resonated with me, and when I was recently cleaning out my bookshelves, I found its originator. "The Best Dictionary for Students by Francis Bacon 1626." It just so happens to say, *Knowledge is Power* on the bottom right front cover. Wow.

Frankly, knowledge is power, and we all know it's what we do with any knowledge that matters. Just like time heals all wounds. What matters is what we do with our time. And I had done a lot in the time I had received all of this information. Yet, there was still so much more to learn and do.

On the first day of the new year I woke up feeling fatter. And technically I was. Over the past three months, I had lost some weight, gained it back, lost it again, and gained it back again. What I had not done yet, was love myself, all day, every day.

She looks at it every day and tells her younger self, "I love you." My friend showed me that photo of when she was a little girl and said she looks at it every day and tells herself—what we all need to tell ourselves. *I love you.* I found a photo of myself at age 13 and taped it to the inside cover of my journal. Front and center. And as luck would have it, my house was full of mirrors.

Whether I tell my younger self looking at a photograph, or my current self into a mirror, I wanted to do that on a regular basis too. I *want* to tell myself the words I long to hear. *I love you.* And if loving myself more is not at the top of my priority list, it needs to be, and it needs to stand strong at number one. *Feed myself love.* Stronger than everything—and everyone else.

I asked each of my kids, "Who is the most important person in your life?" My two youngest were positive they had the *right* answer, and both said very matter-of-factly, "Our parents." I said, "No, the most important person in your life is You! Not to mention 'parents' is plural." The next time I asked, immediately they were proud that they knew the correct and better answer.

January 1st. It's the best, and worst day of the year. The day we take a good hard look at what we haven't done and what we want to do. Most importantly, it is a time to make decisions for the love of our own minds and bodies. The day of resolutions.

The day to create goals, announce desires, and make decisions that hopefully stick around throughout and beyond 365 days.

Knee deep into my love diet—I guess I could consider myself lucky. I had a giant head start on my own Day 90. And I hoped what I create will inspire people to start their own love diets—and begin any day of the year they want to.

A few years ago, I decided to claim one word for the year that is powerful and intentional. One simple word that I could be mindful of. It's so much easier and can have a lot more impact. My word this year was of course Love. But this year's word had more meaning behind it. Wrapped around my intentional and powerful word would be lots of curiosity and questions.

Questions like: How can I feed myself more love today? Could I squeeze in some exercise before getting on that call or computer? Would a new yoga mat spark some motivation or interest? Can I stop several times today to just breathe? Which meal on this menu will immediately love me back? And if my exercise regime becomes stale or monotonous, will I intentionally seek an alternative way to enjoy moving my body?

My questions dove deeper. Like was what I am about to eat, and drink filled with love? Is the fat my body holding on to full of hate? Do I really want to push the lazy button today or every day? Is procrastinating my health, love?

My phone rang, and I saw that it was a friend, so I answered it. It was the most incredible invitation. She wanted to feature a story of me and my reflection cards in her spiritual newspaper column, which happened to be national. I didn't see that coming. Sure, I was anticipating a great year ahead and the call helped confirm and solidify my prediction. But perhaps the karma of pouring so much energy into encouraging other women was circling back to me.

Day 91: Tuesday, January 2nd

I tossed and turned so much throughout the night I wasn't sure if I had slept. It was happening a lot. My mind was racing through the night with all the things I have to do running through it along with my typical night sweats and hot flashes. Regardless of how tired I felt though, I popped a love question. What could I do to love my body today?

Ahh, Meditation. I hadn't meditated or done any yoga in a while, so I kicked off my day by quieting my mind to gain back some clarity and focus. Meditation was in complete alignment with my one powerful love word.

Following my meditation, I looked for something to eat for breakfast. Protein is important to have with each meal and I wondered if nuts were enough. When I have an egg for breakfast, I usually don't worry about the ratio of proteins vs. veggies. I just combine my egg with a side of whole grain toast and a tomato or fruit. Obviously, that includes all three food groups.

When I'm in a hurry, I grab a protein shake or some toast with peanut butter. Both of those are easy and I love topping cottage cheese with some crunchy cereal, honey, fruit, and cinnamon, but what about the cereal thing? Is the milk enough? Nuts are great for a quick on-the-go whole snack, but they have twice as much fat as they do protein. I wondered, how much "nut fat" was "slim safe?"

Albeit the article I found about the top ten things we need to know about walnuts discloses upfront "insufficient evidence," I kept reading. They are a whole food and full of Omega-3's, but there were quite a few negatives I never knew. And what a weird list it was.

The article mentioned BMI too and that weight change could happen with excessive walnut consumption. Who the heck is eating walnuts excessively? The list of negative side effects went on to include allergies, asthma attacks, diarrhea, ulcers, acne, and lip cancer among other things. Digging even deeper I also found anemia, diabetes, eczema, and excessive sweating in the hands and feet.

Needless to say, I wasn't about to eat any walnuts after digesting all of that. I wasn't planning to remove them from my love diet either, but my instinct was to let them go long enough to see if my skin would clear up. When I looked back over the list again, I thought it was interesting that the symptom that bothered me the most was the acne, and not diarrhea or diabetes.

Next, I searched to find more detailed information about almonds. This article stated almonds are in fact, a great source of protein, fiber, vitamin E, and magnesium, etc. But I also read that eating too many almonds can actually cause constipation and abdominal bloating if your body is not used to processing large amounts of fiber. Okay, almonds it is!

It took a lot of searching through my kitchen cabinets, but eventually, I found the little digital scale I purchased years ago. Tucking important things away in *safe* places is something that sure does waste a lot of my time. Finally measuring out one ounce of almonds, the small pile came to a total of 27. Looking at the pile I certainly didn't need that many. And I think one small handful of nuts was an appropriate serving. In my hand it came to about ten, so I added eight to my cereal.

I AM ON A LOVE DIET

After coming home from a Board meeting, I poured myself a glass of wine and sat typing in my notes while I nibbled on some all-natural roasted sweet potato chips that I had made before I left. They were the perfect item to snack on and could easily replace potato chips, especially while watching a movie, or better yet, football. I would be lying if I said I don't still eat chips—and love chips. I had been eating only the kind with under five ingredients though for the past several years. But I wondered if I could let go of the bag for good. Could I do it for love?

My day was almost coming to an end and I noticed something pretty cool had happened. I had loved myself for the entire day. It does sound a little funny, but I began my day with a meditation, drank a good amount of water, and I ate healthy all day.

Despite the typical temptations that are always here, there and everywhere in our home, I chose to feed myself love. And I chose not to eat one of the pastries on the counter that my husband and kids had brought home. It did help to keep their treats hidden in the ceramic cake stand under the cover on the island where I keep all of their junk foods. Out of my sight—and off of my mind.

Day 92: Wednesday, January 3rd

Visiting with a friend, I excused myself when I saw my Gynecologist flash up on my phone and confirmed my appointment. Recently, I had made her my primary care physician too. I was excited about my idea of having one doctor to talk to and consult with. One medical professional all wrapped up into one coaching doctor. If I could have given her the additional dermatologist, mammogram, and colonoscopy titles I would have.

Back to my friend, "But what have you gained?" She asked me when I told her that I had lost zero weight thus far; three months into a diet I was creating for myself. Her positive reaction made me grin from ear to ear. I had gained a lot in these past 92 days. I had not only learned that my body and health desperately needed my attention, but that I needed to love myself more and not eat and treat every other day like it was a holiday. I was asking myself more often, is this love? Am I loving myself right now by doing this, or not doing that? And each day a little more love and care about my own wellbeing was slowly seeping in.

Lunch was long overdue, and I was starving. I left her office and headed straight to a cafe for an afternoon meeting with plenty of time to eat something first. The menu was littered with a variety of deli meat sandwiches, which another friend had told me were chock full of bad energy.

Studying every option, I literally had the one and only healthy meal on their menu for me to choose from—a tuna wrap with lettuce and tomato. It came with a small bag of chips, which I ate, because they were baked. And after a quick getting-to-know-you meeting I drove back to my home office. A storm was coming, so I tucked in as much as I could, and prayed the power would stay with me.

Day 93: Thursday, January 4th

My kids' school had been officially canceled and so were my meetings. Everyone came in and out of the kitchen while I sat at the island typing away. And I loved myself by baking another batch of sweet potato chips just before losing power.

Day 94: Friday, January 5th

The house salad I had at our extended holiday luncheon with grilled salmon and honey mustard wasn't sticking to my ribs. And by the time I got home I was already hungry again. One of the things I had read about was that people with Graves' disease sometimes experience a constant state of hunger. *Interesting.*

Luckily, our chicken dinner was already in progress when I walked through the door. The bone-in, skin-on chicken thighs were cooked, so I plucked them out of our stove-top cast-iron red Creuset, gave them our shake and bake flair, and popped them into the oven for a nice crispy finish. I sliced up some thick round pieces of skin-on sweet potatoes and buried them under the nicely boiling liquid rice. Yum.

Out of pure curiosity, I sat down to do a quick search knowing my annual gynecologist appointment was coming up. I typed something like "Can a Copper IUD cause Graves' disease?" *Oh. My. God.* I hit a nerve. After a near virus attack on my six-day-old new laptop I escaped just in time.

The important article that I found said one of the biggest long-term problems of having a Copper IUD was that it can affect the Copper metabolism, and eventually cause a Copper toxicity issue. *Ho. Ly. Shit.* It went on to say that it might take years for that to happen, but it's something that every woman with a Copper IUD needs to be aware of. It also stated that having a Copper toxicity problem can affect the thyroid gland and can be one of the primary problems when it comes to Graves' disease. *I couldn't believe my own eyes.*

Screaming at the top of my lungs as politely as I could I felt like I had literally won the lottery. Elation and satisfaction worked its way through my body from my head to my toes like I had discovered my hidden secret superpowers for the first time. *It was the epiphany of all epiphanies.*

Over the last few years, the symptoms on top of weird symptoms I had been acquiring could soon be over. I had self-diagnosed and resigned to almost everything being related to aging and menopause and I couldn't believe that quite possibly the Copper IU freaking D inside my body was the reason I was unhealthy. Obvs.—it was coming out. *My health concerns were seriously taking precedence over my diet. But I was so grateful to be learning all that I had—through my love diet.*

Struggling with excessive weight gaining and maintaining it, could be attributed to my body actually going through hell—right here on earth! My body was holding onto every bit of fat from pure necessity, in full-on, fight and flight mode. All this time I had spent worrying and wondering had led me up to this one single moment in time and I finally had discovered possible answers, clarity, and hope. I prayed. My appointment was just two and a half days away.

Day 95: 196.5 lbs. Saturday, January 6th

Stress is not a good thing if you want to have a peaceful body. And I woke up in a panic. I had forgotten to pick up my camera equipment for a video recording and had to make several phone calls and arrangements. After charming my way to a resolution, my husband and I stopped to pick up a tuna lunch and a taco dinner. I had made a conscious decision and openly let everyone in my family know, that I was letting go of pizza.

In the middle of the store, I must have hit low blood sugar mode, which happened to me quite a bit, and I was heading straight into full-out bitch mode. We wrapped it up fast and I bolted toward the car. Tearing open the blue corn chips right away I loved my body straight out of the bag. They helped curb my hunger and immediately brought me back to sanity.

When we arrived home we continued, diving deeper into salsa and guacamole, just before making our actual intended tuna fish sandwich lunch with a good old-fashioned pita pocket. I was stuffed. And after eating all of that food I decided to work in a meditation. It's a good solid expression of self-love and I quietly imagined the Copper IUD easily leaving my body. I'm sure it already had come loose after my polite internet discovery scream.

The chick flick I chose was already in progress, so I let it wash over me as I snuggled up with a consoling glass of wine perfectly paired with a bag of pistachios around nine o'clock at night. I know, but my glass was full. And the bag I purchased at the store was small. And I totally convinced myself I would eat less because of the extra time it took to pry open each powerful tiny little shell.

Portioning out a proper serving is always the best thing to do but again, I was eating straight out of the bag. As I sat there trying to open one of the hardest to open—but I still managed to open them ones—I turned the bag over to read the nutritional facts. It said 170 calories per serving. Servings per bag, four. *Shit.*

Day 96: 197.5 lbs. Sunday, January 7th

My chain gang was getting longer, but a little more transparent. One of the symptoms I had been experiencing that could also be attributed to the IUD, was this crackling thing I noticed happening in my back. Spinal cord crackling. It wasn't anything painful or even a real thing. It was just weird and annoying. My back would crack constantly at the computer when I sat for long periods of time. It happened during shorter periods of time too, like when I balanced my checkbook sitting at my island bar stool and even when I meditated in an overstuffed comfortable chair. I could shift my torso just a wee bit and then, *crunch*.

Two knuckles on my right hand had thick bumps on them too which was also new, and weird. My original thought was it could be attributed to something as simple as arthritis, but I had read that *thick skin* was one of the symptoms of Graves. *Thick skin.* And recently over the past few months, I saw a discoloration in the skin on my neck—similar to pregnancy mask or age spots—but interestingly, not in the area of my thyroid.

Sleepless nights had been happening for over a year, I think even up to three, and most recently some more than occasional lower back pain had appeared. Another symptom that was weird was, of course, the messed up menstrual cycles, which had been going on for years. But in the last few months an unusual increase in cramps and some stabbing-like feelings were happening in my gut. The variety of ailments added up to a fair amount of pain.

It made perfect common sense to attribute almost everything to menopause and aging. The accompanying night sweats and hot flashes. The mood swings, and irritability. The heart palpitations and fatigue. Of course, it was all because I was getting older and going through menopause. I thought it had to be. It was either that or I was becoming a hypochondriac. Perhaps the definition of hypochondria is old age.

Most of my symptoms might even disappear after being free from the IUD. Altogether, everything I was experiencing may seem like a lot to most people or hardly anything to some, but each of my symptoms had slowly worked their way into my body and awareness over time. Which made it feel ridiculous for me to even consider making a doctor's appointment for every little thing, like night sweats, fatigue, and two knobby knuckles.

The most recent symptoms worried me the most. The dizzy spells, along with the joint pain in my hips. The tennis elbow, soreness in my knees, left shoulder and neck too. *Joint pain* worried me that I might have Lyme disease. Lyme was the one thing I was happy to make a walk-in appearance for.

They said at the clinic, "No news was good news," and it had been about a week. Likely I was free from the one Lyme thing. I wondered if the joint pain was the first sign of future hip surgery, or if my body was trying to talk to me. But I had rationalized and self-diagnosed again. My hips were probably just shifting after having children and moving back into their upright positions. Um, thank you for flying hip you. Bub-by.

For my own safety, I had asked my doctor about the Copper IUD back in early October, because it had just past the 10-year expiration date. "Should I take it out?" I asked. She said one more year wouldn't hurt, but only if it didn't bother me. Unbeknownst to both of us...

I had made that educated decision to leave well enough alone and kicked that copper can down the road. A road little did I know, was not too far up ahead in the distance. How could I have known though? Should I have researched it more? Why didn't I take it beyond a conversation all those years ago when I first got the goods?

Was I so busy that I couldn't take a little extra time to investigate the choice I was about to make? And would I have made the same decision anyway? Was I to blame for trusting a medically approved object deemed safe for possibly millions of other women just like myself? It had done its job for several years.

Perhaps it was just a few years too many. After living with an IUD that saved me, and eventually betrayed me—it would soon be gone from my body.

Day 97: Monday, January 8th

The day had finally arrived. The IUD had to come out right away. I kindly let the nurse know. And she said with a great big smile, "Oh ok. The doctor may not be able to do that today, but we can make you another appointment." I firmly let her know—without smiling—that I would be insisting that she remove it, and if she wouldn't for whatever reason, then I would be leaving here to drive myself over to the emergency room to have them do it. I was calm, but serious and continued, "The Copper IUD may literally be killing me, and it may very well be, the cause of the Graves' disease." I added that I would also like to be tested for Copper poisoning as soon as possible. *And I thought to myself; don't mess with a woman who's on a mission to care for herself as though she were her own child.*

    I often wondered why we need to talk about what's happening with ourselves to the nurse first when she doesn't relay any of the said information to the doctor. Because the doctor inevitably walks in and asks the same questions. I regurgitated the story, and frankly, I forgot some of the things that were said on the first go around. I should have minimized what I said to the nurse like I do when I wait for the microphones to be turned on. I could have given her a smaller carrot and saved the bigger stick for the main event.

    Once it was out, I felt my spirits lift immediately. I rebooked my preventative visit and took the long way home. Through the winding roads, I looked around at the beautiful trees and winter scenery, letting some much-needed peace wash over me. I felt relieved and grateful to have some closure. And I was so proud about taking charge and insisting that it be removed from my body.

That teeny tiny piece of Copper that gave me insurance for all those years was out and gave me an insurmountable feeling of hope. I felt so assured that I was in the driver's seat and on a better path. But most of all, what I felt was an abundance of love. Now that it was gone, I was anxious for my future to arrive—free from the toxicity of the IUD.

Day 98: 198 lbs. Tuesday, January 9th

One roller-coaster ride was behind me. I was grateful and envisioned myself seated on a new ride: a Ferris Wheel, looking out at all of the infinite possibilities to come, beyond the copper syndrome. I wondered if I could ever actually live a non-roller-coaster-like life too. And did I even wanted to? I was happy to focus on work though, and not be consumed by the constant fear of the unknown—until my next appointment.

Refocusing, I poured my attention back on building relationships and took myself to a networking event. Then I was off to a presentation of my own and on the way there, I ate a tuna fish pocket with lettuce and tomato in the car. Like some kind of malnourished vulture, I devoured it.

Beginning in the parking lot I started with a nice neat lady-like nibble at the corner, then moved on to full-blown heaping bites at each stop light as it practically fell apart into my lap. It was messy, but it was healthy. I was healthy. I was choosing chicken, tuna and egg salad over the easier and much neater sandwiches filled with bad energy deli meat.

I don't even want to eat deli-meat anymore. I have no earthly desire to put any of it into my body. I don't even want my kids eating it. Yes, even my favorite, the turkey Reuben. Unless it was a whole-breast real turkey carved, I was all set. And I have to admit that my love diet was looking pretty freaking amazing on Day 98.

<u>*My Love Diet*</u>:

1) Feed Myself Love
2) Minimize Sodium
    a. Remove High Sodium Caesar Salad
3) Reduce Animal Fats
4) Reduce/Remove Carbs After 12 or 2pm
    a. (still working on this one)
5) Let go of Pizza
6) Remove Deli Meat

I arrived at my event and while unloading the car, I popped my apple into one of my bags. Strangely, as I started to walk into the building a slight feeling of nausea came over me. I prayed to God to help me get through my presentation.

Day 99: Wednesday, January 10th

Another day Copper-free, a sense of impatience came over me. I was extremely aware of my body and I thought about all of the ailments that I had accumulated, along with the recent feeling of nausea. On my way to another breakfast meeting, I wondered which symptoms would go away, and which, if any, would stay.

The fruit that was served was bright and fresh and was cut up into small bite-sized pieces that made it easy to eat during a business meeting. I loved that! The muffins were the only other option, and even though they were already cut in half, I made one even smaller by quartering it. *I didn't need to eat an entire half of a muffin.* Taking great pride in my choices I poured a cup of black coffee and took my seat. It felt really good to love myself in public.

It's fast, simple and satisfying. And it is the go-to for so many people for a variety of reasons and occasions. The evening meeting that I attended had a buffet laid out. And through no fault of their own they served pizza.

Serving pizza was easy and it's what most people want. But I kept my promise to love myself and took the only safe item, which was a few chicken skewers. My diet was getting kind of specific. Not tricky or complicated, but specific and I needed more vegetables. I have to admit, it was very tempting to scoop up some of the decorative lettuce garnish and pop it onto my plate with a few of the pop-of-color cherry tomatoes for a makeshift salad. Tempting but tacky. Even for me.

Day 100: Thursday, January 11th

Meditation. It is one of the best things for anybody, and I began incorporating meditation beads into my practice. It's very soothing to be still, breathe, and say my mantras while moving each bead with my fingers one by one to the other side—all the while keeping most thoughts out of my mind. And after all, that is the sole intention of meditation. To clear our mind. The how hardly matters.

I was down to one cup of coffee a day, one black cup, sometimes one and a half. And someone had asked me quite shockingly, "How did you do it?" I said, "Getting down to two cups had just happened over time." And it did. But I did have a little help. I had read that stimulants were bad for Graves' disease and that the compromise was one cup of coffee. I think I was able to mentally accept it, and back off of it simultaneously. I have even caught myself washing dishes before taking that first sip, and on occasion, showering before making my first cup.

A luncheon was next on my agenda and I had to choose chicken or fish. For some people, this was a quick and easy decision. But I had forgotten to register and that's where I usually read the details about the choices. Taking a leap of faith, I went ahead and ordered the chicken and rice and asked my server to kindly please put any sauces on the side because of my blood pressure. I didn't dare say "high" blood pressure because I didn't want to be labeled high anything.

The term high maintenance felt complicated—and bitchy too. And I was learning really fast how to talk down my dietary predictions while still working in the proper medical terms. My meal arrived with bright vegetables, saffron rice, and a happy face. A few people watched her hand me my special meal and wondered aloud why mine looked different, better. It was and I took half home.

Watching the staff scraping everyone else's leftovers into a ginormous bowl, in the front of the house for all of us to see was beyond sad. It was such a waste of food and a waste of energy. And those sacrificial chickens paved the way for the colossal brownie dessert topped with vanilla ice cream, chocolate sauce, and whipped cream.

Many women were blatantly indulging, announcing their decision to treat themselves to the enticing decadent chocolate surprise. I asked to take mine home to the kids, and I took only one small bite after peeking, and one more when I got home. The kids ate the rest in what seemed like a millisecond and a few hours later, the unflattering photos of myself I happened upon solidified my incentive to keep my eyes on the prize—me.

Receiving a notice via voicemail, our kids' school informed us that the Board of Health was instructing they close due to a severe virus going around. My kids had just devoured the chocolate cake and appeared to be fine. So, we weren't too concerned, but we kept our youngest home from his basketball practice and were glad we did. It hit him around seven o'clock.

Day 101: Friday, January 12th

Grateful that it appeared to be the 12-hour kind of bug, we kept our date-night plans. I had always wanted to order the beautiful healthy cheese tray with berries, honey, and a funky looking giant cracker, so we indulged. A few people at the bar were ordering fun pink martinis, so I asked for one too, requesting pomegranate juice over the traditional cranberry.

It was my first martini in a really long time, and possibly the best ever. Totally worth the 220 calories too. I chose the mussels appetizer for dinner in their white wine buttery sauce and once again my husband had the calamari plate. We arrived home early around eight o'clock to kid number two starting to feel sick.

Nicole Perry

Day 102: 196 lbs. Saturday, January 13th

We were out of whole grain bread, but I let it go. Giving myself permission to have the white with one egg over easy I made myself a second cup of coffee too. I had a ton of work ahead of me and we all continued to knock-on-wood that no one else would get the bug. It was taco game night and I made mine on a small separate plate, which was eventually followed by another two more during the game. At about six o'clock, child number three said they felt sick.

The energy in our home was full of frustrations and fear of the unknown and of course I ate a few of the shortbread cookies shaped like flowers filled with jelly that were lying around. I topped those off with a couple of oval vanilla cookies filled with dark chocolate too. You know, the kind that melt and crumble beautifully inside your mouth.

My husband and I felt okay, but still we wondered and hoped we wouldn't get it. Optimistic might have been an understatement, but we were nearly certain that we might be immune to the weird bug going around as the day was coming to an end. We were almost positive that the bug stopped there.

When my husband and I had first met in 1992, we caught a horrible bug. It was 24-hours of brutal heaving to the point that I thought it was the end for me. At age 25, I thought I was actually going to die from that flu alone in my apartment. Eventually, someone would find me all gross in my bed, or worse—with a toilet eating my head.

Day 103: Sunday, January 14th

Maybe I could ditch coffee completely? I was switching to water with lemon or green tea after my one cup anyway. And I had already been up for several hours cleaning my closet and reached for my one cup of coffee that was cold.

Over the years like many women, I had accumulated and kept many pieces of clothing that I no longer wear. I do purge my closet often enough and work really hard at only keeping the things that fit, but there were still a few items too hard to let go of. Items of clothing that I dreamed of wearing again. Like the size 12 tan suede pants with the floral design. Along with the two cute pairs of size ten I Dream of Jeannie like palazzo pants that I felt amazing in. I think I was only about 150 pounds back then.

There were plenty of bathing suits of course. But the most recent item that I wanted to fit into was a size 14 taffeta green June Cleaver dress that I purchased at a local thrift shop without trying it on. It was like new and it turned out to be about 12 pounds too tight. It was obviously mislabeled.

I hung my favorite pair of size ten jeans I was able to wear for a fast minute after baby number two on my closet door and got dressed. Before heading to the station, I quickly heated up a small plate of pasta with a little butter, salt, and pepper for a quick and easy light lunch to get me through.

Day 104: Monday, January 15th

Pasta is such a quick and easy fix, but it's such a no-no on the road to good health. I had eaten pasta quite a few times and in the last few days consequently I had no desire to weigh in. Getting myself back on the healthier track, I chose to have a tomato side with my egg. It's one of the easiest vegetables to serve quickly. And I couldn't wait for the summer so I could grow my own tomatoes.

There was so much happening with everyone getting sick, that I completely forgot about my appointment with the thyroid specialist. I was not mentally prepared at all. Basically I forgot to worry.

My oldest son came with me, and we walked into the brand spanking new building together. It was fresh and clean without a germ to be found. As I walked down the hallway, the gravity of what I was about to discover flooded my mind. The nurse asked me a few questions and I was on to her.

I gave her my new standard, minimal reply. When she asked if I was taking any medications, I told her the only thing I took was about 5,000 IU's of Vitamin D a day, if and when I remembered. It was barely a few minutes when the nurse left to when my new thyroid doctor came storming into the room to question me about the amount of Vitamin D I was taking.

She said 5,000 a day was way too much and dangerous. I actually believe that the amount of Vitamin D is very subjective, depending on if you ask a physician here in the states or a doctor in Europe but I hardly flinched since I almost always forget to take it. Then I had to convince her and promise to take only 2,000 IU's a day going forward. No carrot or stick necessary here. I liked them both already.

It was official. I didn't have Graves. And I barely had Hashimoto's. I certainly didn't want either title, but I said, "Are you sure? Look at all the symptoms I have." Flashing her a list so long I was still filling it out. She said very matter-of-factly, "Look at me. You are probably one of the healthiest people I will see all day. And you look smart." I said, "But what about the other doctor, and the list, and the weight gain over the years, and the...?" She asked, "How old are you?" And I said, "I just turned 50." She said, "Congratulations!" with a great big theatrical smile welcoming me into her club and continued, "Look, your numbers are right here. You are within the normal range. You have one number that's a little higher than it could be, and we'll watch it. Even though I don't feel anything in your neck after examining it, I want you to get an ultrasound in about six weeks, along with another set of blood work the same day. Then come back to see me about 12 weeks after that."

Wow. I couldn't believe it. I should have felt happy and elated, and I did, sort of. I said to my son as we walked out the door together in the dumbest looney tunes voice I could muster up, "Well, I guess I'm just a hypochondriac." He laughed.

The last thing the doctor had said to me was, "I'm going to tell you the same thing that I tell my diabetic patients. Eat fewer carbohydrates. Women always say that they feel better when they eat less of them. So, do that." What I heard was—*If you are not careful Nicole, you will become one of my diabetic patients.* She continued, "You know how we women can overindulge with the carbs." I shot her my line. "So, am I addicted to bread?" I left wondering how could I eliminate carbs—without eliminating carbs?

On my way to taking my son back to his dorm, I had to pull over to the side of the road. He was number four and tossed his cookies out the window. *Yikes.*

I didn't see it as a green light to slack off when I was officially undiagnosed. My body was still not where I wanted it to be. And the IUD was not the only thing that was happening with me. The simple truth was—if I didn't keep working on myself, paying attention, shifting and tweaking, nothing was going change.

When I arrived home, I looked at the papers the doctor had given me and there it was in print: "Routine Ultrasound: -Neck: Hashimoto's disease; -Goiter." *Goiter?* What I saw in giant flashing letters was the word Goiter. But what I also saw wasn't written down anywhere. So far, no medication yet.

Later on that night I told my daughter that I officially did not have Graves' disease. And the first thing she said was, "Well that's good, but what do you have then?" In a smarter looney tunes voice, I said, "I have fat."

Family meals had not been a priority since there was always one person missing from the table, especially with kids going to work or at college. And most recently that bug was working its way throughout—keeping everyone down and out.

There were only two survivors left, and our home was becoming an incubator for germs. It was downright depressing. Each new day filled up with hope, then inevitably when we least expected it, another one gets it.

We needed to bring our family dinners back though, not just for the meal, but for the conversations and to lift our spirits. I wanted to be sure we had at least a few family meals per week, regardless of a potential empty seat and we started right away. I served white cod with my homemade breadcrumb stuffing. And later that night my husband became victim number five just trying to stay alive. I thought for sure it would still not hit me. *Mind over matter, Nicole.*

Day 105: Tuesday, January 16th

The projectile movie-like vomiting started around five thirty in the morning when it finally hit me. I barely had enough energy to text-cancel my appointment. I surrendered to my bed that felt like heaven on earth—ready, willing and feeble.

Our bodies heal when we sleep I remembered, but I barely got any. The icicles on the tree branches were melting fast and our dogs barked non-stop throughout the entire day as each one smacked to the ground.

Day 106: Wednesday, January 17th

Getting the flu or any virus doesn't lend the mind to much thought or deliberation. But I finally woke up thinking a little more clearly with the majority of it behind me along with being undiagnosed. I was glad to have some clear answers, and I agreed with the doctor that I do feel better when I eat fewer carbs.

When I look through our freezer and cabinets filled with the kids' junk foods it makes me want to clean up our act, and our house. What's that saying? *A cluttered closet is a cluttered mind.* I wanted my closets and my pantry to be clean and I wanted more peace. Peace, is always there, ready and waiting for the taking. And the food clutter we had did not bring me any peace—or joy. Although taking a sneak peek at a show series about hoarding did bring me a little comfort.

It might be the perfect opportunity to do a cleanse and get a fresh start by eliminating carbs like my doctor had suggested. My body was pretty much empty anyway. And I was still in the mindset of finding how I could remove carbs without removing them. Maybe all I had was a sensitivity though. And digging through my freezer I struck gold. A gold bag of bread that is—otherwise known as gluten-free.

Day 107: 195.5 lbs. Thursday, January 18th

My husband was on his—no solid food prep day—so I ate my breakfast in hiding before going out to a meeting. I ate lunch in hiding too. I had a delicious grilled chicken salad with honey mustard on the side across the street.

For the first time in what appeared to be a couple of days, I opened my voicemail to hear a message saying that my husband's colonoscopy appointment had been canceled and to please call back to reschedule. I had never texted so fast in my life. The poor thing could eat food!

Back at home he was slowly working in some chicken noodle soup and said it tasted like heaven and he moved on quickly to eating pizza with the kids for dinner. I had no desire to go there. My lunch was a late one and I wasn't starving. I opted for apple slices dipped in peanut butter instead. I was determined to live and be healthier.

Day 108: 195.5 lbs. Friday, January 19th

Eating fruit on an empty stomach I learned was a good thing. And just before leaving the house for a breakfast meeting I had a banana. I wasn't sure what the menu would be like and I made a safe assumption that becoming gluten-free would have its fair amount of challenges. So, I ordered something I thought would be easy. An omelet with mushrooms, spinach, tomato and a side of home fries.

Living a gluten-sensitive life didn't seem like that big of a deal. Just before I left to pick up my son from college and bring him back home, I ate the rest of my breakfast and a granola bar to hold me over until his "traditional day of" family birthday dinner. They all had pizza and I ordered myself the grilled salmon with potatoes and spinach. It's so much easier, and cheaper, to order pizza for everyone, but frankly, I was really getting sick of watching my family constantly eat it.

Day 109: 195.5 lbs. Saturday, January 20th

Reading the nutritional information on my favorite cereal box it was full of gluten—and chemicals too. Darn it! Looking for a new one would be an interesting task. In the meantime, I made one egg over easy with some gluten-free toast for dipping.

For lunch, I curled up a raw zucchini with my new curly noodle maker and placed my leftover salmon on top with some red marinara sauce. The kids had pizza. Shocking, I know. This time the homemade kind. And later that night we all had a nice stir fry dinner with rice. Again, eating gluten-free was not that big of a deal for me.

Day 110: Sunday, January 21st

We finally tossed out the fire hazard of a tree in our living room and swept up the mess. I had a banana for breakfast and a small dish of almonds followed by a hard-boiled egg for a snack. For our early Sunday family dinner, we made pasta with red marinara sauce and mussels. My meal was with the curly zucchini noodles again and it was delicious. My daughter even made a gluten-free chocolate cake for my son's birthday so that I could enjoy it too.

I wasn't feeling deprived at all and more empowered than anything else.

Sitting in my sunroom, I looked across the way into our pool table room at the curtains and cornices that had dressed my windows for over 14 years. No wonder it was the darkest room of the house. My windows were drenched in fabric.

Counting out the curtains I had exactly enough to move all six panels into my living room. I'm not sure how many calories I had burned, but it was a productive day cleaning up the rest of the Christmas decorations. And a little redecorating too.

My pool table room was so open and full of light. My living room looked great too and I had snuck in some exercise. It was interesting to see things from a different angle. To open up my mind to possibilities and make an immediate change for the better. I worked up an appetite and sat down with my good ole gluten-free friend, potato chips in my beautiful new living room. It felt so good to be working on one small change at a time.

Day 111: 196 lbs. Monday, January 22nd

Having not a minute to spare, I grabbed a banana for breakfast and dreamt of the day that I would find a gluten-free cereal again that I could eat fast, easy, and guilt-free. I want to keep some carbohydrates in my diet, beyond the complex ones.

For the time being, I had some gluten-free toast with butter and peanut butter. My skinny stylist breakfast was getting a little old, but it was still a great backup. And I am thrilled to say that the gluten-free bread was starting to taste better than it did when I first started eating it. Were my taste buds adjusting or was my body starting to crave what I was feeding it?

Across the street, I had an interview and since my breakfast was small, I was looking forward to eating something there and reading the menu. The omelet looked like it fit into my easy love diet parameters, but holy crap, I nearly fell over when she said they use up to eight eggs in each omelet. Ok, why? Just why?

I ordered one scrambled egg with a side of spinach, home fries and tomatoes. The tomatoes were barely red and practically dead, so I made a mental note to be sure to order cherry or grape the next time with my sautéed spinach. The side of home fries looked like it could have fed a family of four, so I brought most of that home to recycle into another meal—or two.

Our dinner at home was stir-fry and I practically had to beg everyone to keep the soy sauce separate. I would have to look for a low-sodium gluten-free soy sauce another day and for the time being I substituted hot sauce instead. We all watched a movie together and my daughter kindly brought me the bag of lightly salted potato chips. The salt and vinegar ones they were eating were beyond salty and made my mouth pucker close.

Day 112: Tuesday, January 23rd

Before leaving for a recording I made myself a simple one egg over easy with some of the leftover home fries. Driving home in the pouring rain I took some time to think about what I was really doing. I was not only teaching myself through my own living experience, I was retraining my brain in a way that was adaptable. Including testing out a life living without gluten.

I found a ton of information about Non-Celiac Gluten Sensitivity (NCGS), but what if I had a real gluten-sensitivity? I thought it might be a good idea to get tested for Celiac, but you actually have to have gluten in your body in order to be tested.

And I was at a point in time that there was no way I was going to eat any wheat.

I already had almost a month of eliminating most gluten-filled foods from my diet. And after all that I had been through. I did still believe that it was possible to heal my own body—with some help. From my doctors. And from making better choices.

When I got home, I poured some energy into my business and then took my daughter to dance.

Day 113: Wednesday, January 24th

I was having another home office day and began with some old-fashioned Quaker Oats that I found stashed in the back of the cabinet. I added some chopped almonds, cinnamon, honey, and blueberries. I made a mental note to keep some raisins in the house for convenience when I'm plum fresh out of fruit. And for a quick snack, I toasted some gluten-free bread, dipping it into a small dish of turkey Bolognese red marinara sauce. Yum.

Once again, we had the turkey Bolognese for dinner, and I had my go-to zucchini curled up into a nice little nest on my plate while everyone else had pasta. It doesn't even feel like I am eating it raw. And I love using my curly zucchini maker! We almost threw it into the bucket of non-usable slicers and dicers we had accumulated over the years. But then we watched a video on how to use it properly. Duh!

Day 114: Thursday, January 25th

Breakfast was simple again, toast with butter and peanut butter.

After my meeting I drove back home to have a working lunch and made a small salad that was pretty lame with only one hardboiled egg in it, but the homemade honey mustard dressing was great. I mixed equal parts of Dijon mustard and honey and made about one and a half tablespoons. I was doing so much home making, I was practically Plimoth Plantation primed!

Around noon I started making some soup knowing I was going to need some stamina after the somewhat sucky salad. I began with simple leftover diced chicken and broth and added some frozen carrots and rice. Letting the whole thing boil I added chicken base, and a little salt and white pepper. I thought it was good enough until my daughter came home to try it. She doesn't even care for chicken and she loved it.

I consumed plenty to hold me over in case I wouldn't be able to eat anything at the event I was going to. But I got lucky. They served good stuff and I made myself a small plate of cheese, olives, and cherry tomatoes and poured myself a cup of water.

Within my love diet I was cutting back dramatically on cheese because of the cholesterol, however, since I had almost entirely removed shrimp, bacon, pork, and yogurt, I was allowing a little bit of cheese back in.

Day 115: 195.5 lbs. Friday, January 26th

My day began at a café and I was excited to finally meet the gal that I had to text-cancel. It was a great connection and our discussion turned in the direction of vision boards. It was the bonus within our conversation and motivated me to start a new one.

Next on my schedule was a volunteering gig then a luncheon. For dinner, my husband popped in a pizza for him and the kids, but there was no way I was going to eat it, even when he said, "What's the big deal if you just have it for one day?" He truly had no earthly idea how many times pizza had been on our menu. In his mind one day—was literally every other.

≈ ≈

Chapter 6
To Carb or Not to Carb

"Perhaps the real question was: Why did the old me—not want the new me to exist?"

Day 116: 196.5 lbs. Saturday, January 27th

It helps to be proactive and plan out my meals, so I made myself some rice to have handy throughout the week.

For a quick brunch, I placed about a half cup of the sticky cold rice into a frying pan and added some olive oil, ginger, and garlic. I scrambled an egg into the center of the pan and from the fridge I grabbed three stalks of raw asparagus. Snapping each of them into small pieces I tossed them in toward the end just to take the chill out. On the side, I sliced a bright red tomato in half and topped my pseudo-Asian meal off with a little hot sauce.

I used to make that dish all the time for a quick and easy breezy breakfast or lunch. Especially if there was plenty of pasta leftover in the fridge along with vegetables. And to adjust it to my new personalized love diet, I replaced the pasta with rice and removed the sodium-rich soy sauce—adding a hint more ginger. Because I've always eaten way too fast, I slowed myself down by eating with chopsticks too.

We packed up the car and were on our way to a little weekend getaway. It was only for one night actually, but we were excited to spend some time together away from kids and work. It's my favorite kind of escape, to feel like we are in another part of the country, but a quick drive brings us right back home.

The dinner reservations we had in place disappeared after they told us they could only hold it for up to 15 minutes. Still, I was feeling lucky and quickly searched for an alternative. We saw a nearby bar in the casino with two empty seats and jumped into the bar stools fast. Immediately I ordered the pan-seared scallops with sweet potato risotto and grilled brussels sprouts. It could not have been any more perfect for me. And both of our dinners were so good they went right on top of our best-ever meal lists.

It was a mini vacation weekend so just before trying our luck I had a fun chocolate espresso cocktail martini for dessert. It was delicious and later I found out it was only about 285 calories. Not too shabby.

Day 117: Sunday, January 28th

Together we walked down to the familiar continental hotel breakfast. I was hoping they would at least have scrambled eggs from a box and maybe some canned fruit cocktail. I would have even broken my love diet for a little fake bacon.

I had been to a fair amount of hotels throughout the years, but I wondered if they would have enough to offer a person with a dietary restriction such as gluten-free. Still, I was hopeful since I hadn't really run into any issues so far. But I was a little hungover and hoped there would be *something* good for me to eat. The short answer was no. There was an abundance of gluten-filled food like muffins, pastries, bagels, cereal and toast. But none of it was gluten-free. Frankly, there was hardly anything remotely healthy.

While my husband was artistically making himself a giant waffle, I asked the kind woman if she could point me in the right direction. She said in a very lovely voice, "I'm not sure what we have, maybe a hard-boiled egg?" And then she followed that with, "People usually bring their own."

Yes, she said those exact words—out loud. And without any hesitation. It was one of the stupidest things I think I had ever heard. Really? People with dietary restrictions bring their own food down to a hotel continental breakfast. Although, as absurd as it did sound—she may have been right.

My breakfast was barely good enough. And while my husband was devouring his gluten-filled waffle slathered in liquid sugar, I painstakingly peeled an orange I found—immediately noticing a brown spot in the center. Yuck. After taking one hopeful bite of a non-brown section, I did the right thing and tossed it in the trash. The only other fruit I could see were a couple of red delicious apples that looked barely decorative. I would have bet my first unborn grandchild that they were bland, brown, or bruised, just below the skin's surface.

It was risky. So, I took it slow. After a quick glance around the room to be sure no one was looking, I smelled the infamous hardboiled egg. It was funky but authentic, like it came from a rubber chicken factory. I tossed that too and replaced the whole orange idea with some watered-down orange juice. My continental finale ended with a plain bowl of oatmeal that I added one package of sweet and safe jelly to. My breakfast ranked top of my worst continental experiences ever. Except for the coffee. But overall, the challenges were kind of inspiring, because no amount of rubber eggs, brown fruit or plum-out-of-health hotel was going to sway me from loving myself.

Checking in with the kids, one had woken up sick and my motherly instincts told me it could be a ploy to get us to come home sooner. They were likely bored without us. Either way, it worked. We packed up our hotel room early and stopped at the store to pick up some meds. When I saw the long aisle filled with large bags my eyes grew wide and my stomach thanked me. I grabbed a bag of chips and a bag of cheddar popcorn too. To obviously make up for the continental suckfast.

On the ride home, my husband and I made a list of things we could do together each month to continue putting a little fun back into our relationship. Like another casino weekend and dates that would take us beyond the standard restaurant dinners out. Our evening ended with a white cod dinner my husband whipped together, which took us from suckfast to suckfish.

When fish is just tossed in the oven with salt, pepper, and lemon, it's just not very good at all. Especially cheap white fish. Butter would have definitely helped.

Day 118: 197.5 lbs. Monday, January 29th

Turned out my son was actually sick and had a low-grade fever. I had to keep him home and move my mammogram out a few days. With him being sick and so much to do I didn't have any extra energy to get creative in the kitchen. Luckily, I still had some of the rice I made and could make myself another snappy Asian dish for breakfast and then again for lunch.

They say this was one of the worst flu seasons ever. And when I searched, I found an article that said nothing compared to the flu in 1918 which held the record. It had killed more people than the estimated 16 million in World War I.

Day 119: Tuesday, January 30th

Mammograms used to freak me out. Not because of the top half humbling nakedness or the enduring few seconds of squashing torture, or even having a strange woman hold my each of my breasts like a delicate organ unattached to my body. But obviously for fear of the results. And although I wanted to go and love my body with another wellness visit—we were snowed in. I had no choice but to reschedule my appointment again.

We were both home office bound. And I asked my husband a simple question, "Do you want to have a salad with me for lunch?" His response, "Pffft, Hell no!" This came from a man who faithfully took a salad to work *every single day*. I was a little surprised by his answer because he eats healthily, but evidently just not when he's with me. I would venture to guess that given a choice he would easily drop the word vegetable from his vocabulary and happily replace it with a George Jetson pill. But then again, a lot of people are like that.

My husband has never had an issue with his weight, and he eats healthy most of the time. But on occasion and often enough he goes to the extreme opposite. And when he indulges, he eats things like burger plates and fried everything platters. It just blows my mind when he looks at a menu and says things like,

"I'll just have something healthy today like a turkey club sandwich with bacon and a side of fries."

How can a woman eat clean when her other half eats dirty? Sheer will—I guess that's how. I made myself that salad with homemade honey mustard dressing. And I topped it off with a little tuna fish. I looked forward to making chicken alfredo for our family dinner to try out my new gluten-free pasta for myself too. And of course, pleasing my husband with another salad-less meal.

My doctor's office had called and informed me that the results came back from the lab. They found two kinds of bacteria on my IUD, which meant ten days of antibiotics for me. It did feel good to know that removing it was the right thing to do and I was glad to have even more information, no matter how infected it was. I celebrated the great bacteria news later that night with some white wine and popcorn. Knowing it's not smart to eat straight out of the bag I cleverly scissored off the top of the bag for a makeshift bowl anyway.

Day 120: 196 lbs. Wednesday, January 31st

Waiting rooms used to annoy me, and I have never really liked the word wait, but I didn't mind waiting anymore. The annoyance had flipped. If there wasn't a reasonable wait, I would get a little miffed. I was beginning to treasure all of my writing area times.

Hate is a very strong word. But getting weighed in public brought out the anger in me. Especially lately. In the last several months I had already been at the doctor's office plenty of times. Was it really necessary to "hop" on their scale again? It's almost always incorrectly five pounds higher than my crystal. Especially midday, fully dressed, and most likely, after lunch. I wanted to say *just look at my chart and put the damn number from the last time for crying out loud.* When I begrudgingly stepped onto the scale, I was full of jewelry, jackets, and my Jessica Simpson high heel shit-kicker boots. I was so close to holding my purse.

My appointment was a follow up to my blood pressure, cholesterol, and recent thyroid issues. Sitting on the crunchy white paper waiting, I wondered if I was meant to be a fat—but fashionable out of shape older white lady.

The doctor walked in and said, "Your endocrinologist said you don't have Graves' or Hashimoto's. And look here, she added that you are a delightful 50-year-old woman." She smiled, agreeing with the specialists' assessment. Okay great, everybody thinks I'm delightful. I cut to the chase and said, "Thank you, but what are we addressing next? The possible Hashimoto's in my future or potential diabetes? How about that goiter?"

I told my doctor that at this point, my theory was a process of elimination, which quite frankly, I am sure is the standard medical approach. Next on the agenda was the copper poisoning test. I was anxious and ready to get on with my personal discovery to-do list and scooted up the hall to the lab.

Fasting is not fun, but I walked into the lab this time, to a room full of happy people. Why was everyone so happy I wondered? Hump day? Football? My stomach was growling, but I couldn't help but smile.

Their gritty playfulness was indeed infectious. They all threw cute witty comments at each other into the air, no one allowing a single ball to drop. The front desk technician was getting them riled up even more. Having blood work done is love. And these people were all head over heels for each other.

Nicole Perry

Day 121: 196 lbs. Thursday, February 1st

The fever was back, and I said to my son just before walking out the door, "Wait, I need to get my wallet." He said, "What for?" I said matter-of-factly, "It's only free if you're not sick." In the car, I told him what our monthly payment was—for the "free" visits.

Looking around the waiting room it appeared to be hoarding germs from 1973. The power of suggestion can be strong, so as not to catch even a glimpse of another illness, I hurried my eyes into my phone and a photo of me flashed up from a recent event. I actually looked good. It was the best photo I had seen of myself in a long time, outside of a professional photo-shopped, photo-shoot that is. It had only been a few weeks since eliminating the IUD and the majority of gluten from my diet and what a difference a couple of weeks made. My scale may not be showing very much of a change but cleaning myself up on the inside was starting to show on the outside. And I may have just gotten a glimpse of the new and healthier looking me.

Another order of antibiotics was placed. This time for my son. He had pneumonia. We were medicating together and we both felt nothing shy of relieved to be given answers along with supporting—and temporary—medication.

Our dining table is where we usually eat dinner, but we lazily landed at the island this time. And it was nice to have it full of people because someday it will eventually be deserted.

Day 122: 196 lbs. Friday, February 2nd

My husband and I got on the subject of iron after sharing a pan-seared scallop appetizer on a bed of spinach. It was drizzled with balsamic vinegar and the feta cheese was placed on the side.

He said, "Men in their 40's and 50's can't really consume that much iron, so I have to be careful of how much spinach I eat. We don't eliminate it like women do." The conversation was very interesting and sounded like a good point to bring up at my next doctor's visit. Especially now that I was past peri and almost post menopause and I was about to "not be eliminating iron" right along with him.

Looking over the menu on what to have for my main entre I decided to give their gluten-free pizza a try. Why not. I hadn't had pizza in a long time. It was obviously not the same, but it was okay. And it might take some time to get used to it—if I wanted to get used to it. Come to think of it, my taste-buds did adjust to the gluten-free bread. And it was not so great at the beginning. It may just take a little time for my body to crave the new crust.

My doctor had asked me why I had given up pizza and I told her that through my love diet journaling I discovered I was eating way too much of it.

Day 123: Saturday, February 3rd

The Super Bowl day eve was uneventful except for a little anxious anticipation.

We picked up a few fun foods to eat for the entire next day that would revolve around the game and tried not to dip into any of it. Typical foods like nachos and wings. It was a lot of junk to have in the house, but we did one good thing and chose plain wings. There were no added sugars or sauces. And we planned to make our own recipe from scratch.

Nicole Perry

Day 124: Super Bowl Sunday, February 4th

One of the ways I love to love my house again is to move around some furniture. Repurpose, reuse, redecorate or all of the above. And for this project I enlisted my daughter for help and insight.

The first thing we did was move a table away from a large window in my bedroom, where no one ever sat, to the other side of the room in front of the TV. Now there's a place where the table will get used I thought! We shuffled the rest of the chairs and plants around moving everything into their new space. By the time we were done it felt like I had a mini built-in hotel room in my master bedroom.

Once we got everything settled and the final touches complete, I introduced my husband to our new little get-a-way, conveniently inside our own home. I had several visions of quiet little romantic breakfasts, lunches, and dinners for the two of us to enjoy. And I couldn't wait for Mother's Day.

In the kitchen, I began our Super Bowl menu early by getting the chili started with the usual olive oil, minced garlic, and chopped onions. After the ground turkey was cooked, I added the black beans, white beans, and diced red bell peppers before going into my office for a bit to tidy up while it was cooking.

I guess I got a little side-tracked because I heard this weird crackling sound and finally the smell coming from the kitchen smacked me upside the head. "Oh, shit the chili!" Darting into the kitchen to save it after almost ruining it I moved it to a new pot and added in the tomato sauce, zucchini, and more spices. Thank God it was salvageable. Oops.

The day was going to be long and all about football, so I asked my husband to join me for a little romantic pre-game meal in our new bedroom dining area. I served the small bowls of chili on beautiful white faux china plates shaped like flowers, with a side of one of our favorite cop-and-law episodes. I loved this idea of stealing some time away together inside our own bedroom—minus the afternoon delight. And I was so impressed with myself cooking up a great guy meal and serving it with one of his favorite shows, but I could feel his energy shift into a bit of angst. Perhaps torture was a more of an accurate word. The good wife that I am I set my prisoner of love free.

The amount of food we ate over the course of the day was somewhere between asinine and ludicrous. It was just a game. But a game in which everything we ate was orchestrated around the glorified sport. The small ramekins of pre-game chili were followed by several more we continued to eat during the game along with some nachos.

After the main course of wings, we were torn between commercials and snacks and more chips and dips. And toward the end of the game we introduced some popcorn. Finally, we had no room for anything more and threw in the towel. But only after eating like it was our last supper, again and again, and again.

Day 125: Monday, February 5th

Ironically, my crystal scale has the word *thinner* displayed directly above my score. Hmm. To weigh in, or not to weigh in. Was there really a question? I had some cinnamon raisin toast with butter for breakfast and tried to shake the guaranteed dreaded weight increase from my mind.

Continuing to feed my body what it craved, I made a small plate of nachos and leftover chili, topping it off with a tiny dollop of sour cream. Then I had a little popcorn, followed by a little more popcorn. What was I doing? During that game, most of America did the same. But did I even remember the last healthy meal I ate? And if we were all coming down from our football highs, why was I being so hard on myself?

Thoughts of commitment vs. obligation is what kept popping into my head. Either way, it's a good thing to ask myself these questions especially when it comes to the passion I have for my business. But was my health becoming an obligation? And a better question could have been: Why wasn't I more committed to becoming a healthier person? *Perhaps the real question was: Why did the old me—not want the new me to exist?*

Day 126: 197.5 lbs. Tuesday, February 6th

Beginning with some leftover cooked chicken I pulled out from the fridge, I started to make myself a chicken salad sandwich for a brown bag lunch I was attending. I was getting back to eating healthy and grabbed the last roasted sweet potato that was nestled next to it. I thought it would be nice to add it to my lunch. But then I got an even better idea.

Scooping out the innards of the sweet potato I added it to the diced chicken and light mayo. I was tired of boring and dry sandwiches and my idea was looking delicious and moist. Weighing my gluten-free bread options, I landed on cinnamon raisin, toasting it lightly and adding some spicy red pepper jelly I found hiding in the door of the fridge. Slicing it carefully I wrapped it in parchment paper like the gift that it was, excited to open it later in the day. The healthy and unusual sandwich creation had to be one of my best ideas ever!

On my way home from the lunch I stopped at the store to pick up a large bag of carrots to make homemade chicken soup again. I know, I was overusing the word "homemade", but I was reconditioning my brain. Dicing up some cooked chicken, I added garlic powder, onion, white pepper and parsley to the pot. I'm not even sure what the point of parsley is, but it's totally second nature for me to toss it into almost everything I make. I then added in some nutmeg, one of the ingredients in my recent chicken alfredo recipe.

The carrots were not the only thing I picked up at the store for my soup though. I think my husband is the only person on the planet who can walk into any store for a gallon of milk—and walk out with only a gallon of milk. What I also got were some cracked black pepper crackers for the soup as an alternative to oyster crackers. Oh, and a bag of Fritos for a pre-soup appetizer. And finally, I grabbed some incidental sweet potato chips. Everything was glute-free. But it was interesting that by removing the gluten from my diet—other somewhat unlovable things were finding their way in.

Day 127: 198 lbs. Wednesday, February 7th

While I was in the shower, I started to really think about how I had arrived at the 127th day of this journey and how the weight I had lost in the beginning had found its way back in. My body was programmed to receive, but would this fat ever permanently leave?

It had taken me four months to lose exactly zero pounds. But I reminded myself again that this wasn't a real diet. And I'm not sure how many of those other diets out there are even real or safe. All I know is that if I were doing one of those diets—that I had been accustomed to doing for so many years—I would have quit and restarted several times by now. Or I would have lost 30 to 40 pounds, and probably already be on the fast track to gaining it back. With a little bonus weight of course. No extra charge.

My love diet journaling experiment is helping me to change my mindset first by paying close attention to what is going on inside this body of mine and educating myself during the process and my body feels better now that I have reduced my sodium, which has consequently helped to reduce my blood pressure significantly. I am really proud of myself for not just being aware of what animal fats I consume, but also reducing them too.

So much has happened in these past four months and the information was purely positive. And when I think about it, four months is not a very long time at all. In essence, I am working on me from the inside out. It just may take the old me a little longer to help free the new me.

Sometimes I like the motto to be consistently inconsistent because it introduces an element of surprise. But not with my health. It's the one thing I want to be more consistent about. While I whipped up a quick breakfast of oatmeal with granola, banana, and cinnamon, I thought about how the winter was nearly over and soon I would have to be more consistent about shaving my legs.

Wondering what the spring would look like for me I envisioned my long, lean, and slender new body. I could see myself very clearly fashioning a one-piece bathing suit and feeling confident in my coverup flowing in the breeze at the beach. It had been fairly easy to remove the gluten from my diet. And I couldn't wait for my waistline to start showing me the rewards of time spent eating wheat-free. And when that vision would finally come to fruition from bettering my nutrition.

Just like my lawn, I don't need to have the greenest or the most manicured grass in my hood. And it's pretty clear that we don't. But I certainly don't want to have the worst lawn either. That's up for debate. But I would be happy to be somewhere in the upper middle taking great pleasure with a B grass grade. And I would love to be somewhere in the B+ body range. Anyone can see that the grass is always greener on the leaner side.

My new gluten-sensitivity prompted me. There was an evening networking event I was going to attend, so I thought I would let them know and asked if I should bring something for myself. She said not to worry and that they would be sure to have plenty of options for me. She even brought me three gluten-free cookbooks to borrow. That was so nice!

The spread was simple and there were plenty of things I could eat like the grape tomatoes and little cubes of cheese. But I stayed clear from the bowl of corn chips and salsa. When I ate the Fritos, I had gotten so bloated, it was an easy decision to let go of corn chips in general. Giving up corn would mean sacrificing more than Fritos and chips though. I would have to give up nachos and tacos. And more fun things like popcorn and corn on the cob. I certainly didn't want to do anything irrational, so I let the idea wash over me and focused on just letting go of the chips for a little bit.

Looking through the gluten-free cookbooks later I found a ton of great recipes that looked delicious. But interestingly, most of the recipes included a corn substitute of one kind or another. Corn was the common denominator. When something is removed, it's usually replaced with something else and I wasn't sure I would be able to live a life—gluten and corn-free.

Nicole Perry

Day 128: Thursday, February 8th

The special listed on their menu sounded delicious. Mussels that were sautéed in a buttery white wine garlic sauce. But this type of sauce raised a pink flag for me because it's usually too salty. Thankfully, I had gotten pretty savvy talking my way around the waitstaff in most restaurants. Kindly, I asked if they had a gluten-free pasta option and they did. Then I asked if I could substitute the white wine sauce for something less questionable like their red marinara sauce and they did that too. It was so good, but when my husband was scraping the last traces of the marinara sauce out of my bowl with his loaf of bread, I remembered the restaurant where we first met.

It was in Charlotte, North Carolina. I was the waitress and he was the wine salesman. One of the owners was also the chef and I loved watching her cook. Vividly, I remember how they would put leftover crunchy bread into the blender when making gazpacho soup and sometimes they added it into their marinara sauce.

Day 129: Friday, February 9th

One of the symptoms I had been experiencing was hip pain, so my doctor suggested an ultrasound to be sure everything was okay with my girly parts.

Pulling into the parking lot, I remembered the unusual copay I was supposed to take care of two visits previous, so I dialed up my insurance company just before going inside. The gal on the phone was almost too helpful. She must have been bored because the simple question took all my writing area time. When it was my turn, I was still trying to hang up the phone with my new customer service BFF, but I got up anyway and followed two women into the next room. One was showing the other the ropes.

Hopping up onto the table I was happy that I only had to expose a few stretch marks by unzipping for the exam. The one in charge swiveled her deodorant looking stick across my abdominal area and appeared to get all of the measurements she was looking for. She was almost done and smiled when I asked, "Are my ovaries pretty?" I knew they were, or at least without warts considering the expression on her face and her delightful non-serious energy. The exam was simple, and I was relieved until she said, "Okay we're almost finished. The doctor just wants an internal exam as well, so I'll need you to empty your bladder and then come back and remove your clothes from the waist down." Shit, I knew I should have shaved my legs!

Mistakenly I thought the embarrassing days of internal exams ended with my last pregnancy. And the paper napkin I was given to drape over my lower half was just as belittling, and almost dignity free. The two of them came back into the room and I immediately confessed and said, "My dirty little secret is out. I haven't shaved... for a few weeks." It was way beyond stubble. Almost soft and curly. Kindly, they brushed off my hairy legs with compassion as most good women would do, but what bothered me more was that the gal in training had the Tweety-eye-view of my putty-tat.

I am a confident woman, but I didn't want to make eye contact with either one of them. I could feel the energy of the trainee trying not to look toward my paper-thin tissue. And she was about seven months pregnant too, which was amazingly positive all by itself. At age 50 it was a first for me to see a pregnant woman—training for a new position. But whether she got in a glimpse of the position she would soon be in I didn't know. I was a good doobie and inserted the vibrator-less looking wand as gracefully as one could with the gang all there. All I could think to myself was—this is my body—and I'm sticking it up for you.

It was not strange at all. Lying on the half bed, half-naked. Inserting the wand into my va-jay-jay that was attached to a spiral phone cord, attached to a TV monitor. With two other women in the room wearing lab coats with their eyes attached to my reality vagina show. Nope, not strange at all. This was all perfectly normal. We all have vaginas and each of us has to do something similar each year. I just happened to be the only one of the threesome, who wouldn't get to be on the other side of the napkin.

After I put my dignity back on, the doctor came in, looked over my ultrasound pictures and gave me a clean bill of health. So, it was worth it. Casually, she asked what I did for exercise. I held my head up high flashing my invisible half marathon mental image from four years previous, envisioning the medallion hanging on my bedroom mirror. Then I quickly dropped my chin back down when I said I hadn't done much of anything since. She said I probably shouldn't do that anymore. "What, run?" I asked. "No, marathons," she said and suggested I take up something softer like yoga or walking. Which I assumed was code for any exercise suitable for a now out-of-shape geriatric.

Anyone who knows me knows, that I am definitely a woman who is driven. But I could also be described as a woman who is defiant and one who is most likely to succeed by conquering any suggested doubts, fears, or infamous shouldn'ts. Mostly, I was just a woman who was sitting in a doctor's office, annoyed that I didn't have any desire to prove her wrong. I didn't even have the motivation to sign up for something as simple as a 5K.

Had I reached a defiant and energetic plateau? I knew for sure that there were plenty of real people, who were beyond my age, that ran plenty of marathons. What happened to my ambition? And how the hell did she know that the old me had left the building?

Shortly after my appointment, I arrived at a networking event. And it just so happened to be at a local gym. Seriously, I had no idea. The power of suggestion can be very strong, and I believe in the law of attraction theory. It's old school, but it's a good school. With a grin on my face while I walked through the parking lot I thought, how ironic? Well, it was just January, so maybe not that ironic.

Walking through the equipment room I absorbed the positive high-energy and the smell of leftover sweat. One woman said that this type of gym was not her thing. But she looked just like me. We were both a little older and a lot out of shape. I wondered what she did do if anything. And what crushed that thought was that *I still had the desire to do something*. I wasn't looking to find reasons why I couldn't join like she appeared to be. This was way better than running outside and I was already searching for ways I could sneak a trial workout into my calendar.

Popping my business card into the raffle like any other event I openly double crossed my fingers and toes in hopes to win something, and I did. Just moments after my doctor suggested I find an exercise regime, I won two free classes inside the new free gym bag. *Interesting.*

During the event I had another interesting conversation. This time with a friend. We landed on the subject of gluten and I shared that I recently gave it up as of January 15th. She asked if I had been tested and I said, "Well, whether I get tested or not, I will still have to give up the gluten if I have celiac, so what's the point?" She went on to open my eyes further about how there are many other things that people with celiac disease can't consume, like barley, oats, rye, and millet. She knew because her daughter had it.

Getting tested may be on my love process to-do list someday, but for now, I didn't think it was necessary for me. I didn't have any digestive issues at all. I just had fat. It was interesting to learn that I didn't know very much at all about the gluten-free thing, and of course I have no idea what it's like to actually have celiac disease. It made more sense to consider myself gluten-sensitive for the time being and not worry about anything other than wheat.

If I ever needed to get tested for celiac in the future, I'll at least have some of those other items in my body. What I was curious about though, was that thing she called *millet*. And what I found was that the numerous small seeds are used to make flour and alcoholic drinks and it is a fast-growing cereal plant widely grown in warm countries and regions with poor soils. *Sounds yummy.*

What I was comfortable doing was what I continued to do; remove wheat from my diet and my body. "But this has whey Mom, you can't eat that." my daughter said. And I had to explain that some words listed as ingredients can be tricky. The term "whey" is actually dairy. And boy were my kids getting a good solid, real-life education through my love diet.

For lunch I made a simple salad with my homemade honey mustard dressing, adding a few black olives and a little taco cheese. For dinner, we made turkey Bolognese with freshly grated parmesan. I served gluten-free pasta for myself, and regular pasta for the five slender people in my house that had no weight issues.

Day 130: Saturday, February 10th

Almond flour might just be my saving grace. I picked some up to have on hand specifically for breading fish or chicken, but also for baking and yes, pancakes.

The gluten-free pancake recipe I found seemed a little strange and even cumbersome, but there was no way of knowing until I at least tried. The batter turned out to be really thick and I burned most of them. Just enough to not want to eat them, but not want to throw them away either. The next time I attempt a gluten-free pancake recipe it may easier to just follow my gut, along with a normal recipe and simply replace the wheat flour for the almond. I may actually become a pretty darn good chef by the end of this book!

Shortly after eleven o'clock in the morning, I had a small bowl of leftover turkey Bolognese with my gluten-free pasta. A few hours later, I found some black olives and ate them straight out of the can of course standing in my kitchen. I was extremely mindful though, so I did not view the standing and eating as too unlovable, yet.

Day 131: Sunday, February 11th

Consumed with the state of my health, I had lost track of my original intention to become a socially acceptable and average American size eight.

Loving myself more began back in October with a typical preventative appointment at the doctor. My mission hadn't changed, and I was still on a journey to get healthier and be free from anything that wasn't loving me. I am still working harder from the inside out by looking within. And I'm staying clear from the quick fixes "out there" and being lured into tempting, and temporary solutions. So, yeah, I think my mission is still the same—only better.

Shedding the weight was the original idea as if the only thing I was missing was motivation or willpower. But what I had been lacking in was not just about desire. It's about discovering what is actually going on inside my body, educating myself, and taking actionable steps toward better health. My mission is about adapting change that is achievable for me personally, and more importantly—sustainable. It's about continuing to be me but also fine-tuning myself into a healthier version of me. And that me that I long to be—is in here somewhere dying to be set free.

One bite at a time, that's what I have chosen to do. Take in everything one bite at a time. And I was so glad I was taking it slow—to figure myself out rather than just settle for what is or what will be. Accepting myself as I am and loving myself for who I am is one thing. But not trying to change my size or figure out where my health is at is like giving up and giving in. And settling for what was, is a sure-fire path to several unhealthy chapters ahead in my future.

At around 2:30 in the afternoon I used some more almond flour and tried out a new gluten-free fried chicken recipe for dinner. It was right up there with one of the stupidest recipes I had ever attempted. There were way too many steps. Why must people make things so complicated?!

My instincts were shouting at me through the whole process to just do it my way, but I didn't listen. I don't usually follow any recipe precisely, but I wasn't sure about almond flour and how different or difficult it would be to work with in any recipe. In hindsight, it wasn't necessary to have so many steps. I didn't need glue to replace my gluten. The complicated recipe was ridiculous. I had to use three times the ingredients that it called for, and it still came out like shit.

During our family sit-down dinner, the table topics went sour. But frankly, we hadn't sat down together in so long, I think it was the dynamic that went bad. Luckily, my daughter brought us back to life with the gluten-free brownies she made for dessert. *Delish.*

Day 132: Monday, February 12th

It was going to be a really good day and I was excited for it to begin with my rescheduled preventative OB-GYN visit.

Did she really just say that I had lost two pounds with a smile? I didn't have the heart to tell her that she was wrong since the last time I weighed in I was fully dressed in high heel shit-kickers and layers of coats and jewels. I was pretty sure that I hadn't lost anything.

The subject circled right over to cholesterol. It was still not as good as it could be. Which made me wonder how much more I was going to have to eliminate. In approximately three months, I only had two yogurts, sour cream maybe four times, bacon once or twice, no pork for at least two months, red meat twice, and no shrimp at all. Was butter next? Butter seemed to be the only cholesterol challenge that I had left. That and what I considered to be a small amount of cheese.

We have LDL and HDL, and my final combined overall number was higher than it should be. But my body had to have more adjusting to do. Especially since at the beginning I kept making mistakes while cooking and when ordering food. Realistically, my blood work might be more at the six-week mark rather than twelve. Regardless, the information sure did put a fire under my butt and I was determined to come out a winner.

On the ride home I ate my banana and drank the rest of my coffee letting the news wash over me. Later, I had chicken salad for lunch, light on the mayo and without the cheese, which equated to a dry and boring sandwich. For dinner, I remade the gluten-free fried chicken, minus the ten stupid steps. Was this all even worth it? It could be me, but my doctor didn't appear to believe me when I said I had changed my diet and I wasn't feeling any TLC from my OB-GYN turned PCP.

Day 133: 197 lbs. Tuesday, February 13th

There are behaviors that run through both sides of my family, but that didn't mean that those behaviors needed to run through me. I know that loving myself more and accepting nothing short of greatness is what I deserve. If it's what any person deserves, then that includes me.

I am lovable.

My mind shifts. My body is healing.

Self-love breeds more love.

One of those "drive-thru" restaurants caught my eye. The ones that provide fast fake comfort foods, and good old-fashioned crappy consistency. I drove right by that familiar place eating my banana and looking that building straight in the eyes. Did I feel resentful or deprived? No. I felt like a superwoman—wicked full of confidence and power. I drove by reflecting and rejecting that restaurant flashing my invisible Wonder Woman bracelet cuffs. Pshew-Pshew!

Day 134: 196.5 lbs. Wednesday, February 14th

Being high maintenance isn't a title I think woman want unless you are The Sally that Harry met. But I think being moderately high maintenance is now the new acceptable. And I learned how to chit-chat-it-up with my servers fast and downplay all of my needs, tossing my imaginary long hair into the air.

This particular restaurant had blackened chicken on the menu, which I love, so I simply asked them to remove the useless bun. Preservatives are great, if we're hiding in a cellar from a natural disaster or if we were under a bombing attack, but we don't need them on a regular basis. And I asked if they could place the delicious BBQ sauce on the side. I was positive it was filled with chemicals and/or sugars that my hips and heart didn't need. I added a fun side of coleslaw and it came with a bonus of lettuce and tomato. *My lunch was magnifique!*

Day 135: 197 lbs. Thursday, February 15th

I was a day late and a dollar short, but I still wanted to participate and give up something for Lent. But what could I give up? What would I be willing to let go of? It had to be something I loved for the sacrifice to have any validity behind it. And it couldn't be anything I loved too much because I needed it to be sustainable. Ok then, potato chips and white wine it is! Giving up wine altogether would not be realistic and probably make me insane or start drinking more vodka. But I wondered if I could make it the entire 40 days. So, I gave up just chips and chardonnay. How hard could it be anyway?

After my meeting I got into a discussion with a friend in the parking lot and she was telling me about juicing. It did feel good to talk about our health, turning anything remotely negative into positive. She said that juicing gives your body a break from digesting. And I said, "You could give your body a break by getting a colonoscopy too and kill two birds with one stone."

Some of us met for an impromptu lunch and it was lovely. However, I noticed that I was starting to apologize about my gluten-free label. So much so, that I started to say things like, "Don't worry if any gluten gets in there. I won't die or anything like that. I don't have Celiac, I'm just sensitive." The low-sodium and cholesterol labels were easy enough for me to work around, but I didn't know why I felt like I had to apologize. It wasn't love.

Anyway, we're almost at the point where we don't even need menus anymore. All we really need to do is order what we crave according to the ingredients a restaurant appears to have on hand. Overall, my meal was lovely, and I took the baguette home for the kids. But within the hour my stomach had ballooned. Like secondary smoke, did I inhale secondary gluten from the lovely gluten lover ladies at my table? Back at home I realized my initial instinct was probably spot-on. The scallops might have been undercooked.

Day 136: Friday, February 16th

Oatmeal was an easy choice with diced apples, cinnamon, raisins, and honey and it carried me through my morning meeting.

Using the cafe as a business office, I stayed there for lunch and chose the Cobb salad. I was totally okay with having my one egg for the day. And I hadn't had any bacon or bleu cheese for a long time, so I was okay with that too. My husband and I had made plans several months previous for a special date night dinner that we already knew would potentially be high in animal fats. And I figured I may as well get it all in on the same day.

At the register, I asked if their balsamic dressing was low in sodium. Interestingly they said it wasn't. I had no idea all these years I thought I was choosing the smartest dressing of the bunch. And it was the first time in a long time that I was happy to ask for the oil and red wine vinegar. I was happy because what I was choosing was healthier.

Rather than just ordering red wine during our date night knowing that I gave up the white, I thought I would have another fun cocktail. I did have that pink martini that was delicious and that chocolate dessert martini at the casino too. So, I asked for a pre-dinner espresso martini.

It was like heaven in a glass and I couldn't taste the vodka at all. Moving on to a second, this time I ordered a dirty martini. Years ago, I watched a cool friend confidently order an extra dry and dirty double vodka martini with extra olives. I love olives*!* Clumsily, I tried to order that martini like a professional. And my husband added, "I think she wants it extra filthy."

Taking the tiniest of sips, I wasn't quite sure about it. After a second tinier sip and then a third I was positive. It was gross and way too strong for my wimpy chardonnay palette. Our bartender took it away and cleaned it up for me. Much better.

Short story even shorter, I was drunk. You would think that a woman of my size, and the many years of experience partaking in adult-beverages, that I could handle a cocktail or two, but clearly, I couldn't.

One glass of wine has approximately 13 percent alcohol, while one martini has about 40 percent. Needless to say, two martinis pushed me over the edge. And that cleaned up dirty martini messed me up bad. Maybe it was full of cheap filthy millet. Regardless, I think the likes of Chelsea Handler would have had a good laugh out loud if she saw what a wreck I was over those two girly martinis.

The only thing really worth documenting is that the next day I looked like a two-dollar hooker. And I vowed to never drink vodka again. If I ever decided to have another fun cocktail in my future, I will be ordering a Shirley Temple pomegranate martini with a splash of orange juice and make doubly sure they hold the vahdkahhhh.

Chapter 7
Tell Me Something Good

"...and I thought to myself, maybe it would serve me better to swap out my heels for sneakers—and do this outside—faster."

Day 137: Saturday, February 17th

Before commercialism influenced existentialism, food was different and simpler. TV trays and dinners paved the way for even easier drive-thru's that supported our self-induced busy lifestyles. Manufacturers changed the food we ate, and we changed with it. Man got smarter, and consumers fell for it.

Every step of the way, I consumed theory after new theory, hand over fist. And it all led me to more questions and endless confusion. A recipe destined for disaster. What I wanted was to sift through the necessary information and still embrace a life full of simplicity around what foods are best for me to eat. And I wished I could follow my own gut instincts and listen to that old-fashioned thing called common sense. But it was buried far too deep inside layered years of questioning.

Outside of fitness fanatics and noble nutritionists, I wondered how many people actually knew what is good for us anymore. I wondered if most people have simply surrendered to absorb the paragraphs of ingredients served to us because it's easier. I wondered how many are caught between the chemical—and the clean.

Once upon a time, every meal was made from scratch. And oh, how I would have loved—to have lived—100 years ago with my ancestors when growing vegetables was necessary and churning butter was exercise. I'll never know that life, but I can go beyond imagining. I can work toward eating cleaner today and lean toward the healthier side of the extreme.

I used to think I was eating, and serving healthy meals, and that I was just eating too much of it. So, I did the smart thing and chose smaller plates and smaller portions. For a little while. But week after week my attempt at change was meek. Months turned into years of making small changes that literally amounted to next to nothing. Ultimately, I gave in to the next dress size—and sizes.

When the muffin atop my waistline was too large to hide, and my spare tire grew her twin, I gave in. I bought new so I could physically breathe. I allowed my younger and skinnier self to be replaced by the older version of me. Over time my closet sprinkled little hints of panic into my psyche. And after finding a fair amount of frustration, full-blown desperation arrived. Ahh, but only after I had already settled into an unwanted and unhealthy lifestyle.

The word healthy is overused and underappreciated. Chemicals, dyes, preservatives, and additives have all pushed their packaging envelopes too far, and I was one of the people who did the expanding. We adopted the suggested and helpful structure of the Food Pyramid. Some may even remember The Basic Seven.

Now we live in a world filled with labels while we struggle to un-label ourselves. We followed suit and learned how to read the nutritional information that, since its inception, has turned on a dime into a sea of science. *The average person needs to know how to interpret and decode the facts that we read. And after we read it, some of us still eat it.* And to find our way back to a simpler life, we have to resort to being high maintenance.

If you came to my home, you would find a lot of simple foods in my fridge. I have the basics on hand like milk, juice or cider. Eggs and butter too. We have the typical parmesan cheese in its original hard form, and now "light" sour cream. Of course, we have zero percent plain yogurt for us, and the individual ones with added fruit for the kids. We stock a variety of potatoes, carrots, tomatoes, onions, whole garlic and crushed, mushrooms, box lettuce, berries, and an apple or two. You would definitely find condiments like yellow mustard, Dijon, ketchup (now organic), jelly with only six ingredients, beef and chicken bases, a variety of hot and soy sauces, and light mayo.

We always have bread and bagels on hand for the kids which I constantly have to move out of my way. It used to tempt me to see my old favorites like the cinnamon raisin or the everything bagel but not anymore. I had finally arrived at a place where bagels are always at my fingertips and I have no desire to put them in my hands or in my mouth. Since I no longer eat bagels my body doesn't crave them—and my eyes don't see them.

We definitely don't have a lot of inventory either. What you would not see is a jam-packed freezer because we only buy what we will eat in a short span of about two weeks because inventory is money. So I try to feed an entire family of six, on a budget of less than $200 a week, maybe $250. We keep some frozen veggies on hand, lean ground turkey, and a few different types of chicken and fish. There are plenty of accidental bags of frozen spinach, a few half bananas for shakes, and frozen berries in our freezer too and I tend to hoard crusts of bread to make my Grandmother's bread pudding with or bread-crumbs from scratch, sort of. There might be an earless chocolate bunny from a year ago that no one cares about that I eventually toss. But only after a respectful amount of abandonment.

In my pantry, there are many typical items on hand. The so-called "junk" food is on the bottom two shelves out of my vision, including but not limited to: Cheez-its, sugary cereals, hot cocoa and yes, cookies, crackers, pretzels and popcorn. I hide all of my gluten-free cookies way in the back up top behind the baking section, where no one ever looks. Yeah, they're that good.

My daughter and I both love to bake, and we are slowly weaning out the regular flour for a variety of gluten-free choices. I don't encourage my family to eat gluten-free, but if there's one thing that I think they can live without, it's a home-baked item made with regular flour.

I always try to have a few large cans of tomato sauce on hand too and some sick soup for the kids, black beans, black olives, taco shells, artichoke hearts, regular and gluten-free pasta, basmati rice and risotto. All the basics for our family meals. If there's one thing I do right, my house is generally packed light.

It was the weekend and I wanted to cook an old-fashioned shepherd's pie recipe but tweak it into my own perfect healthier version. I combined the recipe from my childhood brain file with a few new ones I found online, including a scalloped potato side. It was fairly easy to prep, and I whipped it up in no time. I'm not the type to measure—unless I'm baking, then I pretend a little—but I wrote down the basics on an index card just in case it was worth making into round two.

Nicole's Gluten-Free Shepherd's Pie

Browning some lean ground turkey into a pan, I added olive oil, crushed garlic, onion powder, parsley, salt, and pepper. When it was fully cooked, I layered it at the bottom of a large casserole dish, adding a bag of peas next. Then I peeled about eight large baking potatoes and sliced them scalloped-potato style, layering them on top of the peas.

Separately I made the creamy mixture. In a large bowl, I was going to add 6T. of potato flour to 4T. of melted butter and 2c. of milk, but I had buttermilk in the fridge leftover from the gluten-free pancake recipe. So, I added the buttermilk to the flour instead. I sprinkled in some white pepper and salt, and about 1T. of onion powder to the creamy, thick mixture, spreading it over the top of the potatoes. I baked the dish at 350 for about one hour covered with foil then another half hour without. My son Duke said it was amazing. There was hardly anything to change.

Day 138: Sunday, February 18th

We were planning a slow-cooker, whole-turkey family meal so I asked my husband to find a new recipe. When it was about halfway done, my entire house smelled like a Mexican fiesta. It was not the typical smell that went with turkey, but it was interesting, and we had high hopes that it would be better than the standard spices we tend to reach for. Overall, it didn't turn out that great. What that turkey really needed was my French flair using similar ingredients to a roast like potatoes, carrots and baby onions, adding a hint of rosemary and thyme. We managed to salvage the meal though after adding rice to the pot and hot sauce at the table. It was one of those bad memory meals that had my OCD redo written all over it.

When I was pregnant, pick any child, if I had a bad meal or lack thereof, I would let my OCD take over and go out of my way to recreate the meal experience. It didn't matter if it was a meal at home or in a restaurant.

One time I drove up to my favorite fast-food deli to order a seafood pocket with light mayo, shredded lettuce, and a side of chips. It was the perfect baby craving combination of fake fish and slight salad. What was that spice I had craved and grown to love? Old Bay Seasoning? MSG? If I had time, I would savor every bite while people watching—from a table meant for four. If I was in a hurry I would wolf down half of the pocket in the car and the other half about an hour later when the flavors evaporated from my body. In my opinion, there was no other restaurant that could ever replace that chemical masterpiece. Not a one.

When I drove up to that restaurant one day to order my lovable seafood pocket—the deli was gone. The look into my soul that day must have been somewhere between shock and emptiness and my seafood pocket craving grew stronger. I searched for what seemed like probably weeks—ordering replacement pocket after pocket. Everywhere I went nothing came close. One arrived in a hotdog roll, another on a bulky, the innards just as lame, different, wrong. Very wrong. In hindsight I know I was being silly, and my obsession was ridiculous. But still, it took weeks—and the birth of a baby to get over it.

I AM ON A LOVE DIET

Day 139: Monday, February 19th

I had a meeting at a local cafe and ordered one scrambled egg, a side of broccoli, home fries and splurged with a slice of lower calorie swiss cheese. Clearly, they used three to four eggs, not one—and after the initial shock wore off my face, I discreetly measured out what I wanted to eat by drawing a half-imaginary line into my plate.

We all know that restaurants serve way too much food. And my ordinary breakfast was the perfect example. I couldn't even finish the portion I carved out for myself and continued to work my leftovers into three other meals at home. Drawing that imaginary line on my plate was love, and I'm glad I have at least gotten myself to the point where I wasn't looking for excuses to overindulge—just because food was there for the taking.

Kicking off my kids' school vacation week, I took them to a dine-in movie. Practically everywhere I go, I seem to get a little worried if there will be anything safe for me to eat. *But I can't live in a shell. I have to figure this out—in real life terms and situations.*

The popcorn is usually safe, but it's still saturated in butter and sodium, which was risky for me. And I actually thought about sneaking my own grilled chicken into the restaurant to add to my salad. Would anyone even notice if I pulled a breast out of my purse? I could still be respectful of course and order plenty of junk for my kids.

Movies and dieting can often make me feel like a deprived failure. But what was I going to do? Never go to a movie theatre ever again. That wasn't realistic. And who goes to the movies and eats nothing at all—while watching everyone else pass their ju-ju beads, eat chocolate covered everything's, and shovel in heaping amounts of that deliciously necessary movie popcorn? If I were to be so bold as to sneak in my own vegetable snack from home, I can only imagine how royally stupid it would sound. What was once, "Get your candy, popcorn and cigarettes here." Would be replaced with: "*Get your carrots, nuts, and celery sticks here!*"

The other danger for me other than consuming the unwanted chemicals and calories is that if I am not eating food during a movie—any movie—I am usually eating my fingernails. It's gross I know. And it's not love either. Many would even go so far as to say it's a form of self-injury or dare I say even cutting. But what it does for me is to help process my emotions. I am aware. And I came up with a great solution that had been working. Flossing*!*

Why not, right? I floss and drive, why not floss while watching a great movie? It only works though after getting in at least a half hours' worth of crunching and munching first. Which is equated to at least half of an extra-large bucket of the golden-saturated butterless-claiming popcorn. And as unhealthy as I know it is, rarely, if ever, did I let any of my kids hold it.

After studying the fit-for-a-heart-attack menu, I found the perfect thing. Curly fries! I couldn't eat the pizza, so I thought if I were going to suffer through the movie and watching them eat one of my favorite junk foods, curly french fries would be somewhat suffer-less.

Suffering succotash, I don't know why I was so surprised at the size of my side when it arrived. It was plenty big enough for me to share and when the movie was over I left feeling fat, bloated and derailed from love. And being new to the gluten-sensitive life, it didn't occur to me until after, that the fries were likely cooked in the same fryer as all the gluten-filled fried foods.

I AM ON A LOVE DIET

Day 140: Tuesday, February 20th

For breakfast, I had some simple raisin toast and for lunch some shepherd's pie. I snacked on some pistachios later in the afternoon and munched on some corn chips just before dinner. No wonder I wasn't thrilled about weighing in. I was eating like there was no tomorrow—everyday.

We sizzled up some chicken for dinner with peas and the last of the restaurant breakfast broccoli into a wok. I diced up some red bell peppers and threw those in too. People keep telling me that we do need some salt in our diets, which has made me add a little more to my meals at the table and back into my cooking. Still, I was being mindful. Only this time, I threw caution to the wind and added some light soy sauce into the stir fry, which was hardly lighter than the regular anyway. What was their point?

Day 141: Wednesday, February 21st

Giving up something we love doesn't always work and isn't easy. If we love it, then it feels like a sacrifice to it let go. Which is a little different from that saying, "If you love someone set them free," because if they do come back, maybe it was meant to be. Everything is a choice though, whether to eat this or to drink that, regardless of whether what we choose—is a potential mistake or not.

Last week was Lent and I chose to give up potato chips and white wine. I thought about giving up wine completely, but I also wanted to give up something that was achievable. I wanted to give up something that I loved—temporarily. And I did. I do love a nice oaky chardonnay, but I live with an amateur wine connoisseur and I am very aware that there are not a whole lot of redeeming qualities in a glass of white wine. At least red wine has antioxidants.

Anything consumed in moderation is a good thing too. And people who drink two-to-three glasses of alcohol each day live much longer than those who don't drink at all. I wasn't about to go in the direction of complete abstinence, and with some hesitation, I gave up the white to devote 40 days to the healthier choice of red. My body would be happier even if my teeth were not.

Letting go of chardonnay was a small lost love and didn't seem like it would be that challenging. But potato chips—that was a whole other story. Especially now that I was living gluten-free. Potato chips were my new bestie. But again, I wanted to choose things that I loved so that it was a modest sacrifice of some kind. There was no point in giving up pizza. It was already off the table. And burgers were already on the downlow. Potato chips seemed like the natural appropriate next item of choice to give up. Or to take it a step further and set free. Maybe they wouldn't come back to me. But at the first opportunity—I caved.

Bullshitting myself and my husband I rationalized by saying that corn chips were the real item I needed to let go of. And while I was giving in to my favorite rippled kind, just a few days into my lent experience, I drank the last glass of the open bottle of chardonnay in the fridge that I swore I was going to cook with. After just six days, my attempt at Lent was complete.

Day 142: Thursday, February 22nd

Running late, I was grateful the kids were home and asked my son to pop in some gluten-free toast for me while I loaded the car.

I slapped on some peanut butter in a rush and chugged my coffee on the way to my appointment. With school vacation almost over, I went back home to do a little work and then took the kids to another movie. I didn't eat a real lunch, just another bucket of popcorn followed by the dark chocolate covered craisins that I tucked in my purse. I double dared and took a few sips of my kids' sprite, then root beer and was shocked at the taste of their "medium" sized sodas that were practically two liters each.

Later that night I drove to Quincy for a networking event. They graciously served three ample appetizers and I couldn't eat any of them. I was a little hungry though, so I gave myself permission to have the lesser of three evils—the scallops wrapped in bacon. It was the only gluten-free option and I was okay with it. Bacon was no longer on my love diet list because they were in fact, an animal fat and I was considering them to be in the deli-meat category too. A double no-no. They were bite-sized portions though, so I only took six. Sometimes there is no other choice.

Halfway through the event, I saw someone passing out plates of burgers with fries. Yum. It was so nice of them to do! The gal in charge asked if I wanted one with such a hopeful smile that I would accept her gracious offer. And I actually felt bad saying no thank you. But I let her know that it was because I couldn't eat the beef, the cheese, the fries, or the bun. Did I feel empowered? Not really. And at that very moment I couldn't say that I felt proud either.

Back at home, my husband was watching a movie, so I poured myself a safe glass of wine before sitting with him and ate two of my emergency gluten-free chocolate chip cookies.

Nicole Perry

Day 143: Friday, February 23rd

The end of the bread loaf was large enough to serve as a piece and a half and I needed something fast. I toasted it with butter only and quickly grabbed my bottled water and coffee and bolted out the door.

Keeping the promises that I make to myself has become more important to me. Even though the free afternoon work-out class that I was scheduled to attend was canceled, I took an open spot in an earlier class. It was my first time back to the gym in ages, so I was ready and determined to still go. On my way into the building, I heard two women on their way out talking about how hard their class was, laughing and smiling. *Ut-oh.*

I didn't want to do any of the burpees. I was out of shape and older than everyone else there and I was embarrassed to be so uncoordinated. The new way to exercise was hip and I was out of touch. At my age and my current size, I didn't enjoy "hopping" onto the floor—only to get back up—again and again and again. The only time I ever got down on the ground was to organize books—or once in a blue moon fall while skiing. My brain was conditioned to tell me to get the hell up fast, stay up, and to be more careful to never let that happen again.

Was I the oldest *and* fattest person in the room? Did it matter as long as I was there? Yeah. It mattered. I felt the invisible shameful looks of those around me. Not shame on you for getting yourself into "that situation," but the look of, "now there is a good example of what to avoid." I felt like their muse. I was outnumbered by those whippersnappers and embarrassed to be amongst them. I worked hard to not let the smell of judgment in the air deflate my inner confidence balloon in its first stages of gestational growth. But I swallowed my pride and did everything right along with them anyway.

The wall mount thing and weights brought me back to a place of dignity. And the rower and treadmill were where I was both clueless and comfortable. They were already running and walking so the plea I gave to the guy next to me was more of a beg. "How do I get this thing started?" I said. He happily reached over and pressed the "on" button for me. It was so simple. Left side incline, right side speed. Ok, I thought, I've got this. I started out walking slowly to get a good feel for it since the only running I was accustomed to doing was outside, and that was over four years ago. I found my magical safe numbers for the brisk walk and alternated that with a slow jog. I was burning calories in the here and now and learned I would continue to do so long after I left. Nice!

It did scare me a little to be exercising my heart, but I knew I could actually be *the fittest and oldest* in the room if I so desired. I could be their envy if I wanted it badly enough. But could I pour all of my energy into working out and becoming fit, instead of constantly looking at the number that wasn't budging on my scale? Could I be the one who gets addicted to strength training instead of weight weighing?

We have to crawl before we can walk when we first enter this world and evidently many times throughout. And I got through that workout. It was my first time at a gym in more than 20 years. I am not young anymore and I needed to be realistic about how old I am, and what my current body is capable of. This first experience back to the gym—in my eyes—was almost 100 percent complete success.

On my way out a woman said to me, "Don't you feel great?!" My reply: "My legs feel like Jell-O, and I think I'm gonna puke." I'm usually not negative like that—at least not out loud. But she couldn't have smiled any faker or walked away from me any faster. Her body language told me she needed to get as far away from my bad energy as quickly as possible so as not to crush her feel-good moment. *Note to self, it was a fast and easy way to shed a skinny fit person.*

I worked up a hypothetical appetite. The chicken tenders cooked up fast and I placed them on top of some gluten-free spinach pasta, adding red marinara sauce and then real parmesan cheese. This was my simple lunch after my first workout and dinner was lighter. Toast with peanut butter, followed by some gluten-free crackers, red-pepper jelly, sliced parmesan, cabernet, and a quick diet review.

My Love Diet:

1) *Feed Myself Love*
2) *Minimize Sodium*
    a. *Remove High Sodium Caesar Salad*
3) *Reduce Animal Fats*
4) *Reduce/Remove Carbs After 12 or 2pm*
    a. *(still working on this one)*
5) *Let go of Pizza*
6) *Remove Deli Meat*
    a. *Including Bacon*
7) *Live Gluten Free*
8) *Exercise.*

Day 144: Saturday, February 24th

There's a restaurant that we love to go to for date nights which is conveniently close to home, but it's Italian. And that means the options are a variety of carbs: pasta, bread, and stuffing. One of my favorites is their stuffed mushrooms smothered in cheese that I reluctantly had to let go of. Someday, I'd love to come up with a lean, low-sodium, gluten-free spinoff. But would it still taste good? I wonder if they could make it taste good.

It was not a surprise and I had called it. Their marinara sauce was not gluten-free. So, I ordered their gluten-free pizza since that sauce was safe. This time, instead of getting black olives, she convinced me to get pepperoni. Another item I was placing under the deli-meat category. But heck, I wanted to treat myself after the workout.

Day 145: Sunday, February 25th

One of the things that makes me fall off the wagon quickly is when everyone around me is indulging. I feel deprived. And it's a fast ticket to saying, "screw it."

My daughter was whipping up some waffles for everyone which I couldn't eat, but instead of saying screw it this time, I tweaked it. I took my gluten-free bread from the freezer and made myself some warm and comforting french toast. I took back my power and topped off my toast with a little butter and honey.

We needed more recipes though. I was getting tired of making meals without one. Meals that we chuck together and assume will come out amazing, and inevitably they don't. We need better fish too. Cheap fish just isn't worth it.

I grew up in the '70s and was raised by a single mom, so it's realistic and understandable that I prefer my fish square, breaded and from a yellow box. It's what I grew up eating. Protein that vaguely resembled where it originally came from. Now, as an adult, I still like my chicken boneless and my fish skinless. My ancestors are European and Canadian, but I'm American. And I like my protein in its least barbaric form— which is as far from the original version of the animal as humanly possible.

Growing up we had a neighbor that frequently made gourmet Portuguese meals and I remember one in particular was red sauce based when I was there playing. The aroma in their kitchen smelled like heaven, but when I stood on my tippy toes to look into the pot and saw the giant whole octopus that had stopped swimming, I changed.

Sautéing some mushrooms in with our salmon steaks we included a side of asparagus and broccoli, skipping the carbs altogether. We thought the steaks would be better than fillets, but my daughter graciously pointed out during dinner that they looked like they had little mini spines.

After that discussion, we agreed to go back to purchasing fillets. Even though none of us cared for the skin-on version and later we made up for the carb-less meal by eating some corn chips with some leftover guacamole and mixed in a touch of sour cream to stretch it.

Day 146: 197.5 lbs. Monday, February 26th

I was committed to my new gym workout routine and was excited to have that first class behind me. After popping in a couple of french toasts, I left for workout number two. I started to feel like I was almost a regular at my second visit, except when it came time for the floor exercise.

At my age I found myself reaching for simpler moves from my memory bank like yoga stretches and prayed I didn't look like an idiot. I brought new meaning to the word modification. Keeping what was left of my pride intact, I got down on the floor and did some air bicycle moves I remembered from the '80s.

After the second workout, I felt better when I left. I was excited to get the really cool numeric results about my heart rate and the number of calories I had burned. I am such a visual and it helped. I popped a gluten-free cookie in my mouth on the car ride home to sustain my blood sugar levels and reflected on how proud I was that I achieved another successful workout.

At home, I whipped up a healthy salad with grilled chicken, a few black olives and some of my homemade honey mustard dressing. *Delish.* For a snack, a few hours later, I made a bowl of fruit with some granola, cinnamon, and honey. It looked and tasted so good I wasn't feeling deprived at all.

Day 147: Tuesday, February 27th

Exercise. It's what we know we need to do. We have to move our bodies. We all know this. And finding something that gets us motivated can be a challenge. I had tried many different types of exercise throughout the years, but I'm not as young as I used to be. And thank God our muscles have a memory.

In my 20's I could work out for like two weeks at the gym and have a rocking body in no time. I barely had to jump on a few machines or pick up some weights here and there. With little to almost no effort, the workouts worked. And frankly, I put more effort into my leotards and body thongs.

Before and after birthing babies in my 30's, it took a little longer to see my body bounce back and take shape. During pregnancy, I attempted a little prenatal yoga once or twice too and in between births, I spent most of an entire decade doing at-home VCR yoga during nap times, along with a little driveway jump roping at yellow bus drop-offs and pickups. But the need to have my old body back was slowly replaced by the desire to focus on the new family we were creating and that, "Oh shit it's now or never" mentality finally hit me in my 40's. I panicked but stepped it up by taking up running. Jogging really. And one of my neighbors had asked me what made me decide to do it. I just said it came to me one day. I was in my basement doing some exercising that resembled aerobics on my stair stepper with little two-pound weights in my hand...*and I thought to myself, maybe it would serve me better to swap out my heels for sneakers—and do this outside—faster.*

I was really getting into my new Shake Weight too, but I grabbed my pretty little pink two pounders instead and took them outside. I just did it. My neighbors may have had a good laugh that first time or two. Or perhaps they quietly cheered me on. Either way, I was filled with so much desire about my new idea that I didn't care who drove by or who mocked me.

Running my first 5K I felt pure joy, accomplishment, and pride as I crossed that finish line. I think my time was under 30 minutes, but it didn't matter. I was so proud of myself, even though I ate that doughnut just before the race started.

Now that I'm in my 50's, I was sort of looking forward to how this next decade would unfold. And this new way of measuring each small success at the gym by knowing my heart rate and how many calories I burned did help. It helps for me to see something. Especially when on the outside there hardly appeared to be anything happening. It helped to have something to hold on to—to keep me holding on.

I made myself a green protein shake that looked and smelled delicious. I started with eight ounces of almond milk, a heaping scoop of protein powder, a hunk of frozen spinach, one half banana, and a little frozen pineapple. It was plenty satisfying to keep me focused on my presentation and to share I brought some homemade gluten-free blueberry muffins, a few bananas, and bottles of water.

One of my guests hugged me when I told her the muffins were gluten-free and showed her the photo of the box I took as proof. She was also a friend, but she did say that it almost never happens. Hardly anyone offers something as simple as gluten-free. It's amazing how many people are gluten-free, but why was the simplest of the dietary restrictions not embraced by the masses? I was so happy to be serving something delicious that anyone could eat including myself, and I did. I gloated a bit too, over the fresh blueberries I added to the recipe.

Afterward, I met some friends for lunch. There were plenty of things on this menu for me to eat and the abundance of gluten-free choices almost made it harder to decide than when I usually have hardly any choice at all. I settled on the hummus and veggie plate which arrived on a gigantic platter. I knew right away that I would get plenty of additional meals out of it—even after sharing. And around three o'clock I enjoyed round two. Round three came after coming home from a board meeting.

Day 148: Wednesday, February 28th

It was around 10:30 in the morning when I finally decided to break my fast. I found a fresh zucchini and curly noodled it onto a plate with some turkey Bolognese, freshly grated parmesan, and a few red-pepper flakes. It was on a small plate, but it was a good-sized portion and even when I was plenty satisfied, I kept on eating. It was more along the lines of shoveling than anything else. Nothing remotely graceful about it. Just one more bite I kept thinking, again and again. Perhaps it was just a little extra fuel that my body needed.

Later that night my husband met me at a networking event that I planned to transition into our date night. It was so crowded, that I could barely work my way over to even see what they were serving. So, I snuck out early and my husband arrived at the same time. We found seats at the bar and I ordered the gluten-free pita triangles with Camembert cheese and fig. It was delicious, perfectly portioned and nothing left to take home.

Day 149: Thursday, March 1st

March 1st is one of my favorite days of the year because I know spring is just around the corner. I chose to go home for lunch and whipped up an egg over easy with a side of tomato slices and raisin toast. I opened the door to get some fresh air with my lunch plate and sat on the deck with the dogs by my side. Soon my yard would be full of green grass and outdoor rooms.

It was Day 149 and I was still practically the same size as I was on day one. The idea of creating my own diet was great, but the thought of accomplishing this in one year was starting to feel more like a burden than that of self-discovery and change. We ordered pizza for the kids and a gluten-free one for me again with some not-so-slender pepperoni.

Day 150: Friday, March 2nd

Grazing the entire day was not my intention. Or subconsciously, maybe it was. I began with a simple protein shake for breakfast with cocoa and peanut butter. And at around 10:30 I had a small slice of gluten-free pizza and a small plate of roasted veggies from the day before. Shortly after that, another slice for lunch and more roasted veggies, this time eating straight out of the container while standing in my kitchen. Around four o'clock I had one slice of raisin toast to hold me over until dinner. Like I even needed it.

Dinner was a roast, a bloody well right roast. It was beyond rare, and I simply couldn't bring myself to eat it. Even after they tried to cook some of it longer. Changing my own mindset had taken a lot of work but getting my close family members onto my new healthy train seemed to take even more effort. Once we had settled into our dining places, it occurred to me looking around that the raw meat with extra-large pools of blood on each plate might be unsafe for my youngest kids to eat.

Like a king to his throne, my husband practically guarded his plate with his utensils as did most everyone else. I took two no-thank-you bites from the outer-edge and snuck my meat onto my husband's plate when no one was looking. I was surprised when my youngest son said it was good, but even more surprised when my daughter said out loud that she didn't like the feel of the meat in her mouth.

Day 151: 197 lbs. Saturday, March 3rd

Before eating and leaving for the gym I stripped down most of my clothes and weighed in at 197.5 lbs. Then I weighed in again. FYI, a pair of small earrings, undies, one workout bra, and a pair of socks weighs in at a half pound.

It was snowing, but I was determined to go have my workout. As I pulled into the empty parking lot, disappointment flooded my face because they happened to be one of the nearby towns that had lost power. Driving home I thought about what I could do on my own. I felt like I *needed* that workout. But did I need the group coaching and enthusiastic support every time?

Rather than figure out some kind of traditional exercise, I tackled the mountain of Christmas decorations that I had been meaning to take care of for weeks. And I moved my body beyond the chair to the fridge. I got on a roll redecorating and cleaning and even organized the magazine rack by the toilet, multi-tasking while I sat on it.

I was exhausted and had worked up an appetite. Pouring myself a much-deserved glass of wine and grabbing a bag of corn chips, I settled into a chick flick.

Day 152: 196.5 lbs. Sunday, March 4th

It was the second consecutive day I looked up from my desk and saw a runner passing by outside. Was that a sign to ignore? Could I consider becoming a slow jogger again? I thought about timing myself for 15 minutes as I run out of my neighborhood and then turn around and come back. Thirty minutes is a very good workout regardless of how many miles it turned out to be. Maybe I didn't do it because it was cold and wet. And maybe I shouldn't because of my age, and my knees. Maybe there will always be a reason and another maybe.

When I was a runner, I was so proud to talk about my time and ask others about theirs. Technically, runners only compete with themselves, but I found it interesting to listen to what other people did, what they avoided, what their goals were and why. I thought for sure when I asked one particular neighbor what her time was, she would tell me that she ran five to eight miles a day and was a seven-minute-miler. Nope. She laughed and said she can barely run two to three miles a few times a week at nine minutes a mile. Back then I thought to myself wow, she's in great shape. Maybe I should back off trying to climb such huge five-mile mountains every day. I wasn't a real runner like her, why was I trying to act like one?

We wanted to come up with a better idea to cook white fish for dinner and I found an awesome fish cake recipe. I substituted my own homemade gluten-free breadcrumbs and served the fishcakes with asparagus and broccoli. Variety is so good*!*

Day 153: 197.5 lbs. Monday, March 5th

I woke up to the sound of the trash can dumping over in the driveway for the second time in about four days. It's interesting how something so small and insignificant can get under my skin.

I tried my best not to let it get to me, but my son gave me a hard time about helping to clean it up. Then my daughter picked a fight with me just before getting on the bus about something I don't even eat, Oreos.

I felt like a tiny fish swimming against a massive current—in a race where no one wanted me to win. Everything is a choice, so I coached myself and put on my just-do-it attitude and settled into my meditation. Which did help, a little.

Day 154: 197 lbs. Tuesday, March 6*th*

Beginning my day with another meditation I was starting to feel like me again. I made a simple protein shake and ordered a healthy unsweetened green tea at my meeting. On the ride back to my office I quietly ate a banana. I was starting to see a shimmer of light.

My body was adjusting to the new copper and gluten-free living quarters. It took years to pack on all that weight while my body cocooned that copper in its wheat-filled home, so I convinceed myself it was understandable that my body needed more time to heal. I enjoyed a simple grilled chicken salad with honey mustard for lunch and a few strawberries with Nutella for a little sweet afternoon treat before taking my daughter to dance.

Day 155: 197 lbs. Wednesday, March 7*th*

I heated up some peas and baked potato cubes into a pan and tossed in a scrambled egg in the corner for an early lunch. It was a challenging day in a few different ways, so when the kids got home from school, I took them out to dinner.

Their root beers reminded me of when I was a kid. The size seemed like the only thing that had changed. In the early '70s, we still had one of those hanger-on restaurants where they placed the tray of food onto the window-sill of our car. It was so cool. At home, I showed my kids the size of that little glass root beer mug they gave us back then. It must have been like three to four ounces and was gone in no time at all.

We hated that ridiculous child-sized torturous mug. My goodie-two-shoes, little-girl-self failed every time I tried to savor the flavor throughout my meal, but boy did I try. My son Duke said, "Yeah but you would get free refills, right?" I laughed out loud! "No, we didn't, and when I was your age, I had to walk two miles from the summer camp bus stop home every day too."

Day 156: 197 lbs. Thursday, March 8th

Another spring snowstorm was in full force. And as I sat down to my computer and snuggled up to my morning black coffee I wondered if I was truly on the right path.

Questioning my direction is a good thing. And I was almost 100 percent certain that I was exactly where I was meant to be. But sometimes a spark of doubt does appear. It's normal. I get it. We all have it. To a degree. But would I be able to snuff the doubt out? Or would that spark of doubt ignite into a flame for me to continually blame?

No matter where I go it's the same. Regardless of the quality of the restaurant, the salmon is always delicious. Whether it's a chain or an independent one, the salmon is served to me skinless, thick, and juicy. Restaurants don't serve "skin-on" salmon. And I wished I could make it like that at home. Anyway, I planned to try again. This time resorting to one of my favorite recipes that would surely be a hit. Blackened salmon with garlic mashed.

Chapter 8
Too Little, Too Late

"Before I even considered opening that heavy door, I had to take a big giant step toward forgiveness."

Day 157: Friday, March 9th

They say that moderation is key; As long as anything is consumed in moderation, right? But the word moderation itself has practically become an acquired state of mind. Most people are capable of being moderate at one time or another. But living inside moderation at all times can feel like residing in mediocrity. Especially when we live in a world filled with overindulging. And having more practically equated to winning. Obsession arrives only after innocence meets customary and then morphs beyond routine. I can think of endless ordinary examples.

The shake I made for breakfast was fast, delicious, and satisfying. The paragraph of ingredients on the label—that I still can't pronounce—doesn't sit well with me. But the company is highly reputable, it's protein, and it's gluten-free. It has many other bells and whistles too that would satisfy any nutritionist and even the highly aware, amateur foodie detective like myself.

Depending on my mood I can turn my protein drinks into fun treats that practically taste like candy bars, milkshakes, and even a virgin pina colada! Now that's moderation I can live with. The one I made got me to the other side of my hair appointment and into a lovely quiet lunch.

Fast food isn't made with love—or from love I should say. But I wasn't looking for a *farm-to-white-table-cloth* place to eat either. I wanted comfort. So, I chose a familiar chain because it had just the right amount of consistency and I was curious. I hadn't been there since I let go of the gluten, so I was prepared to have limited choices. It does feel pretty good though. That the limitations I have, are the ones that I actually want.

Surprisingly enough they had a gluten-free menu. I started with a glass of cabernet and a salad but completely forgot to ask for the dressing on the side. There's enough waste in the world so I let that go and ate it anyway. Forgiveness is something we need to give to ourselves and I forgave myself for forgetting.

My food runner arrived with part of my meal, but the large white plate she held only had a piece of grilled salmon on it. That's it. A ginormous plate with a salmon fillet nestled to one side and nothing else.

I hesitated to take the plate with all that negative space when she tried to let it go into my hand. Thankfully, *my* server appeared and steered her in the other direction. Why did I feel like the thorn in my own side? When the runner came back, my garlic and parmesan broccoli was missing the garlic and parmesan. But I ate that anyway too, this time I forgave them. It was more delicious than I could have ever expected though. My salmon was grilled to perfection: perfectly pink, juicy, and about a half inch thick. This meal was so good I actually savored every bite, no wolfing around. It's so frustrating that I can't seem to cook fish like this at home. Was I the only person that was fish-challenged?

Watching the kids come and go with their Friday night snack meals, I picked through my playlist while my husband and I sat at the kitchen island enjoying a glass of wine together. A softer side of Pat Benatar, some '70s, then a little Fergie. We were discussing a fair amount of challenges we were facing with our first child in college.

It was all still very new to us. Our family and our marriage were both shifting into new chapters. When Bonnie Raitt came on, my husband took my hand and we slow danced in front of the fridge.

Day 158: 196 lbs. Saturday, March 10th

Before leaving for another casino getaway I wanted to get in a workout. It was my last freebie class before I had to decide whether or not to join the gym. And it was so good I was highly motivated.

I bought enough passes to keep my ass moving for several weeks. And I hoped to discover some moderation within my new routine. Joining the gym to begin with was a big step for me. Considering I was more of a workout in private via VCR kind of gal. I had only joined a gym once in my early 20's, and then a second time shortly after my second marriage kicked in. I'm in my 50's now, and most of my peers at this place were young eager millennials. Maybe if I hung around them long enough, I might start to look like them. You know, like when people start to look like their pets.

Our pets like to take an occasional poop in our home gym. It is in the basement, but it's more ideal for my husband who has accumulated quite a bit of equipment over the years. It's got a lot of man weights in it.

We tried the gym thing together like many other couples or even individuals, but that trend came to an end. Especially after we found out that the monthly membership fee was still coming out of our bank account almost two years after we gave up going. Naturally, that was the end of us ever joining another gym. In my husband's eyes, it was a waste of money and all gyms were thieves.

I had purchased a fair amount of equipment myself over the years too. My first piece was back in 1995 shortly after we tied the knot. My Health Rider is still a part of our home gym today and I have to say, to this day it was the best $600 dollars I had ever spent. I was sold right away when they demonstrated people using it that had an injury to one shoulder or an ankle. Why I was convinced at the age of 27 by the potential future injury I had no idea, but I used that piece of equipment, off and on, many times over the years. Mostly off. But I did pretend to be injured once or twice just to get my money's worth.

Shortly after buying into the infomercial, I bought into another: The Ab Cruncher. I didn't get as much use out of that, but at the time it seemed perfect and totally worth the two or three $25 payments. I even have photos of me using it in my nightgown on Christmas morning. At age 28 and pre-children, did I really even need it?

Of course, I do have a few Suzanne Somers' items and books. Who doesn't? One of my favorites was the stair stepper I inherited several years ago from my aunt. What a bonus that was—and it was free! I loved it so much I practically danced on it. Well, as a matter of fact, I did dance on it a couple of times—in heels. And last, but not at all least, one of my favorite infomercial purchases of all time for only $19.99 was the Shake Weight, which of course still stands the test of time—every time I wipe off the dust.

Someday I imagine we'll sheetrock the walls and make our basement gym a little more pleasing to the girly eyes than just good enough for the guys. At this point in my life though, I surrendered to the community-driven millennial motivation to keep my ass moving and shrinking in the right direction.

Something old, something new, something borrowed and something blue. Our new area rug had arrived, and it was time for me to shuffle some of our somethings around. I was excited to change things up and use some of my muscles that tend to get ignored. I love it when I get so into decorating and repurposing that I accidentally get a bruise or scratch myself and not even notice I'm bleeding until significantly later. I feel so alive when I'm dialed in like that and living in the present moment. Those days are the best!

I whipped up enough protein shakes for at least three of us and started to prep the area. And by prepping the area, I mean do almost everything I possibly can so the actual help I need to enlist anyone for is little to none. It keeps the complaining down to a minimum. Like a game of chess, the first move began. The old rug came out before the new rug could go in. And of course, in the middle of the rug shuffle, I opened up the clockworks from the back of the brand-new clock that I bought which was broken, saving myself a trip back to the store. We moved another rug and then another, finally taking the least favorite down to where it would be loved again—to my son's room on the good side of the basement.

I had accomplished not one but two workouts and finally went upstairs to get ready for our date night out. Just as we were leaving the house I whispered to my daughter and youngest son, "Hey would you guys mind continuing the decorating and organizing in the basement while we're gone?" Their eyes lit up excited like I had just given them money. Perhaps they had recently learned the word patronize at school. Or they liked change. It was a scratch-on-the-head moment for me, but I knew they would be home alone, and I thought a team project would be a good way to keep them busy for at least a few hours.

Within the hour they sent us a video of the completed organized space. Wow! All those years of them watching me tackling any given room in no time at all had officially paid off. I couldn't have been prouder! Until we got home. And I opened the closet.

The last trip we made to a casino was our very first one together, which we had driven to and stayed overnight. This time we took a bus with a group of other individuals. They allowed us to bring snacks and booze too if we wanted. Clearly, we were amongst the pros. Once we were seated, we immediately dove into our cooler bag and ate—snack after snack—and drank, drink after drink.

Moderation was nowhere to be found. I think we took their cooler suggestion to an entirely ridiculous weird level.

Chips and dips and cabernet oh my! After reading the labels of each dip, I discovered there was one that I would no longer be able to eat. It had some kind of wheat dust in it. I wondered, could wheat be just as addictive as sugar or cocaine?

Coke or any other kind of no-name brand soda was one sugary substance that we never had in the house growing up and as I became an adult and I thankfully never got hooked on it. I've managed to live a life free from Coke and cocaine, even in high school. One time I actually sat at a house party where they passed a glass tray with many white lines on it around the room. I let that tray pass right by me to the next person. My friends always agreed with me that I didn't need any more energy. Plus, it was more for them.

What came in perfectly handy for the trip were my plastic stemless wine glasses with the thumb imprint. I enjoyed my white chardonnay while my husband enjoyed his scotch and cabernet. We arrived at the casino and just before we pulled into the red-carpet service entrance, they called the raffle winner. Holy shit I had won! My husband was beaming with great lucky-charming-wife pride hoping my luck would continue inside.

We walked straight into the heart and center of it all. And regardless of the endless amounts of snacks that we ate, as well as having had plenty of adult-beverages, the first thing we did was find a restaurant to order more drinks and more food.

Entering the fast-paced hurry-it-up atmosphere, and snap-to-it energy, we had to order quickly or risk losing our server to the next couple. I opted for a simple burger with lettuce and tomato, minus the bun and a side of asparagus. And it was so good I was really glad I saved the red meat opportunity.

It is interesting how our bodies change as we get older though. During our blast-of-a-fast date night dinner, I was ready to take a nap! We chugged some coffee like the older lame couple we were before taking to our slot machine positions and tiredly tried to make some magical money appear.

The whole night was fantastic, but there was just one thing. During the course of the evening, the two workouts I had done earlier started to kick in. My legs were so sore that I could barely walk up or down any stairs. Sitting on any given toilet was challenging and standing back up was even harder. The muscles in my calves must have been asleep for decades!

We were so grateful to be sitting on the bus again at the end, ready for a quiet ride home. We didn't win big at the casino, but they drew more raffles on the bus, and I won again, and again. It was almost embarrassing to the point that I started to cross my fingers hoping they wouldn't call my name. Overall it was exhausting but we both agreed that it was so much fun we would easily do it again.

Day 159: Sunday, March 11th

Slowly coming back to life with a cup of coffee I opted to get back on track and start the day out healthy. I had a small bowl of berries sprinkling it with some granola, cinnamon, and honey. Enjoying the extra daylight savings hour and quiet breakfast in my sunroom, I noticed that the rug under my feet was fighting with the new rug just a few feet away. As exhausted as we were, we shuffled them one last time.

We lounged around all day recuperating in our pajamas and got into a discussion about comfort foods. When we become adults—I think I can speak for most—there are plenty of foods we still reach for from our childhoods.

One of my favorites that I got to enjoy a few times when my kids were little were Spaghetti-O's sandwiches. Another was the traditional peanut butter and jelly sandwich, but we would add an extra layer of chips inside. It was something I learned at camp—Doritos were even better. I loved orange Creamsicles from the ice cream truck too. I believe there's a shake for that!

In my 20's I was devastated to find out that my favorite fried food shack diner was closed. They had the best fried clams and clam cakes that we would dip into mounds of tartar sauce and ketchup. They had the good old-fashioned hamburger and hotdog too. And when we were kids, we claimed our condiment choices by ordering red, yellow and green.

My husband's most endearing childhood love was of course, macaroni and cheese. As an adult, he'll order it in a restaurant, especially if it has lobster in it. The conversation stopped there when my husband and daughter decided to make their own homemade rendition of mac and cheese and I let their idea get a hold of me. I had a frozen gluten-free mac and cheese meal I was saving for just the right moment. And this was it.

Several hours after, I had already devoured my meal for one and their non-healthy ginormous version with crunchy bread-crumbs on top came out of the oven looking delicious and smelling like heaven. I wanted to join in—but not that badly and I made myself a small bowl of gluten-free pasta and sat with everyone while they oohed and ahhed over every yummy morsel. Quietly to myself I hoped that there would be nothing leftover to tempt me.

Day 160: 197 lbs. Monday, March 12th

The radio station I work with was being recognized as a leader in the community for their efforts to bring awareness about suicide prevention and I was invited to attend the award ceremony.

It was held at the State House in Boston by the Massachusetts Coalition for Suicide Prevention (MCSP) and many of us contributed in large and small ways. My part was small, raising awareness by participating in a dance competition and featuring one of my shows on suicide prevention. I also aired my own personal story at the end of that show. I was really grateful to be invited and proud, but still a little nervous about attending. It's a pretty big deal to come out about being a suicide attempt survivor because it's still a subject no one wants to talk about.

Lord only knows what I was going to be able to eat during the event if anything, and it would be a long day. So, early in the morning I had a hearty two-scoop protein shake and tucked a few Kind bars into my purse along with some other just-in-case essentials. I met Mr. Ed Perry at a nearby plaza so we could drive to the State House together and hopped into his jeep with my now 20-pound purse.

It was bumper to bumper getting into the HOV lane as he pointed out the fast-moving non-HOV traffic. He said it can be very tempting to go that route because it *looks* faster, but he added that the best course of action was to stay where we were, and he was right.

What began as an idle start for us, was soon smooth sailing, and to our right was a sea of red brake lights. It was a really good sign and I was grateful to be by the side of a smart man, sharp as a tack, who some even considered a legend.

We found the parking garage, walked up the stairs, and then hiked up the hill to the State House. My body was still sore from the weekend workouts and I regretted lugging my practically useless 20-pound purse. But time was of the essence, and there was no time to complain or slow down.

Ed said very matter-of-factly at one point, "The good news is, on the way back it's all downhill." We both laughed and then again as we entered the "General Hooker Entrance". During the ceremony, I discovered that WATD (my radio station) was up against 30 other nominees, only to be recognized amongst six and I was so proud to be a part of it.

Day 161: 197 lbs. Tuesday, March 13th

Another storm had arrived, and we were homebound again. I got on a quick phone call early after making some simple raisin toast in case we lost power. Our lights flickered a few times but luckily that was it.

The kids each found their ideal leftover options for dinner after they politely declined the mushroom, green pepper, and tomato omelet with a side of home fries I was making. Enjoying a second round of gluten-free cookies in the semi-late evening, snow day number two was confirmed for the morning.

Day 162: 198 lbs. Wednesday, March 14th

Journaling what I eat has been an interesting process, especially if I forget to write it down for a day or two. If I don't write it down, poof it's gone. Poof, it didn't happen. And on occasion, I've had to ask several people in my house what we actually ate at any given lunch or dinner before the light bulb finally would go off and I'd remember it.

I used to roll my eyes at the simple suggestion to track what I ate. And it didn't matter whether I recorded everything into an app or wrote it down in a notebook or journal. It seemed silly, especially at the start. One cup of coffee; two eggs over easy; toast with butter. *Blah, blah, blah.*

At the beginning of this book, I was adamant about not measuring every item, every ounce, every everything. I wanted my love diet to be easy: the easiest diet for me to ever possibly follow. But taking care of myself takes effort. And rolling my eyes at the mere suggestion to start with something as simple as documenting what I was eating was, dare I admit, *pure resistance. And complaining about paying attention, was not love.*

Stating out loud and proud, that I didn't have the time to track anything wasn't love either. *It was more like an underlying confession that I didn't want to find the time, because finding the time would mean I would have to look at what I was doing.* It would mean I would have to do more and possibly work even harder. Saying that I didn't have any time was admitting that I wouldn't want to be the one who had to do the looking or the actual changing. Not finding the time was putting my health and my wellbeing at the bottom of my own priority list.

If I didn't write down what I ate, I wouldn't have to change. Changing was hard. Changing is hard. Changing can be hard. I had already tried to change so many times but failed again and again. Simply put, if I didn't change what I was doing, it would be easier than facing the truth. If facing reality was too scary, not writing anything down would be safer. *It would suck to stay stuck, but it would be easier. And there was far more support on the easier roads.*

Most people would agree that we can't change what we won't acknowledge. But I believe there are many steps to take first, long before leading up to that giant room of acknowledgment. *Before I even considered opening that heavy door, I had to take a big giant step toward forgiveness.*

What I had to do was forgive myself for every "not-so-great" choice that had led me to where I was. I had to forgive myself for allowing too many "I deserve this" choices inside. And let's face it, forgiveness isn't that easy. It is a choice, but not an easy one. Before I could forgive myself there was another step, a giant leap of faith, into vulnerability. I had to do more than just embrace it, I had to *be* vulnerable and admit that I was the one who was in control of my own control center. Only then could becoming vulnerable lead me to quite possibly one of the hardest things to do of all. Taking action.

Lights, camera, action. The act of doing would have to be ongoing, and possibly never-ending. But at this stage of my life, I wanted to stay real in my house of love. I wouldn't be able to act unless I invited my old friends Will and Desire back in. In the end, Will and Desire would have to be invited by love.

In theory, it wouldn't be realistic for me to say that I could start with something as simple as an acknowledgement or as difficult as forgiveness. Forgiveness was only going to happen after love kicked Will and Desire in the pants and shoved me straight into the arms of action. I would have to tear down the walls that were holding me back from the center of my own soul and stand directly inside vulnerability. Where the cameras are always waiting. Where forgiveness was holding the light.

Forgiveness was the light worth following. Forgiveness would help me to finally open the door to that giant room of acknowledgment or even better, help guide me to the entrance of my own heart. *Where love was patiently waiting for me—where love was holding the key.*

Change can be love. Change can be whatever I want it to be. Change can be as soft as I need it to be and full of possibility. I know I have the power to do anything because the truth is, it's never too late to make a change. And change could actually feel good.

Without any hesitation, I can say something very different and confidently on Day 162—louder and prouder. That it is better to write or journal what I am doing. But not just writing down three ounces of chicken, or one piece of birthday cake. Just as important as writing down what I eat—is writing about when and why.

After my breakfast shake, I had the rest of the mushroom and pepper omelet for lunch with a side of home fries and went straight past the ketchup to a little healthier hot sauce.

Sushi was a spur-of-the-moment option for dinner, with a low-sodium soy sauce of course, which I planned to do some more research on. I expect my love diet and my life will have the occasional sushi dipped in soy along with one of my favorites, wasabi!

Day 163: Thursday, March 15th

Arriving at a local diner for a breakfast meeting, I sat down and ordered something simple. Black coffee, one egg over easy, and a side of home fries with fresh fruit. It was reasonable and I steered clear of the special apple filled waffle that most everyone else was ordering. I was still happily in love with the direction I was going on my love diet, and proud of my choices, even though I wasn't seeing the weight coming off as fast as I wished it would.

One of the women that arrived had very noticeably lost a significant amount of weight. "I'm down about 30 pounds," she said. And she did look great. But she lost that weight fast. What's your secret someone quickly asked, to which I chimed in, "There is no secret." And I mumbled under my breath, "It's diet and exercise." She said, "Oh yes, there *is* a secret, and I can tell you about it." I assumed it was another fad diet because fad diets are typically the diets that help you drop weight the fastest.

Later she let us know she was on a plan. And that the plan had her removing all processed foods, with a few other interesting twists, one of which allowed berries. And then I overheard her saying, "We have to *shock* our bodies."

She was clearly feeling and looking fantastic. And it was very tempting for me to go down that road again. That road that appeared to be faster. But that road would bring me right back to where I started. And that was a dead end for me. I knew the best course of action for me—was to stay in my *LOV* lane.

Just like everyone else, I want to feel and look better yesterday, but no longer at any expense. I want an entire life of smooth sailing. And I wondered, was removing all processed foods—all at once—a good idea? Would it be sustainable next week or next month? Would she still be doing this diet, at this same time next year? *More importantly, I wondered, would it be sustainable for me, for the rest of my life?*

I brought half of my potatoes and fruit home and bounced our breakfast conversation off of my husband later that night at dinner. He told me that he had recently read a few Biggest Loser articles on the theory of "shocking our bodies" and learned that once we lower our metabolism, our "resting" metabolic rate gets messed up, and can't be reversed. One article he read was about a man who, long after the competition was over, was seeing the weight slowly start to come back, and he was still following the program after his initial reality show experience.

What does that mean? I didn't know, so I skipped right past his article and did a little search about how—and even if—yo-yo dieting can mess up our metabolism. The article I read went on to say that each person's individual resting metabolic rate is different, and as such, diets will never work.

Then I found both an online Basal Metabolic Rate (BMR) and Real or Resting Metabolic Rate (RMR) calculator and tried to figure out the difference between each. My BMR was 1590 and my RMR was 1849. But what did the numbers mean to me? Where did my numbers need to be?

A little more searching told me that both the BMR and RMR for women is about 1,400, which equates to calories. While for men it's roughly 1,800. So, was 200 points over the average too high for my BMR? And what about my RMR coming in at 1849? Even for these amateur eyes my RMR seemed way too high. I wasn't sure how empowering any of this information was. I did have some answers. But did I really have any solutions? I guess I could have kept digging for more links and reading for several more days.

Studying to become a nutritionist or an expert at any rates wasn't my goal. Learning about my metabolism was interesting, but what I was discovering on my own through my love diet journaling—was more powerful to me than any new diet trend, metabolic-rate calculator or rabbit-hole link.

What I know and understand is that depriving myself of everything I had been accustomed to eating over my lifetime was not realistic. Dramatically lowering my caloric intake could be dangerous. And it's been scientifically proven that shocking our bodies will drive them straight into survival mode. What I want to do is to make better choices—slowly.

I want to be so sneaky about getting healthier that my body is so unaware and practically clueless about what I'm doing and knows that it's nothing to be remotely concerned about. *I want to steer my body into a better direction where there is nothing to fear and every step that I take is effortless. So my body not only accepts what I'm doing—but also appreciates it—and can let go.*

The fact remains and is simple. I need to keep it simple and not let outside information cloud my clear thinking or worse, get in the way of my progress. Yes, I am progressing, and I aim to keep my love diet achievable. I know that if I want my blood pressure to come down naturally, I have to reduce the amount of sodium I take in. I don't need to read labels anymore to know how salty something is now. I can taste it. Now that I've lowered my sodium, I can tell when something is loaded with it. And my taste buds are savvy enough to happily reject it. The short answer for me is to stick with my love diet plan.

It isn't easy to resist what will persist. There will always be someone, somewhere, trying something new. But trying out another diet is too risky for me now. And it's something I am not willing to put my body through, ever again. If it took me about six years to pack on 40 to 50 pounds—as well as maintain it—it might take the same amount of time for me to let it go. Hopefully less time, but still, it will take more time.

More journaling is what it will take, better decisions, and shifting or changing my mindset. And I would rather stay on my mission to loving myself more, one small step at a time, even if it takes a year or two. In the long run, a year or two isn't really that much time at all. Creating a plan that I can live with every day and achieve anywhere, for the rest of my life, naturally and effortlessly is the way to go.

Perhaps the diet my friend was on was a natural one. And it very well might have been effortless. But to me it appeared to be another fleeting fad diet. And I couldn't risk it. My love diet is one revelation after another. The plan I am creating and building—is based on love—from love and for the love of my body. What I am choosing to create for myself is just for me. My love diet is personalized and customized and albeit my love diet is realistic and achievable, and some might even consider it to be "vanilla," I don't want other people doing my love diet. However, anyone can create their own customized version of their love diet simply by introducing and eliminating things slowly through love. Under the supervision of their doctor of course too. Just like I'm doing.

I have shared my thought process of what I am doing by revealing a concept of how building upon one decision at a time is possible and achievable. Slowly, I am conquering one small personal challenge after another, and that's how I intend on taking control of my body, my health, and my future. What I am doing is personal and I am doing it for me. I am creating my own love diet that is practically a personalized experiment.

Who am I to say that a gluten-free lifestyle is best for everybody? Who am I to tell someone else that they can't have soup or put cream in their coffee? How can anyone claim that one diet is perfect for thousands or even millions of people? *A grapefruit diet is not realistic. A love diet is personal.*

I believe it is possible for me to create a plan that suits my individual lifestyle, the environment in which I live, and the ethnic traits that make me who I am. A plan that is so personal that it's extremely easy to remember, based on what I like and dislike, and easy to accomplish by incorporating one achievable change at a time. A plan that can be entirely adaptable during any season of the year, at any given family function, or at any facility or restaurant. A plan that I can stand.

My love diet will confidently lead me directly into my healthier future where I can potentially live years longer than anticipated. My intention is to create a plan, that is filled with personalized and individualized sustainable love. My love diet is meant for me, but the concept of how I am creating my love diet is what can potentially be adaptable to anybody.

Back to the conversation I was having at breakfast. I did openly share that I had removed deli meats from my diet but kept pepperoni for my new gluten-free pizza that I'm in love with again. And one of my friends said, "Oh but pepperoni is the worst!" With my face in my hands, I let out a regretful sigh, because I had eaten my new lovable pizza at least twice in the last week. And I couldn't help but wonder what it would feel like to permanently let it go. I want to love myself with healthier options, but would I have to eliminate pepperoni 100 percent?

There are simply some things that I want to keep in my life and eat once in a while. Having a healthier gluten-free option for pizza made me feel less deprived. And adding pepperoni to it was making it deliciously greasy again. Dreaming of my tender pepperoni got me to thinking about the linguica that I grew up eating. The occasional thin crust pizza, with the amazing locally made linguica topping is practically a weekly requirement to have if you live in New Bedford.

It isn't readily available where I live now, and it doesn't make its way into my life very often. But that pizza was so good growing up and having it on occasion through-out my life was pure heaven. So how often could allowing the greasy gift be considered acceptable or qualify as love? Could I commit to letting go of pepperoni again, and only letting it or linguica back in, every once in a blue moon? And how often was an actual blue moon? That phrase "once in a blue moon" is so overly—and incorrectly used. A blue moon is something that happens very rarely.

The phrase refers to the appearance of a second full moon within a calendar month, which happens only once every 32 months. And the number of times I have heard people say that phrase, I presume they were not thinking every 32 months. So, could I own that? Could I let it go and get my pepperoni consumption down to once every 32 months?! I could see myself *including it* once or twice a year, but once in almost three years was definitely unrealistic. Hell, to the no—I don't think so. I think keeping it in my diet, once or twice a year is love. And that is something that I can totally stand by.

On my way home, I stopped to pick up a loaf of bread for the kids and snuck over to the specialty aisle. Red curry with Thai rice noodles sounded really good for dinner.

Cooking up some fresh cod in the pan first I then added more olive oil, garlic, salt and pepper. The curry package said it was gluten-free, but it still had quite a few ingredients that were unrecognizable. Hence, it was highly processed. But I still added the paste into the dish and a little cream. It might be a good idea to try and make it from scratch the next time, or maybe I could find an organic kind.

Nicole Perry

Day 164: Friday, March 16th

After my recording, I popped into one of my favorite chain restaurants for lunch and instead of ordering the salmon, I tried the grilled chicken this time with marinara sauce and a side of broccoli.

Overall, it had taken several months to work on this new mindset of mine, and I was embracing and accepting my new life more and more, little by little. I am happier living with my love diet. *I have learned so much more about myself, taking my own LOV lane than I would have ever learned on any faster fad food fiasco road.*

For our date night dinner, I ordered the gluten-free pizza with mushrooms, green peppers and sausage. I was still learning and later found out that the sausage wasn't gluten-free. Lunch was a better choice and definitely guilt free. Eventually, I would have to find a new topping to help me get beyond pepperoni and sausage. But letting these types of foods go, one at a time was a better approach. That much I believed.

It isn't the best plan to remove all the yummy good stuff all at once, just as it isn't a good idea to eat tons of junk foods all of the time either. Like doughnuts, fried foods, soda, fatty foods, french fries, potato chips, baked goods, and desserts. I remember watching a documentary a few years ago that starred a man who ate junk, fast food style, all day and every day for 30 days. That man was sent to the ER eventually and almost died proving a point.

Removing all of the foods that I had been accustomed to eating throughout my life would inevitably invite feelings of deprivation, and the yo-yo dieting would obviously continue.

After all, history is the greatest predictor. And just because I remove those types of foods from my diet, doesn't mean they would be removed from the planet.

I needed a plan that I could and would want to stick to. That way if and when other people in my life were eating the very types of food I chose to let go of—my body would be okay with it and my mind would be able to handle it.

Day 165: Saturday, March 17th

Consistency is a good thing. I wanted to ditch the workout, but I chose to go to the gym anyway. It was one of those "just do it" kind of days and I didn't push myself too hard. It was an okay workout and I gave myself an imaginary pat on the back for showing up.

When my husband arrived home with the groceries, I carefully opened up the package of salmon and pulled each piece apart with kid gloves thanking him for having the skin removed as well as asking them to pre-slice it. I placed parchment paper in between each chunk before freezing it too, determined to overcome being fish challenged. I was manipulating everything I could in my favor and setting myself up for seafood success.

Chicken is far less challenging and practically effortless. Whether oven baked, slow cooked, sautéed or grilled, cooking chicken tends to be pretty easy. Vegetables aren't very challenging either, as long as I don't overcook-out most of their nutrients, they can be served simple or a little more creatively.

Measuring is hardly a challenge at all, especially with spices. Proper portions have been made even easier too by simply visualizing my fist or a tennis ball. *One for the protein, two for the veggies, three will make me heavy, now go, fat go.* And I don't want to skip over the fact that with each meal, we need to have fat and our thumb is the visual for that. Makes me wonder how much avocado is too much. There could be six thumbs in there!

Day 166: Sunday, March 18th

I popped some frozen brussels sprouts into a pan with a little olive oil and salt for breakfast, adding in one egg over easy with a slice of gluten-free toast on the side.

When my husband said, "Wow." I asked him if he wanted me to make him some too, to which he replied, "No, that's too heavy for me." I said, "Too heavy?" "Too heavy?" I said again. Then he added, "And I don't usually like to eat vegetables with breakfast unless it's in an omelet." While enjoying my very lean and modest healthy breakfast, I looked over and saw him eating cheap pie straight out of the box. But again, he doesn't have any issues with his weight.

We were all excited to play with our new fancy rotary cheese grater that arrived and built our family dinner around it. Parmesan cheese is something we all love, and hard cheese is the better kind according to my doctor. We made a red sauce with mussels and clams for dinner with our two kinds of pasta, regular for them and gluten-free for me. I rinsed the clams thoroughly too, to reduce any extra possible sodium.

Day 167: 199 lbs. Monday, March 19th

Since joining the gym, I noticed that I was starting to feel better about myself. Just in general. I could sense the old chatter of negative tapes working their way out. Things like, "I must be the oldest and fattest person in my class." But those negative thoughts were slowly being replaced with new thoughts after I wiped off the dust. Things like, "Keep up the good work, Nicole." And "Your muscles are remembering. You can do this!"

Seeing visual numbers had really helped to lift my spirits and my confidence too. Knowing how many calories I had burned and how much of my heart's capacity I was using was helpful and kept my interest. My incline was getting higher as well as my ability for speed and I was gaining a positive mental attitude by being able to spend more time on each machine too.

Also sifting its way back into the forefront of my mind was remembering proper form. And the muscles I was using hadn't been flexed for years. It felt good to see myself progress, especially when I wasn't seeing very much happening visually on the outside. And what we see on the outside can change the way we think about ourselves on the inside.

Day 168: Tuesday, March 20th

From the age of about 24, I've had rosacea. And when it first appeared, it was cute to have flush or pinkish cheeks. Then, when I was pregnant with my first baby at age 30, it became full-blown rosacea instigated by hormones.

After experiencing a miscarriage and then almost two years of trying to conceive, I didn't give the extreme acne too much thought. I was finally having my first baby and the acne was manageable. It easily took a back seat to being pregnant and becoming a first-time mother. But still, what happens to our bodies on the outside, can be a huge indication of what could be happening on the inside.

When the first signs of menopause kicked in, that rosacea kicked into overdrive and I assumed it was hormonal again. It got so bad at times; I couldn't go anywhere without spackling on a thick layer of makeup, relieve my pores mid-day and reapply makeup between networking events. It was so gross I know. I wore makeup on the weekends too. That way my family wouldn't have to look at me. And I wouldn't fall into depression looking at myself.

My skin was beyond pimply or even red. It was dark purple. Almost infected. And there were many times I cried looking at my reflection, begging my husband to help me search for solutions. It was not easy to live with, and it was not easy to love myself through. But I did.

In hindsight, the severe acne or rosacea that I was experiencing may have been an indication that something more was going on. Beyond hormones and beyond auto immune. My skin was looking so much better now, and it made me wonder if the Copper IUD had anything to do with how severe it had become.

To say that I felt relieved to have the IUD removed was an understatement for sure. I was blessed and grateful, empowered and free. I was the one who made that change happen. Change is good... And I was dedicated to loving myself into a healthier body and state of mind.

Day 169: Wednesday, March 21st

My kids were watching me navigate through our highly processed world and I talked with them in detail about every choice I was making. In turn, they were receiving a real-life education.

More than ever before, I want them to be equipped with any knowledge as they grow into adulthood. And I hoped my experience would help to keep their health at the forefront of their minds. Even when choices that are not-so-great manage to sneak their way in. Whatever they decide to do in their future, their minds are being fed today with reason, compromise, and solutions.

My kids are absorbing the importance of choosing foods that are less processed and switching to organic. They are learning firsthand and understanding more through my personal trial and error. The healthier foods that I was switching to were all working their way into our family meals anyway.

As a parent, I do turn the other cheek at the many foods they reach for, the very foods that I reach for less. But they are kids. And kids will still want burgers and fries dipped in ketchup.

When I first started searching for information about how I could reduce my blood pressure, the most common item suggested to immediately let go of was ketchup. But forcing my kids to live without ketchup is downright un-American. Ketchup is one of the main condiments we never run out of. And it's not a good day if we do.

Removing things entirely hasn't worked for me. When I remove the foods that I am accustomed to eating and had been for centuries, those items eventually boomeranged their way back in. Bread is a great example of that. For me, a better compromise is to slowly switch some of those items over and replace them with newer healthier versions. *There are plenty of alternatives.* And the great compromise when it comes to ketchup, is to purchase organic.

I want to be realistic. And all I can do is be mindful about what I bring into our home. I can practice what I preach, and I can keep taking it several steps further. I can choose organic, all-natural and less ingredients. I can be consistent with my choices and openly communicate to my kids everything that I learn. *I can love them by educating them with real-life visuals wrapped inside stories and memories.*

By sticking with my new gluten-sensitive label, I was in fact, loving myself to a higher level. It's a level that I had trouble holding on to previously, because I don't have celiac disease or any allergies. That I was aware of anyway.

Without having an allergy there was no real incentive for me to remain gluten-free. That label had no reason to stick with me. And I had let the wheat back in at every opportunity. Until now. Until I was able to weave it into my love diet when I was ready. When taking the actual step seemed necessary, achievable, and full of possibility. Rather than feel like an obligation that I could only carry—until it got too heavy.

Day 170: Thursday, March 22nd

Sometimes I don't even realize that I give my own power away. It's a powerful statement, but it's true. And Deepak Chopra said something in one of my meditations that helped me understand it even more clearly. It was something like, "If you allow yourself to shrink at others' suggestions or opinions, you are giving your power away."

What I thought to myself was: What is it about me that made me invite the opinions of others and shrink when I received them? What was my payoff? What am I afraid of? We all have moments of contemplation and I was having several of them that lasted most of the day. And the deeper I fell into reflection—the clearer my thoughts became.

I AM ON A LOVE DIET

Day 171: Friday, March 23rd

I had a protein shake early for breakfast, followed by a meditation and then around 9:30 in the morning I had an amazing asparagus omelet drizzled with hot sauce and a side of raisin toast. My idea about only needing one egg at any given meal was a good one and led me to think that maybe I could transition to only one slice of toast too. It was a pretty simple thing to slim down from two to one.

The luncheon I attended was fantastic and refueled my fire. I had the cobb salad, with oil and vinegar and one of my favorites, bleu cheese crumbles. I was continuing to be mindful about sodium and cholesterol, so I left most of the bacon bits off as well as half of the bleu cheese. I would love to find a healthy bleu cheese dressing. Or someday just create my own.

Looking over the menu at topping choices on our date night we got frustrated with what to put on our gluten-free pizza. Struggled was too strong of a word. But I was teetering there. Our server was slammed and had already come back to us three times to see if we had decided. I was letting go of pepperoni again, confident that I could indeed live without it. But what could I replace it with? And did I need to replace it?

Obviously, I was giving far too much power away to pepperoni, but I do want my pizza to be delicious. One of my old favorite topping trios was sausage, mushroom and peppers. But their sausage came under my love diet deli meat category. And the trio wasn't the same without it. It wasn't gluten-free either or healthy. I had never heard of anyone putting wheat inside sausage before, but then again, it's a filler. Heck, they even put gluten into Twizzlers*!*

When our boss lady came back around again, I asked for sundried tomatoes, but they didn't have any and I finally settled on black olives.

Day 172: Saturday, March 24th

Before heading to the gym, I had a carb. I had a protein shake the last time and it wasn't such a good idea. During the workout I burped a couple of times on the treadmill and almost had a tiny throw up in my mouth. So, this time I had whole grain gluten-free toast with peanut butter.

When I got home, I was still pumped and shared all of my successes with everyone. Even the funny parts where my form was a little off and how the teacher had to correct me. After a quick shower, I asked if anyone thought I was starting to look slimmer, lifting up my sweater ever so slightly. They all said yes with their bright lying eyes. But numbers don't lie. And what I was loving to see were the calories burned. I know that my body was shifting and that I'm gaining more muscle. The numbers are just a good pacifier. They help me to see what is happening on the inside until my outside can catch up.

After the awesome workout I had at the gym, boy did I want to eat! I placed a large portion of my gluten-free pasta on my plate and noticed it was about the same size as my husband's. But I had worked up an appetite.

During dinner, our new handheld rotary cheese grater had been passed so many times, we could have purchased one for each person. How much cheese did we really need? I was very proud to only have been able to eat a little more than half of my meal. Leaving some lovely leftovers on my plate.

I AM ON A LOVE DIET

Day 173: Sunday, March 25th

Planning meals takes quite a bit of conscious effort and desire too. When I don't have a plan, it leaves the door wide open for me to make decisions that go against the outcome that I want to achieve. Decisions like ordering takeout or delivery. If my intentions to eat and live healthily are met with actionable steps, how could I not create my own recipe for success?

Success to me means stocking the cabinets with better choices and defrosting the fish in a timely manner. It means having fresh and frozen vegetables on hand and plenty of pantry foods with fewer ingredients. It also means to have lots of whole food in my house and at my fingertips. Essentials that do not include chemicals or even dessert.

Before my love diet, I had let chocolate go. I used to eat chocolate every day after lunch. Sometimes scooping a few squares into the peanut butter jar. But after letting it go for a few weeks I completely forgot about the old habit and craving. I did get some chocolate for Valentine's Day and had some small indulgences. But the chocolate in my pantry seemed to sit there now. I wasn't drawn to it like I was before. Perhaps it was because I was drawn to so many other treats. And I was skipping over the better of the bitter sweets.

Day 174: Monday, March 26th

My car had to be towed to the shop after I pulled into the driveway and saw a huge cloud of smoke coming out the rear end.

Stuck in my home office for another day, I made a skinny shake along with some cinnamon raisin toast for breakfast and some fish, broccoli and sweet potatoes for lunch. For dinner I served good old-fashioned open-faced tuna melts with sliced tomato and Swiss cheese. American cheese for the kids.

Day 175: 197.5 lbs. Tuesday, March 27th

There was some kind of cosmic shift happening. New energy washed over me while fresh new perspectives were sprinkled with crystal clear ideas. There was so much that I wanted to do and tackle that I popped some cinnamon raisin bread into the toaster to get breakfast off my plate, just so I could get back to work.

Rocking and rolling, my thoughts poured out of the pen in my hand and onto the giant paper, flipping page after page. It's amazing how I can pour my heart and soul into my work and forget about food. But I could not ignore the growls coming from my stomach any longer. Grabbing some leftover fish and stuffing from our dinner the night before I used the healthy food to fuel my body. I was eating to live, not living to eat.

Day 176: Wednesday, March 28th

To be overwhelmed is a choice and I could have easily fallen into that space. But I had two important events back to back to prepare for. I spent the better part of my day preparing, knocking out one small task after another, while feeding myself when I had to.

We all agreed to surrender to a quick fix for dinner and popped in a gluten-free pizza for myself and a regular one for everyone else and our evening ended early after kids' activities.

Day 177: 196 lbs. Thursday, March 29th

Rolling out of bed I sat in my chair first thing to meditate. Before coffee. I had a big day ahead of me and I wanted to respectfully keep my meditation routine. Ironically enough I was able to do twice as much.

On my way to my first event I ate a banana in the car. And when I arrived, I took small portions from the buffet. I passed on the bacon and took one scrambled egg, three to four small diced potatoes and about a cup of fresh fruit. And after the meeting, I had a second helping of fruit at the suggestion of our server when she was cleaning up.

By the time I arrived at the luncheon, I was starving. I ordered my salad before anyone arrived, just to nibble a bit. It was a delicious baby iceberg with grilled chicken, bacon and Roquefort dressing on the side. The cherry tomatoes and bits of bacon were good enough to hold me over until everyone else arrived. Bacon, I know.

I wasn't entirely sure if their tea was organic, but I ordered it anyway and cut it with water. I only needed to eat half the salad and I was off to another meeting.

It was a long day, so I picked up sushi for dinner and did a quick wasabi search while standing in line. Luckily, it was gluten-free. I asked the extremely polite lady behind the sushi counter what was in the light orange spicy sauce that she decorated the sushi with, and she pulled out the exact sriracha hot chili sauce bottle that I have at home. Ahhhh, the taste of home. My home. She said she mixes it with mayo to make it creamy and it was gluten-free.

Nicole Perry

Day 178: 196.5 lbs. Friday, March 30th

We tried out a new restaurant for our date night and hoped it was a new one to love. Mindfully we talked about our cholesterol.

My husband discovered his cholesterol was not as good as he thought it would be. He was in shock but disappointed in himself really. He makes such great effort to eat a Mediterranean diet, take turmeric, baby aspirin, mega-3's, and vitamins. But as much as he was doing, it was not enough. And it wasn't foolproof. He had to change some of the food in his diet.

He was only a few points over, so I said, "Your diet has changed though because of the things I am doing, so you're already on the right path. We let go of shrimp, red meat and pork, so our numbers are declining." His doctor asked him if he eats starch and said to cut back on whichever he ate the most of, which happened to be pasta. And his doctor also said that pizza was the worst.

Pulling together as much compassion as I could I put myself in his shoes. I had already gone through all of the same emotions he was going through. Discovery, rejection, frustration, disappointment, guilt, shame, and blame. He grumbled, "Now I can't have rice?" I said, "Who said anything about rice? Just look at the menu a little differently and feed your body with love. I know it's easier said than done. But of all people, I know. I've been working on it for almost six months! You can keep working on the sour cream, the cheese, the burgers, fries, pizza and pasta. We don't purchase red meat or pork anymore, so you are already ahead of the game. And we are some people's goal weight for crying out loud!"

When I mentioned that the eggplant tower appetizer that he loves to order was probably high in cholesterol he rolled his eyes. He said, "But eggplant is healthy." I said, "But we have no idea what a restaurant does to a healthy eggplant."

In the end, we agreed that if he needed to drop 15 points from his cholesterol, and I needed to drop 50 pounds of fat, the fact of the matter was, ignoring our numbers was not love. And the sooner we forgave ourselves and took the necessary action steps, the better.

We looked over the menu together and found many delicious healthy choices. Scallops, peas, and risotto for me, and salmon and sweet potato fries for him. Baby steps. Our meals were once again at the top of our best ever lists. But more importantly, we were caring enough about ourselves to want to choose healthier meals—not just because we had to.

❧ ☙

Chapter 9
Taking Back My Power

"Just when I thought I was about to discover what was wrong with me—there was nothing wrong with me."

Day 179: Saturday, March 31st

I let the positive energy from my two meditations carry me to the gym and I gave myself a little pep talk along the way. Move my body: that's what I needed to keep doing. Every day or almost every day. Just like they say, move it or lose it. Whatever was working for me, I needed to keep doing it. Each time I do, I will be one step closer to getting back into shape. I don't have to prove anything to anyone. And I certainly don't need to try so hard to keep up with the millennials that I push myself straight into an injury. That's not love.

But the weight of desperation crushes rationalization every time. Each time I arrive at that gym, something happens. I get so excited and absorb even more of the positive energy from everyone there. I get a glimpse of the machines and go for the gusto, knowing that I was getting one step closer to gaining back the muscle that was once mine.

To those millennials, what they probably see is an old try hard who will eventually, and very sadly, stop showing up. But I don't care anymore about what I think they think of me. I want to give it my best shot every time and that's a good thing. And it's a really good thing—that it's never too late.

I had let myself go for far too long, so I was on a mission to go to the gym—for me. I know I don't have to prove I am some kind of superwoman or something. My husband loves me no matter what. My family loves me regardless of what I look like from one holiday to the next. And my kids love me just the way I am. No one cares if I've gained or lost ten pounds. What they care about is that I'm healthy, happy and here.

The reality is—my family would be devastated without me as I would without them and I'm certain they want me to live a healthy life. My kids are definitely healthier when I am healthier. And frankly, what I'm doing at the gym—is working on the biggest muscle I have, my heart.

I want to exercise my heart muscle because I wanna stick around. I want to be here for my children and see them grow old. The bottom line is—exercising while I age—has become more about what I cannot see—than any silly pair of skinny jeans.

When I got home, I was famished and excited to add an egg to my leftover date-night pan-seared scallop dinner and turn it into a fancy breakfast for one before running some errands with my daughter.

If there's even a hint of me stopping for lunch while I'm out and about, she's right by my side. And after several hours of running around, we sat down for lunch. My daughter ordered one of her favorites, their mozzarella sticks with marinara sauce and I asked for something not listed on their menu; gluten-free pizza crust cut into pita triangles with a side of pizza sauce for dipping. Enjoying something fun and similar felt good.

Luckily for me, our server had Celiac. She was a bubbly and confident young gal eager to help—which made me feel so relieved that I was ordering the right things, the right way, at a place I go to all the time. Trust can be a wavering term to the gluten-sensitive, and after getting the inside scoop from someone legit, I couldn't imagine what it would feel like to be her—to actually be allergic.

Day 180: Easter Sunday, April 1st

While I was getting ready for Easter, I took a moment to look at my skin. I may not have lost any weight yet on my love diet, but my body was starting to show signs of good health, *in my face.*

My skin was looking fantastic! I was almost in shock at how much it had cleared up. Was it because I had removed the IUD—or was it because I was living gluten-free? I almost didn't have any signs of acne at all. It could have been a combination of both, but it could also have been because my hormones were settling down. Regardless of what was it was, I was keeping the new label of gluten-sensitivity just in case it was the change that was working.

Eating gluten-free was a little tricky—in the beginning. But once I got the hang of it, my life has been way less complicated. It's like a no brainer everywhere I go. Living a gluten-free or gluten-sensitive life takes the guesswork out of everything. At our non-traditional family Easter buffet, I didn't even have to think about whether or not to put the pasta or the roll onto my plate. The bright flashing signs of typical temptation that once were there, were no more. I was free. Now it was easy. I simply couldn't put any of it into my body. What appeared to others as a dietary restriction—was in fact, for me, love diet freedom.

When we got home from our family Easter gathering, I was hungry. And it wasn't because I didn't eat any bread or pasta. I was hungry because the amount of food that I did eat with our family was completely reasonable—and it was dinnertime.

What I didn't do was stuff myself so much that I couldn't even think about eating another bite of food. I even ate one of the gluten-free brownies my daughter made. What I ate was normal for me. So normal, that shortly after arriving home, the thought of dinner came naturally.

No one else in my house was even thinking about food. And my husband cringed at the thought of it. They had all overindulged and eaten anything and everything in their line of sight until they couldn't eat another bite. And so, I sat there at my kitchen island smiling. I was happy and proud of myself—eating my leftover grilled chicken salad for dinner—alone.

Day 181: 198 lbs. Monday, April 2nd

Opening the fridge or cabinet can be so automatic. We can turn on the autopilot, mindlessly eating the easy without a single thought of curiosity.

I was going through the motions myself looking in my fridge and I stopped to think. What do I want? Was I just bored or was I actually hungry? How often do I hear myself say that I'm starving? Was that an accurate description or an exaggeration?

Exaggerations can be playful. Like saying, I could eat that whole buffet; or he looks older than dirt; or I have a million things to do. We can find plenty of hidden meanings in some of those exaggerations too. If I say to someone out loud or even to myself, "I'm starving," what I'm usually thinking—is that I'm willing to eat almost anything. Saying the words, "I'm starving" was giving myself permission to eat whatever I wanted.

If I hear myself saying things like; "I do most of the dishes" or "I'm the one who cleaned the kitchen three times today." What I'm really hoping is that someone will catch a clue. If I say I have a million things to do depending on who I say it to, what I am actually implying—is that I might need help.

Talking between the lines isn't direct at all or perhaps even clever. But whether it is a behavior I learned or one that I created on my own, it is acknowledging how I feel. Albeit in a roundabout kind of way. It could also be old-fashioned passive-aggressiveness, a couple's code or family phraseology. I don't know if I'd call it the latter, but I do know that I'm not alone.

Some exaggerations can be a little scarier. I overheard my daughter Greenleigh saying to her brother, "Duke you just killed yourself in our Minecraft game." I ran into the room saying, "What? Who killed whom? Why did you kill your own guy Duke?" Of course, they rolled their eyes at my cluelessness to their gaming ways. But no matter how in jest or casually it can come across, to hear that statement or any statement similar thereof, I am not clueless at all. And it's something I can't ignore. I can't let it go without asking the question. Any question.

When I hear anyone say something as common as "I'd rather kill myself than go through that again." Or "Just shoot me now." Or how about the infamous way people describe an event or conversation so horrible, and they make an imaginary gun with their index finger and thumb and point it at their own head.

It makes me cringe and I worry about the person. I think about their future. Immediately I have to stop the conversation with *worried eyes opened wide*. My mind is dialed in and I have to ask the question. I have to. It's too hard for me not to. I can't let any type of statement in question go untouched or let it die. I can't bear to hear even just a hint of a person wanting to take their own life. And there are far too many statements being said out loud—and going untouched.

I can't let any of those statements get past go in my game of life. I don't think it's a big deal to ask, and it's not a big deal to press pause and take notice. It's simple. Frankly, it's easy. It's easier to touch it than to dodge it.

If someone I'm with says anything remotely in question, even if it's over the phone, I ask questions. It's not an obligation. It's a kind gesture. I ask because I care, and because every person matters. Because asking the question has proven to save lives. Any question asked from love will do.

Day 182: Tuesday, April 3rd

Before I left for my thyroid specialist appointment, I had a fruit bowl with a little granola, cinnamon, and honey.

My new doctor said to me, "Why did you remove gluten? Don't do that." When I asked her why she was asking why, she said, "Because out of my three patients that removed gluten, all of them came back with weight gain a year later." Ah-hah, but I was different. I was not one of her ordinary patients I thought. And her patients were definitely not following a love diet. She said, "When we remove something, our tendency is to replace it with something else. And my three patients that removed gluten are all eating far too much rice and potatoes now."

I would also venture to guess that her patients could potentially be indulging in many of the packaged gluten-free foods that are all over the market in the dry and frozen isles too. Foods that have the gluten removed but are injected with other chemicals to recreate the traditional flavor and consistency of a flour-filled muffin, doughnut, coffee cake, or cracker. But in any case, when we eliminate something, our tendency is to replace it. So, she was right. We are human and it's just our nature.

The manufacturers proved that theory when they created "fat-free". And they're doing it again with "gluten-free." I wasn't sure how much my doctor knew about living a gluten-free life, but I knew nothing was wrong with rice since it's a staple in the Asian diet, so I asked her, "What's wrong with potatoes?" My mind immediately wandered to the Idaho potato commercial gal. "Too many calories," she said.

When I got home, I searched and found that potatoes only have about 110 calories. They are free of cholesterol and have three grams of protein. They are also a good source of potassium providing 18 percent of the daily recommended allowance. So, I disagreed with her assessment and knew right away that it's likely what we put on top or beside them that's the real problem.

It's amazing how much information can be exchanged in a matter of eight minutes, and that I had to wait 38 uncharged minutes to do the dance. I didn't have Graves, and I didn't have hypothyroidism or hyperthyroidism. What I had was barely there Hashimoto's. *No medication required.*

It was good news because she told me it was fixable. I could fix it by changing my diet. And if I did fix it by changing my diet, it would mean that it would not escalate. Basically I could reverse it. At the end of my drive-thru doctor visit, she said the best diet to follow is the Mediterranean one, and of course, to cut back on carbs.

What I heard, was: *the American diet is the worst diet to follow.* Luckily, we do eat somewhat Mediterranean in our home already. And I was willing to look into it further. Interestingly, the subject of cutting back on my carbs seemed to keep popping up. But I was already removing gluten, and I wasn't overindulging on rice or potatoes. I was eliminating baked goods, pasta, bread, and desserts. Plus, my skin was clearing up.

My thyroid specialist is smart—and funny. And I do love listening to smart women. But I'm smart too! So, I thought it was best to stick with my plan. I walked out of the building a little relieved, but also a little frustrated. *Just when I thought I was about to discover what was wrong with me—there was nothing wrong with me.*

At home, I looked through all of my cookbooks and found an essential Mediterranean one. I couldn't wait to create a few special meals over the weekend with salmon and chicken, but when I finally had a moment to open the book, there were no pictures. *Bummer.*

Before leaving for my board meeting, I tossed some white cod, butter, salt, and pepper into the oven. It was a lame attempt at dinner I know, but I figured the least I could do was to give them a head start with a main attraction and they could figure out the rest. I had no time to wait for the cod myself and would have to eat mine the next day.

On the way to my meeting, I looked for a restaurant to grab a quick grilled chicken salad. No telling what I would find inside the questionable place I pulled into, but one never knows. And wouldn't you know, it was a Greek restaurant, perfectly Mediterranean. One of my favorite salads is the Greek salad and when I was in my 20's I used to enjoy a gyro every now and then.

The grilled chicken had some unrecognizable spices on it, but it was okay. Their dressing was heavier on the spicy mustard than it was honey, but I thought that was okay too. It was a good salad, but I was glad that there are well over 20 other countries in the Mediterranean to be inspired from.

Day 183: Wednesday, April 4th

Stopping at a local coffee shop before going into the station I wanted to get a little something to eat before my recording to be sure my stomach wouldn't start growling during the interview.

They didn't have any premade salads left, but the endcap had many gluten-free choices. I'm not a huge coconut fan, but I grabbed a bag of organic chocolate coconut cookies because they looked really good. And when I took the first cheesy bite of the orange crackers, I was pleasantly surprised and practically blown away that they tasted just like Cheez-its! They were amazingly similar.

Back at home, I suffered through my leftover grilled chicken salad lunch from the night before and then was off to my final networking meeting of the evening where they served some gluten-free foods especially for me. It was so nice not to worry if I was going to be able to eat! The grilled chicken was pierced with nice little bamboo skewers and tossed in a sweet and sour sauce. There was a cheese tray with thoughtfully pitted kalamata olives too, so I made myself a small plate, followed by another.

Day 184: 197.5 lbs. Thursday, April 5th

Carbs are everywhere. Let's just face it. So, learning to live my life with some carbs, and living my life without most of them was going to take some more practice.

Removing carbs entirely from my home was just not realistic. Especially since I don't have Celiac. My husband and my kids have no issues with their weight or with wheat. It wouldn't be fair to them and they are already doing their best to accommodate me—without inconveniencing themselves.

Pasta, potatoes, rice, bagels and bread are some good examples of what they love to eat. Along with all the other fun foods like cookies, pies, cakes, and donuts. They love ramen noodles too, chips, and tacos and nachos. So, *I need to practice seeing the carbs that I choose to remove. The ones that no longer serve me—because I can't control the entire world around me.*

It worked for me with the bagels. I don't even see them anymore. I move those bagels around my fridge daily, and it is interesting that I have no desire to pop any of them into the toaster. I don't crave them at all. So, it is possible to remove one carb item at a time*!* And my body could adjust again and again. Not all at once, but I could remove one more item, and then another, and then another.

There's a local cafe I had been going to for meetings that have plenty of carbs in a glass case right when you walk in the front door. The carbs are the breakfast bakery kind like giant muffins with the crunchy shiny sugary bling on top, jelly and lemon filled Danish with sweet sparkly swirls, blueberry scones too, and a variety of bagels and buttery crisp croissants.

Could I remove all baked goods I wondered? I think I had been doing it anyway. Their showcase was filled with comfort foods for the average comfort food lover and it didn't seem to faze me to see those delicious baked goods since removing the gluten from my diet.

Their glass stage was filled with all the carb stars *and they were practically invisible to me.* I even complimented them once or twice at how delicious they all looked. But I never had to look back after that. *Beyond training my mind, I was training my eyes.* Removing gluten was easily helping me to remove most baked breakfast goodies.

I looked past the case and ordered one scrambled dairy-free egg with a quick-and-easy side of tomato and cucumbers. With my doctor's words about potatoes flashing in my mind, I didn't get the home fries this time.

My meeting was fantastic and just before it was over one friend said, "I have one question I want to ask you. Do you love yourself?" I said, "YES!" Loudly, with a great big smile that came straight from my heart. It felt so good to be unprepared for the question and to respond honestly without hesitation. It felt good to really mean it.

For lunch at home, I grilled some brussels sprouts and reheated some of the white cod I had baked while I contemplated the theory of one day at a time. Perhaps I could also lower my carb intake one meal at a time. Similar to the way I had just let go of those home fries.

I AM ON A LOVE DIET

Day 185: 196.5 lbs. Friday, April 6th

After my hair appointment, I squeezed in a bikini wax to make my pee-pee pretty. Then I went upstairs to the premade comfort deli food diner to see if they had any gluten-free wraps.

The only gluten-free bread they had was a cross between a bun and an English muffin. It didn't sound very appetizing at all from the way they described it, so I opted for their salad with tomatoes and carrots and added humus to eat mindfully the Mediterranean way.

They didn't have my favorite honey mustard dressing, so I thought I'd try their sesame ginger. And I took two giant chocolate chip cookies for the kids to go. No wonder restaurants get confused when people say they are gluten-free and then turn around and order dessert. In the car I started to eat some of the salad, but the dressing was terrible. I couldn't taste any sesame or ginger. Just thick liquid sugar. *Yuck.*

Later that night we had a comedy show to attend so we splurged on a nice dinner beforehand and we ordered an ahi tuna appetizer to share. I usually love it pan-seared slightly with sesame seeds and soy sauce, but the little half-inch 100 percent raw cubes served in a bowl was just too much for me.

It looked beautiful, very chic and gourmet, but their version of tuna went against every ounce of my frozen and breaded, square fish from a yellow box upbringing. I had to pass. I got their beet salad instead and it was not only beautiful, but also delicious. They kindly put the feta cheese on the side for me too, which I'm sure went against their upper-class culinary institute chef training.

Overall, the menu didn't have much to choose from for a person with dietary restrictions. And since their roasted chicken was not gluten-free, I had what I hardly get to eat, the steak.

Day 186: 195.5 lbs. Saturday, April 7th

It's certainly not a good idea to go too long without eating anything during the day, but it does happen. I made myself a protein shake for breakfast then forgot to eat lunch before leaving for my appointment. And I wasn't hungry again until much later in the afternoon around three o'clock.

Patterns. It's amazing when we can discover them for what they are. I didn't have a pattern of not eating for long stretches, but my eyes had been opened wide to a pattern that I did have. During the session with my life coach the light bulb went off about a behavior that took a lifetime to create and very likely will take the next chapter of my life to try and eliminate. The pattern I was made aware of is that I can tend to go into a certain mode. A defense mode. And I'm empathic too, which can trigger the pattern.

For years I had been looking for convenient ways to create layers of any kind that could protect me from the emotions of others seeping into my skin. I feel too much is my problem. And trying to keep other energy from getting to my heart by purchasing "things" was in fact, searching for the "out there" rather than looking at the one thing I had, which was right here. Me.

To have empathy is one thing. But to allow my own ability to be empathic take over my mind and change the course of my own direction was leaning toward pathetic. In my efforts to constantly avoid falling into the depths of empath, I was falling deeper into my own pattern. And what I discovered during my session was that all I had to do was *decide* whether or not to let anyone else's emotions graze me, or any directional daggers stick me. *In the end, it had always been my choice. All along, I have held the power.*

Day 187: 197 lbs. Sunday, April 8th

Caffeine is not good for someone with Hashimoto's or even the *barely-there* diagnosed like myself, so I had been thinking of switching back to decaf.

 I did it for years during my pregnancies, so I knew it was possible for me to live without it. And I do have a lot of built-in energy anyway, but chemicals have to be added in order to remove caffeine. Hmm, caffeine or chemicals? It wasn't much of a debate. And it was another no brainer for me to choose coffee with caffeine over a beverage that I was already living without, that come to find out, is filled with chemicals. I hoped my now grown children were not indirectly or haphazardly affected.

 My thyroid doctor had told me that drinking one cup of coffee a day was fine, especially since I preferred to drink it black and American style, which meant fairly weak. European coffee or espresso is too strong for me and tends to kick my ass into overdrive.

 One cup of regular caffeine can actually cancel out one cup of water. Which was something I learned years ago from the nurses when I was having my first baby and water is something most of us know we need to consume more of, but still continues to have its challenges.

 It has always driven me crazy to think about it. Having to drink eight, 8-ounce glasses a day seemed almost unachievable. And each time I tried; I would fail shortly after. Water is not the first choice for most, even though most of us know, that the human body is made up of mostly water.

Many articles state that up to 60 percent of the adult human body is water, which was interesting because my public-school education had led me to believe it was more like 80 or 90. Evidently, the brain and heart are composed of 73 percent, the lungs alone are about 83 percent, the skin is 64 percent, our muscles and kidneys are 79 percent, and even our bones are made up of 31 percent water. It was all good knowledge to think about and be made aware of, but still, was *I* drinking enough?

A great formula I found to calculate how much water for me to drink was to take my weight in pounds and divide that by 2.2. Then I had to take that total and multiply it by my age and divide that number by 28.3, which would give me the number of ounces appropriate to drink each day. I divided that final number by eight to see my results in cups. OMG, I am supposed to drink 20 cups of water each day!?!!? That's like 6-8 large bottles of water! It was so much more than the eight, 8-ounce glasses I thought I had to drink, which was likely over 50 pounds and 25 years ago.

This was exactly the kind of information that feels unachievable to me and is very discouraging. Especially to a person my age and size. Trying to count seemingly endless glasses of water throughout each day and then having to start from scratch the next seemed monotonous and daunting, and when something feels unrealistic, I tend to go straight into stage fright mode and do nothing, which isn't love either.

In this 21st Century I want to be more mindful about water and feeding my body plenty of it. And there were plenty of things I could do when I started to think about it. I could add a splash of orange juice or a slice of lemon to my water to help me to drink more of it. Just a splash or a slice. In a restaurant, I can ask for sparkling to make it a little fancier. And in the afternoons, I could reintroduce tea into my day. Without cream or sugar; not even honey. And decaf of course, so it would count as water, but organic, because organic tea means it's chemical-free.

I think all of these choices are good and better suited for me. I would be drinking more water, in unique ways and frankly, I would rather simply follow my gut instinct and watch my pee color just like Dr. Oz and Jennifer Lopez talked about. When it's light, I must be all right!

Still on my mission to create my own bleu cheese dressing from scratch, I found one online with the standard ingredients to start with. Sour cream, mayonnaise, lemon juice, bleu cheese crumbles, salt and of course, I added a little water. Ideally light products would be better and luckily, I had both. But I wondered, was mayonnaise really gluten-free?

I knew it wasn't chemical-free, and I read that some mayo brands are not safe for people with celiac, but what I had in my fridge was gluten-free and that was good enough for me. I used my light mayo and light sour cream and it came out pretty good. As a dip too. It could still use a little tweaking, but I was excited to enjoy one of my favorite salads, the Iceberg wedge. Minus the bacon, of course. And I know, Iceberg is the McDonald's of lettuce. But eating a salad made with Iceberg is obviously better than eating at McDonald's.

Whether large or small, regular or noteworthy, when I was growing up, the memories we shared with our immediate and extended family were everlasting. And my husband and I carry forward at least a hint of those traditions.

Holiday family meals on my mother's side were the best. As many of us as possible getting together for a day filled with food and laughter, visiting and reconnecting. And of course, performing. And when I was growing up on my father's side, our day revolved around the preparation of an amazing family Sunday dinner, usually French or Italian, which was followed by a delicious leisurely nap for myself on the couch with the dog and the sound of a Patriots game on in the background. Or my childhood crush Elvis Presley.

For this particular non-monumental occasion, we made grilled salmon, mashed potatoes, broccoli, and grilled zucchini. The simple dinner we created was made from a foundation of many previous that would someday—collectively accumulate to our own treasured tradition.

Day 188: Monday, April 9th

My body was definitely changing. And I could tell because I was feeling less bloated. But I could also see a dramatic change happening in my face. It had been about three months of living mostly wheat-free and it was finally starting to show. Perhaps living my life gluten-free was a good thing. The human body is resilient, and my body appeared to be recovering from years of excessive wheat consumption.

In a conversation I was having with my son Duke, I listened to the words as they fell from my lips. I said, "Just think about what you need to get done today. Focus on today. Because if you allow your mind to wander to all the work you need to get done tomorrow, next week, or even how much next year's grade will be harder than this year—you could send yourself straight into overwhelm mode. But, if you live in the present moment and focus on what you can do today, and you do that every day, you will get to where you want to be."

Huh. It's exactly what I needed to hear myself. I could focus more on what I want to achieve today by living in the present moment. And I'm already doing that most of the time. Then I thought about the words I learned from my Deepak-Oprah meditation series, *"Awareness IS the change."*

Day 189: Tuesday, April 10th

In a fully caffeinated early conversation, I said, "You are so lucky. We're raising you to be completely independent and yet you also have a mother that is accessible and at your fingertips whenever you need her. I'm so conveniently here for you that I'm around practically all of the same times that you are." Later that day in another conversation I asked the same child, "What do you want? Tell me what you do want—not everything that you don't.

Sometimes it's easy for me to discover what I do want simply by acknowledging what I don't want. But ultimately, I have to circle back to what I do want—in order to receive what I want. I love to say this out loud and ask myself the same question often. What do I want? It can be so powerful and empowering that most people would agree that the ancient Chinese proverb is an important lesson in life; *Be careful what you wish for.* I like to be mindful of what I do want often—and get ready to receive!

My home was spotless and organized when I arrived. And I am so grateful each month for the three days that it lasts. Ironically, the meeting I had come from was all about organizing and how some tactics just won't work with our personalities or our life structure.

I walked away from that meeting with so many great ideas on how to get myself organized and of course I took it one step further metaphorically with my health, leaving with a sense of optimism and eagerness to do more. I saw the meeting as an opportunity to shift my mind and try, try again.

Day 190: Wednesday, April 11th

For lunch I made myself an easy peanut butter sandwich to take with me and brought a bag I hid in the back of the baking cabinet with the last two gluten-free cookies in it.

Like any mom or environmentally conscious person I look to reduce, reuse and recycle anything I possibly can. And after eating the cookies in my car, I noticed the pot of gold sitting at the bottom of the bag—the crumbs. Those seemingly little meaningless crumbs that when put together could make an entire baby bite of a cookie. I taught my kids to never let those golden morsels go to waste and make their way down any drain or into any trash can. I showed them how I sprinkle that deliciousness into an ice cream bin for a bonus creamy and crunchy treat. I wasn't about to toss the gold just because I wasn't at home, so I saved the bag.

When the ice cream container I held in my hand was empty, I had no regrets. It was almost empty anyway and I put those crumby carbs to good use. I wanted a little treat. And the key word here was *little*. If I had to quantify how much I had eaten during my recycling cookie crumb and ice cream binge moment, I would guess it was about one cup or less.

I do have to admit that I felt a tinge of guilt at the first bite. Not a lot, but a little. And that guilt left just as quickly as it arrived. I'm not an ice cream fanatic. I only have it a few times a year. And when I do, there's little-to-no guilt involved.

After taking my daughter to dance, my night ended with some crackers and Swiss cheese while watching TV, along with an extra, probably unnecessary glass of wine.

Day 191: 197.5 lbs. Thursday, April 12th

I woke up thinking about the yo-yo thoughts in my head and the yo-yo numbers crystal kept showing me. Two pounds up; one pound down. The yo-yoing decisions to eat clean and healthy and then finding myself snacking on cheese and crackers just before going to bed.

If I had to put a number on it, it would be somewhere around six crackers and two slices of cheese. Which makes me wonder even more, why do I beat myself up over such small amounts of food? Was it because it was after nine o'clock at night? Was it because it was in addition to eating ice cream and recycled cookie crumbs?

According to my Deepak-Oprah Shedding the Weight meditation series, I was not actually "being bad." I was hungry, and I chose partially healthy gluten-free cookie crumbs and a very small amount of ice cream. And then a few gluten-free crackers and cheese. It wasn't a giant slice of chocolate cake or even an entire bag of Doritos. It wasn't even several slices of pizza. It wasn't bad. And I wasn't being bad. They were just small snacks.

Nicole Perry

Day 192: 196.5 lbs. Friday, April 13th

Most of the time in the mirror, what I see in myself is not what other people see. What I see is a skinnier person and I think I'm actually skinnier than I am. But then reality sets in when I see myself in a photo. When Rosie O'Donnell admitted this about herself on her talk show several years ago in her organically witty fashion, I laughed out loud. But it totally resonated with me. She said that she had the opposite of anorexia and I felt the same way.

Of course, whenever I mentioned my newfound theory and epiphany, my friends would be supportive and say that it was a good thing because we have to imagine something first, before we can become what we believe. But I think there is a name for what I've seen in my mirror all these years, and I think it's called denial.

Day 193: Saturday, April 14th

I opened the fridge to find my Iceberg head was dead. But my craving for a wedge salad was not completely shot. Taking the remainder of the spring box mix we had, I added diced tomatoes and drizzled my homemade light bleu cheese dressing on it, topping it off with some fresh cracked black pepper.

It was the simplest of salads without a whole lot of umph and when my husband walked through the door with the groceries, guacamole was the first thing we made. Delicately, we took turns scooping our chips into the dip. I had no desire to eat the corn chips and I was happy to switch to a gluten-free cracker. Eating corn-free was working its way from the back of my mind to the frontline.

It was getting easier to let go of it, because whenever I ate corn of any kind, my stomach blew up like a balloon almost immediately. And the only exception I was willing to make was popcorn and the colon-cleansing corn-on-the-cob kind. As long as they remained exceptions.

My son was kind enough to point out that the ground turkey they brought home was in fact, gluten-free. Clearly, he was several steps ahead of me. I was avoiding chicken with antibiotics, but I hadn't given a second thought about whether our chicken was being wheat-fed, grass-fed, or corn-fed. Or if our fish was farm raised or ocean caught.

I wasn't sure how much investigating or research I would have to do in order to be well informed. But, if I were to be honest, I wasn't ready for any of that. Because placing too many rules or restrictions into my life or facing too many challenges could easily throw me off track. I certainly didn't want to paralyze my own progress. I was not going to ignore the elephant in the room, but I wasn't ready to hop onto it either. Not just yet. And I have plenty of OCD in me to go around so I knew I would get there.

My daughter cooked up the ground turkey and taco seasoning for our impromptu non-Tuesday taco night. And after replacing the corn holding shells for lettuce wraps, the only problem I had—was the quantity I ate.

Day 194: Sunday, April 15th

My husband made me an asparagus and parmesan cheese omelet with a side of raisin toast before I left. I was going live at the radio station followed by a card reading, so I had no time to eat in between. I took a banana along for the ride to the station and a peanut butter and jelly sandwich on raisin bread for a quick lunch in the car before the event.

When I arrived home at the end of my long working Sunday, my family had a nice baked chicken dinner with red bliss mashed, carrots and broccoli ready when I walked in the door.

It's important for me to take time for myself on the weekend and recharge with my family. But once in a while, I break my own rule. And during the weekend I broke that rule on both days. *Note to self-love.*

Day 195: 198 lbs. Monday, April 16th

I silently stood staring at my scale. I was getting cleaned up from the inside out and I had shifted and changed, but the number I saw was just not budging. When I look in the mirror, it feels like I might be shrinking, but clearly, that's part of my problem. What I'm still seeing is that skinnier person. And what I actually am is different. Cameras and numbers don't lie.

Maybe it's stress. The stress of working all weekend. The stress in general. I had been meditating for several days, even weeks, though. Faithfully, it had become my "me" time, filing my fake-less nails and sniffing my sassy oils, getting into my meditative routine grabbing a blanket and taking the last few sips of my coffee until finally placing my glasses down just before closing my eyes. Each day I was clearing my mind from clutter. I was going to that still quiet place even if the thoughts of yesterday or the next day came my way, I was reducing my stress breathing and releasing. But was it enough?

It was just past nine when I looked at the clock, and still had not had breakfast, so I ate a banana while making myself a shake. I met a friend for lunch and had the Cajun grilled chicken salad. We easily got into a deep discussion and she said to me, "When you think you can't, you must. And when you think you must, you can't." Her words clung to me and I was trying to hide how speechless I was.

When I use the word "can't", I'm usually very mindful. I love to use it if there's something I simply don't want to do or won't do. In that scenario I grab the words easily and say, "Sorry, I can't." On the flip side, I do teach my children if they want something to happen, not to use the word. Even something as simple as opening a jar of jelly. Like any good parent I say, "You have to have the 'I think I can, I think I can' mentality *while* you're twisting the jar open. No matter how hard you try to twist, if you are thinking to yourself 'I can't get this damn thing open,' you will be right—and it will stay stuck."

During our lunch, the word very unintentionally slipped out and I had said, "I can't believe I haven't lost any weight yet." I was using the word 'can't' like a crutch and it was spilling out of my mouth all over the place.

Day 196: Tuesday, April 17th

Probably somewhere between four to five times per week I do eat out. Whether it's breakfast, lunch or dinner. And since I have become more mindful of my diet, I have had some pretty awesome and delicious meals. I was practically a professional food critic, but this lunch put a kink in my restaurant chain.

The American grill style place had plenty of salads to choose from and the one with brussels sprouts caught my eye. But it came with bacon so I asked if they could put it on the side. It was already mixed in though and I ordered it anyway. I love brussels sprouts and I was excited to have them in my salad.

It looked dry right away and it was raw and bitter with far too much baby kale. The raspberry vinaigrette it came with was so sweet I couldn't bear to ruin my meal further by trying to drench my salad in it. And the oil and vinegar I asked to replace it with was no help. My last and only saving grace was their bleu cheese dressing. It turned out to be one of, if not the, worst salads I ever had. But I took the rest home—just for proof.

Day 197: Wednesday, April 18th

I had a very early meeting to attend so I made myself a coffee shake for breakfast and grabbed a banana for the ride. It was a good meeting and afterward I had a quick peanut butter and jelly sandwich before my recording and just enough time to stop at a local coffee shop. I wanted to snag my new favorite knock-off Cheez-its and maybe a few other gluten-free goodie items to tuck in my purse for the movie I was taking the kids to.

There were plenty of gluten-free snacks to choose from, *but was I doing just what my doctor had said? Was I replacing all of my gluten-filled food with something else?* Taking a closer look at the ingredients at home, there were far too many chemicals in each of the easy, on-the-go pre-packaged gluten-free bags. And they all had some type of corn in them, or soy—or both.

On the ride to the movies, I talked with my kids about my struggle with whether or not I "should" eat the popcorn when we got there. It's something they don't think twice about, but I was communicating my thoughts, milestones and struggles. I knew I was giving my kids a priceless, real-life education.

They were paying attention. And I hoped what I was sharing and teaching them would sink in and actually be of value to them today, and in their future. I want them to love who they are—more than just enough. And I want them to figure it out when they are at their youngest, so they don't find themselves trying to figure it out later in life—like I was doing.

The venue was definitely not gluten-free, and I was sure if I did have Celiac, I most likely would not have been able to enter the building.

When our waitress came over, I ordered the grilled Cajun chicken sandwich, without the bun and honey mustard on the side. I kept the fries "for the kids" and ordered them a cheese pizza along with some curly fries and popcorn.

Their popcorn was drenched in butter—by accident. We usually don't get the extra butter and it was a disgusting greasy mess all over my hands. I said to my son, "Maybe we should order our popcorn *with butter* more often so that I won't eat as much." I didn't eat as much as I usually do, but I still ate more than I wanted to.

Later that night, my daughter said out loud, "I love carbs!" Pffft. I said to her, "Yeah we all do. But someday you will love yourself more than the empty-calories." I told my husband that I felt so stuffed and bloated and his response was kind and supportive as usual, "You'll be fine," he said. "It just takes a day or two to get back on track after eating at a place like that."

Day 198: Thursday, April 19th

Was I still 198 pounds on Day 198? Or was I more? Mustering up as much compassion for myself as I possibly could, I tried very hard to not beat myself up over what I chose to eat at the movie. I had given myself permission to indulge. It was just with a little fun junk food with my kids during their vacation week.

Looking at a lunch menu later in the day, I didn't see anything that appealed to me directly, but I came up with a great plan. When the waitress came over, I gave her the heads up that I was a little high maintenance. But she was pen-in-hand cool with it and ready. I asked for the chicken salad sandwich without the bun. And then I asked if she could please put it on top of a bed of romaine lettuce and add some tomatoes. I asked for honey mustard on the side, for when I finished eating the chicken salad part. My skinny friend loved it and ordered the same thing! And she dove right in when it arrived. When she was almost finished with her meal I looked down at my plate and my salad was practically untouched. I said, "Wow, this is a great measuring tool for me, just eat less than the skinny person I am with and I'm bound to shrink."

After dinner, we caught up on some TV and had a fun night hanging out together. I didn't binge on any junk food, but I did eat my leftover salad a little late in the evening and had an extra glass of wine. In hindsight, both the salad and the wine were completely unnecessary.

A funny thing happened during that lunch though, I noticed that after only having a couple of bites of the chicken salad, I felt full. When I was eating the rest of my salad that night, it occurred to me that the chicken salad may have had gluten in it. But why would they add wheat to chicken salad? Perhaps the chicken wasn't free-range or wheat-free eating chicken.

Then the bigger light bulb went off. The reason I was still feeling full at lunch—was because I was! All of the curly fries and popcorn I had eaten the day before at the movies with the kids was in my body processing. It was still in my blood.

Chapter 10
I've Only Just Begun

"I was taking too many steps back in the wrong direction and what felt even worse than that, was that each new day felt like I had just begun."

Day 199: Friday, April 20th

Weight unknown.

A one egg dairy-free omelet with green peppers, mushrooms, and parmesan cheese is what I asked for and she was one of the few people that actually listened. She said, "But that's not dairy-free?" So I confessed. I told her that I just didn't want the milk.

My requests were getting a little trickier and there was a fine line between giving clear instructions so my food would be prepared the way I wanted it to be and overthinking it. My love diet had layers of meaningful decisions that I had made along my journey and required a degree of translation almost daily—inside my home and out.

At the top of this chapter, I wrote "weight unknown" because I hadn't weighed in for several days. I didn't want to know. What I did know though, was that in the last 20 days I had dropped down about three pounds and was pretty sure I had climbed my way back up again. I wasn't on a good path and I was afraid to see the number.

My husband said, "It all comes down to calories Nicole, if you eat less…yadda, yadda, yadda." And I know he is right to a degree. My problem could be simply eating too much—period.

I don't eat junk food every day, but I do still eat it. In documenting this journey there had been a fair amount of junk foods that made their way past my lips. I had shoveled in handfuls of popcorn from giant bottomless paper buckets and I had piled on heaping amounts of guacamole, chip after endless chip. I had eaten countless slices of pizza and numerous amounts of french fries. Foods that are high in calories, sodium, *and* fat. Foods I ate mindfully in the present moment, but with very little thought about love, let alone what those foods would do once they made their way inside my body. *As clear as the light of day, I knew that continuing to indulge in any "on occasion," unnecessary, loveless, junk food binging—was, and is—no longer serving me.*

On this nearly 200th day—I was very aware that I had lost next to nothing. Except for some blood pressure points, which was a pretty big something—that sat next to that nothing. And to lose those points by myself in a short couple of months—just by changing my diet was nothing shy of amazing, because I was keeping my numbers there.

Medication was not necessary for me, and so far, through healing my heart, I didn't have to start. I knew my cholesterol was on its way there too. But regardless of the accomplishments I had made on the inside, or any junk food binging hiccups, my original intention to love myself more had taken a side-step because of the health issues and desperately needed to take the stage again, front and center.

I had made a few other internal strides, but I was subconsciously ignoring that I was the one making the bad decisions about the food I was eating, school vacation or not. Stepping on my scale was not going to bring me joy. I already knew that the number staring back at me would have been well over 200. And letting that thought wash over me was not easy to absorb. I didn't want to admit anything, and I certainly didn't want to see that flashing bright red number solidifying the choices I had made. The choices that were not moving me in a healthy direction.

Just a few days previously I had weighed in at 198 and just a few days before that I was 195.5. I thought hard about what it felt like to be a 200+ pound woman and furthermore, what it would feel like to be that size for the rest of my life. Lugging around an extra 50+ pounds of weight was not good for my back, my knees, or my heart, not to mention my mental health.

When I woke up, I felt heavy with shame and guilt. I was tired of disappointing myself almost every time I stepped on crystal. And she was getting sick of me too. *I was taking too many steps back in the wrong direction and what felt even worse than that, was that each new day felt like I had just begun.*

On Day 199 of my love diet I was knee-deep into it. And the truth was, I had only just begun, and each day was a rerun. The love I was finally pouring into myself had barely touched the surface of what my soul was longing for. *I do love myself and I have loved myself throughout the years, but the love I was feeding myself was not enough.*

So how could I let myself fall so deep, barely able to climb out on my own? How could I ignore my body's need for more care and self-love, and *not* more curly fries? But asking myself how is to insinuate that I wasn't smart.

I stopped asking my kids "how come" they didn't do their homework because I realized that simply by using the word *how* was inviting shame and guilt—when what they really needed was attention and guidance. To ask them how, implied they were not smart either, when in fact they are only human.

I am human too. And we don't know—what we don't know. And all I had done—was do what I knew. All I did was live my life *and* in the midst of doing the best I could, my metabolism slowed down, and I got older. So, I let go of the how and asked myself why instead?

Why did I not have the desire to give myself more love and care with proper nutrition and exercise? Why was I continuing to blame the manufacturers, my environment, and the self-induced stress? And why was I escaping any real ownership? I am smart. But did I feel worthy? *What was it about me—that the desire to be healthy—did not come naturally?* Clearly, I still had a lot more healing to do.

Still, the how's and the why's are practically irrelevant. What matters is the here and now. Questioning how or why I had gotten to this place was moot. What mattered more was where I am. *Because when we know better—we do better. And staying stuck looking in the rearview mirror wasn't providing enough of an incentive to propel me into my future.*

Learning a few years ago that awareness is the key to everything was so eye-opening for me. And I had been extremely aware; I was constantly curious, and I was being present in every moment that I possibly could. I was making every effort beyond all efforts I had ever made.

Even on this day, when I could have easily walked toward any excuse of an exit sign, somehow, I knew that everything I was doing would work. Even though I knew I had jumped over the number 200 on my scale, I knew deep in my heart that everything I was doing was different. I don't know how I knew, but I knew that my body would eventually adjust. Then, in my Deepak-Oprah meditations, again I heard: A*wareness IS the change.*

This path of awareness was key and would likely take me several steps closer to becoming the healthiest woman that I can be. Continuing to focus my attention on my love diet is the best thing for me. And my love diet might just be the conduit to my own freedom. I can see myself shrunken down to the size that I think I am not the size that I actually am. I can see my body smaller, and the reason I want my body to be smaller—is because it will automagically be healthier.

In my mind, not my mirror, I have a vision of my healthier self, down to the glowing sun-kissed skin, and the organic smile and laughter. Inside that vision of mine, I am surrounded by my loving family. I can see it often in a conscious state of mind and in my meditations. The sun is shining. The grass is green. The gardens are manicured. Everyone I love is with me. There are even new little ones in my vision—with fuzzy lenses hovering over their little unborn faces. Ironically, there isn't a single potato chip, slice of pizza or glass of chardonnay insight. Isn't that interesting. My vision is just me and my family. Wholesome, clean, happy, and healthy. Thriving, energetic and worthy me. *I want to help myself become—that free.*

Rushing home after an amazing meeting to get a quick bite before our last school vacation movie, I looked in the cabinet and then the fridge for something healthy—stat. I was running behind, but I was still being proactive. I grabbed a blackberry yogurt, which is low in calories, sodium, and cholesterol. Perfect. It was a good idea to eat something healthy before the movie, so I wouldn't eat as much *during* the movie.

I tucked a perfect little dark chocolate peanut butter cup into my purse that I had picked up from the coffee shop, and we were off to get our tickets. I still ordered a bucket of popcorn for us to share, a medium soda for my daughter and Twizzlers for her too. The fun chewy red candy that was one of my old favorites invoked not a single hint of temptation for me ever since I found out they were not gluten-free. They really do put that wheat dust into almost everything.

My husband was making a lovely pan-seared scallop dinner with risotto but forgot one thing, the vegetable. It's one of my biggest pet peeves when he cooks. But I took care of it fast and threw some broccoli florets into the microwave.

He was still adjusting to my dietary needs when he wears the chef hat in our kitchen and got a little carried away when I saw him asking about—and searching for—the little orange box from the spice cabinet.

Stopping him mid-reach I took the box into my hands to examine it. I said, "If you add this to our meal, we won't be able to taste the expensive scallops or anything else. It's just a box of chemicals pretending to be flavor. Trust me, in this meal, less is more. And I'm pretty sure that removing most of the chemicals from our regular everyday cooking will eventually add up for all of us." Praise God he caved.

Day 200: Saturday, April 21st

The two of my workouts in a row had sucked. It was like each class had that "start/stop" feel to it and I couldn't get into a good rhythm. I went from thriving on intense energy rushing through my veins to falling flat and wishing the class was over—twice.

I didn't care for that style, but this time, I didn't let the deflated aura consume me. I focused my attention back on my intention. I kept the bigger picture in the forefront of my mind because after all, I was shifting like never before. My latest workouts were menial, but my vibrations had been turned back up on high.

Day 201: Sunday, April 22nd

We were positive there would be a feast at the family event we were attending. But I can no longer treat every event like a holiday.

Otherwise three holidays a year can easily turn into six. In no time at all I'm "celebrating" something every month, which I practically can find in every weekend. Then my weekends start to last longer and longer, until finally they are kicked off with a more than occasional hump day. So, it's not too far from the truth that Mondays and Tuesdays can easily become the only two days a week to stick to any diet. And I can easily forget about the whole idea when there's a holiday on a Monday.

What I want is to care about what I eat every day. And what I had was a good healthy breakfast nice and early and just before we left, I made myself a small sweet potato with butter, salt, and pepper. It was already close to lunch and I knew there would be plenty of chips and dips when we arrived—as with any holiday or party. So, I didn't want to show up starving.

It's not like I can't have a good time unless I'm munching on chips and dips. I can still have fun *and* honor my commitment to myself. And living it up, as they say, does not necessarily equate to eating bad foods or drinking to excess. Living a great life can be had—by respecting my body, including when I attend a party.

They served one of my favorites: steak tips wrapped in bacon. Two delicious items rolled into one. Double no-no's. When I said out loud that I had given up bacon, everyone within listening distance shouted with smiles, "But why!?" After that reaction, and without making very much effort at all, I easily caved, enjoying a few small bites of the delicious bacon one last time—again.

The salad I scooped up for myself was delicious too, but while I was eating it, I realized the candied walnuts were probably not gluten-free and full of sugar I'm sure. In my defense, I was making fewer mistakes than when I first started my love diet. And overall, I did my best. When I got home, I thought it was the perfect opportunity to give my love diet a fresh look and see if there was any room for improvement.

My Love Diet:

1) *Feed Myself Love*
   a. *Is Love on My Plate, In My Bowl, In My Cup?*
2) *Minimize Sodium*
   a. *Remove High Sodium Caesar Salad*
   b. *Remove or Reduce Soups, Dressings, Sauces, Gravies and Dips.*
3) *Reduce Animal Fats*
   a. *Red Meat, Pork, Shrimp, Yogurt and Soft Cheeses*
4) *Be Mindful of Carbs*
   a. *Remove or Reduce to Size of Fist*
5) *Let go of Pizza*
6) *Remove Deli Meat*
   a. *Including Bacon, Sausage, Linguica, etc.*
7) *Live Gluten-Free*
8) *Exercise at Least Once a Week*
9) *LOVE My Body as It Is Today.*

Day 202: Monday, April 23rd

My sister gave us a jar of some amazing homemade honey from her own personal beehive. We have so many bees in our yard that we wondered if it would behoove us to broaden our horizons by engaging in some backyard bee-hiving too. But she told me that the investment was about $800 at first—and if you lost the queen bee—you would have to replace her. Wow. I wouldn't want to be replaced. She also said there were no guarantees that the queen bee would stay—or that the existing bees would welcome the newbies. So we put the bee idea way on the back burner.

I made honey chicken for dinner with a side of green peas and reheated some leftover rice and pasta. It's funny how my husband and I were starting to fight over the rice ever since his doctor said to reduce pasta from his diet.

Day 203: Tuesday, April 24th

The saying popped into my head again. "If you love someone, set them free. If they come back, they're yours; if they don't, they never were."

Most of us have heard that saying once or twice in our lives and some of us have experienced the metaphor firsthand. But sometimes we are happy to let go of some things—beyond food or our loved ones. And when some of those things don't come back, it is meant to be—and we settle into a new normalcy.

I was approaching five solid months of missed cycles. In the absence of it, whether consciously or subconsciously—I was half-heartedly almost free.

Day 204: Wednesday, April 25th

Watching TV with my family, I walked over to the cabinet and complained out loud. "How come you guys have plenty of fun snack foods and I have none?" No one replied of course and I ended up getting nothing and sat back down.

Was I resisting the inevitable? Was it too risky to keep carbohydrates *in* my diet and in my home? The subject is so subjective. That pain-in-the-ass thing called carbohydrates. We

I AM ON A LOVE DIET

have all come to love them or hate them. And it's a full-blown struggle for a lot of people.

Where I stood was still in question because I was still questioning. All in all, it wouldn't be realistic for me to remove carbohydrates 100 percent from my own love diet. It wouldn't be sustainable or worth it mentally, to set myself up for that kind of failure. And to do it temporarily felt like a waste of time.

Day 205: Thursday, April 26th

When my day began it was pretty uneventful. I ordered a simple breakfast: oatmeal, craisins, apples, cinnamon, and honey, with a fruit cup on the side and the usual small black coffee. For lunch, I had my typical grilled chicken salad with honey mustard on the side. The dressing was a little spicier than usual and I wondered if my stomach was still capable of handling spices the way that it used to.

I was craving chocolate and in need of a small snack to hold me over until dinner, so I dipped my spoon into the creamy chocolate jar, alternating it with peanut butter. It was not a huge binge, which made me wonder, was I binging or was I having a normal snack? And why did I think *everything I ate* outside of a regular meal was a binge?

It can be challenging to do what's best for me and my body in a public setting such as the one we were at. And with well over 300 people there I was prepared to make the best of it.

Dinner was plated and the sit-down meal was not easy to work around. Beginning with the first course it was a Caesar salad with croutons. The lettuce was drenched in dressing too. So I took my three "no thank you" bites and left the rest. Glancing over at my daughter's plate, she devoured hers lickety-split.

When the main course arrived, the chicken, roasted red bliss potatoes and green beans looked delicious at first. But then I noticed a very light layer of moist breadcrumbs that were covering the breast along with a puddle of gravy. It was a meal fit for serving multitudes of people. And it was easier for me with my gluten-sensitivity, to scrape the gluteny layer off and hope for the best. Sometimes it's just not worth asking for a special meal or even an adjustment.

Dessert was a chocolate mousse. I ate that without a single thought of consideration or hesitation. Especially since I had already presumably consumed a small amount of gluten from the chicken entrée. I gave in to the chocolate dessert temptation easily and imagined it was made from Cool Whip or egg whites, with shaved chocolate and the like.

Later I did a simple search to see what a typical mousse was made of. The initial ingredients that were revealed sounded delicious: Whipped egg whites flavored with chocolate, coffee, caramel, pureed fruits, and various herbs and spices such as mint and vanilla. *Yum.* Reading further the mousse is generally served as a dessert or used as an airy cake filling—sometimes stabilized with gelatin. *Yuck.* Gelatin: a protein obtained by boiling skin, tendons, ligaments, and/or bones with water, usually obtained from cows or pigs. *Ew.* The more I read, the more thought I gave to the vegan way of living and how it was appearing to be more appealing.

Overall, I considered myself blessed to have had a wonderful dinner with two amazing women in my life: my offspring and upline. Interestingly, my daughter and my mother were born on the same day and I pushed really hard to make that happen. They are both very different from each other, but at the same time very much like me. I really hoped that what I was doing through my love diet research and efforts would eventually rub off on them.

Of all the people in my life, they were standing strongly by my side on my path to more self-care and love. And they both had front row seats to my inevitable transformation.

Day 206: Friday, April 27th

The acne that was deep under the surface of my skin was all but gone. It was proof that loving myself from the inside out was making a difference and it was showing in a subtle way. People, not just friends, were complimenting my skin all the time, and it felt genuine.

I knew a real major change was happening on the inside too. My stomach felt like it was shrinking. Not the kind of shrinking that happens after fasting into a new diet, but the kind of shrinking that doesn't go back. I was getting fuller, faster, longer. And I noticed that it was happening after eating things as simple as the tuna melt I had with tomato and swiss. I continued to feel full for what seemed like more than four hours afterward.

Nothing was speaking to me as I searched the restaurant menu that I had all but memorized as a regular. The dinner choices had too many sauces and too much pasta. I do love to eat with my eyes, but sometimes I like to think about what I want to eat and run with my own gut instincts.

It's something we do instinctively anyway. Think about what our bodies are craving when we look over a menu. So, I said to my husband, "I'm in the mood for grilled chicken. I think I'm going to ask for that, along with a side of asparagus and cherry tomatoes." They obviously had all of those ingredients in their kitchen from reading their menu. And for a simple appetizer, I asked for a gluten-free pizza crust toasted, and this time with a side dish of olive oil, garlic, and parmesan for dipping instead of marinara.

My husband looked at me and sort of rolled his eyes at my decisions. He said, "What's the point of eating out if you're not going to order a real meal on their menu?" With a smile, I said, "I want to eat something healthy and they have all the ingredients. Why not make up my own meal? Their chicken is delicious and much better than what I can make at home. My meal is being served to me and we are enjoying our date night."

I forgot his point while he went back and forth trying to figure out which meal to order and was leaning heavily toward the seafood pasta—claiming he would take some home. I said, "You and I both know that you won't take any of your meal home—and that you will eat all of it." But then I lured him in and said, "I know how you can guarantee taking home half."

Sarcastically, he took the bait and said, "What, draw a line on my plate?" I said, "No. I learned a trick from a friend that when you place the order, ask them to put half of it into a box first—before they serve it to you. Most restaurants are serving double the size portions of what our bodies need to eat anyway." He rolled his eyes and said, "Isn't that something a woman would do?" I said, "No. That's what a smart person would do—especially if they were told they had high cholesterol by their doctor and to eat less pasta. That is something a person could do if they love themselves enough to start making the changes that they say they want to make. I'm no angel, but I do make the effort a lot. You just need to start."

After all that discussion, he asked, "Should I have the pasta or the eggplant?" This time I rolled my eyes and sighed. I said, "Just have the eggplant. It's breaded and drenched in lord knows what, but it was the first thing you wanted to order anyway, and it's healthier than the giant bowl of pasta." In the end, I took all of that going back and forth as a positive. He was starting to make the shift and let go of the pasta la resistance.

Day 207: Saturday, April 28th

She wiped the sweat off of her face with her tiny workout tank top. Lifting it up slightly, her light brown semi-taut skin was exposed. For just a millisecond I looked, but not long enough to see if she was equipped with an eight pack or even the desired six.

Under my "extra-large" shelf-bra tank-top, what I had was beyond an eight pack. I had thousands of little packs of fat hanging tough with their sidekick cellulite. The thought that raced immediately across my mind was how I wish I could do that casual lifting it up thing. In my world, I was always tugging my tops down—far down—as any garment could stretch. Ergo the thoughts of a 50-year-old woman, standing next to a 25-year-old gal. Both of us filled with different types of will—on the infamous treadmill.

Day 208: Sunday, April 29th

I had gotten deep into my meditation and one turned into two. I blew out my hair and applied a minimal amount of Sunday morning makeup. Then I started trying on some clothes. I was loving myself as is—and I pulled together several outfits for the week that were complementary to the trajectory of my aging body.

I am aging, but my body was changing. I was getting cleaned up and toned up. And beyond drying up, I was excited to be using my muscles again. It was shortly after ten in the morning and all I had was a cup of black coffee. So, I made myself a small bowl of berries and sprinkled them with granola, cinnamon, and honey. It was good enough to hold me over until our delicious Sunday family dinner.

Everything we cooked came from love. An impromptu appetizer was easy too using cooked chicken from the fridge, reheating it and serving fresh honey mustard for dipping. We planned a mussel meal with pan-seared scallops and reminisced about the bread we loved from the restaurant where we first met. They took the baguette rolls from dinner the night before, sliced them lengthwise and drizzled olive oil and minced garlic before toasting and dusted them with parmesan cheese hot from the oven to serve at lunch. It was a nice touch to our delicious pasta-less mussel meal. And I gave myself a gluten-free version.

Later for a simple snack, I sliced some strawberries and dipped them in creamy chocolate sitting outside, followed by an afternoon nap with the warm semi-spring sun shining on my face.

Day 209: Monday, April 30th

Everyone said it was going to be a hot week, so we brought back the outdoor rooms. It was almost May and I couldn't wait for the warm weather to arrive. I took my cinnamon raisin french toast outside to our bistro table on the deck and sat there freezing in my eager-beaver summer shorts.

One of the dinners that we all loved was the grilled pork chop dish we used to make with minced garlic, olive oil, Dijon mustard, light brown sugar, butter, and a splash of orange juice. We all loved it and there were hardly any leftovers.

Any vegetable was easy to pair it with as well as potato, pasta or rice sides. It was just one of those meals we missed. So, we gave it refresh and swapped out the pork for chicken. And it was still a good hit.

Day 210: Tuesday, May 1st

Before heading out to my event, I made myself a quick protein shake for breakfast. The meeting space was different than what I was used to, but full of great energy. It's amazing how the mind and body can adjust.

Several hours had passed in what seemed like the blink of an eye. It was approaching two in the afternoon and the only thing I had eaten was a protein shake around eight o'clock. My stomach had shrunk, but I was downright running on empty.

Arriving at the restaurant, I was starving and ordered myself the grilled chicken salad with my usual honey mustard. The chicken was so juicy and cooked perfectly it turned out to be one of the best salads ever. Perhaps it was because I was hungry, or perhaps healthier food was tasting better, and my body was craving it. After eating such a late lunch, I wasn't hungry for dinner. I didn't feel like cooking either and luckily everyone was okay with scrambling for leftovers. Later that night I snacked on a small amount of my gluten-free favorite Cheez-it knock offs along with a couple of cookies.

Nicole Perry

Day 211: Wednesday, May 2nd

<u>Love Is A Gift</u>

Living with love comes respect, safety, and compassion
*   and there is no need to ration.*
Living with love breeds kindness, hope, and desire
*   and it feeds my soul's purpose and fire.*

With love comes many things, that only love can bring.
In love, there is healing and beauty. In love there is me.

Love is a gift I want to unwrap every day.
Love is what I found and it's where I want to stay.

Lovely are the people who walk with me,
*   together we are free.*
To those who have walked away—in their dismay,
*   I send love their way.*
Where there was once darkness and despair,
*   love is strong and fills my air.*

Love is where I want to start,
*   if there is an emptiness in my heart.*
I found love in my reflection and I faced it.
*   Love looked back at me—and I embraced it.*

I deserve to be loved. I am worthy of love. Love is a gift.

I AM ON A LOVE DIET

Day 212: Thursday, May 3rd

Sometimes I feel bad sending food back, especially when I know that it's prepared with love. But I won't eat anything blatantly that isn't in alignment with my love diet plan at my own demise.

The salad looked lovely, but I had added corn-free to my dietary description—and they simply forgot. When they handed the salad to me, it was covered in corn confetti and I didn't want to eat it.

I imagined removing corn from my diet would not be easy. There is such a variety of corn everywhere and—like its little buddy wheat—it can be found in almost everything! In its whole form, yes, it's clearly a vegetable and some people like me might even call it a healthy colon-cleanser. But in my humble opinion, corn in its finest form has over-extended its welcome. Corn has been used as a primary filler repeatedly—and for far too long.

A plethora of corn has been added to our American-made and manufactured foods—hidden in plain sight. And we can find all sorts of corn-like ingredients when we take a moment to cast our eyes in the direction of the cultivated kernel.

The list is long and substantial, but the least I could do was remove things like corn syrup, corn starch, cornmeal, corn oil, and corn flakes whenever I possibly could. After reading the list, removing corn seemed downright impossible. But I wanted to remove it whenever possible. Especially if it wasn't on the cob—slathered in salt and butter, or in a bottomless paper bucket.

I would venture to guess that corn syrup is the best of the refined, and they made it even more superior by taking it to its higher fructose level. In my opinion, corn syrup in its purest form is heaven right here on earth poured straight from the bottle onto pancakes, french toast or even the waffle.

When I was a kid, and my siblings made the last few drops of our favorite 1970's liquid brown sugary gold disappear at breakfast, I happily reached into our baking cabinet to pull out the thick and sweet clear alternative that shined like a diamond. I wouldn't feel slighted at all. In my eyes it was practically an upgrade.

My husband and I met at one of our local favorites for a quick date night and once again, I created my own meal. Pan-seared scallops, asparagus, and creamy risotto. It ranked the top five on my best-ever meal list, again.

Day 213: Friday, May 4th

There were no gluten-free symbols on this particular menu which I knew was a red flag. But the hostess assured me that they had options. When she pointed out some of the items that one of her gluten-free customers came in for regularly, she had me at stuffed peppers.

They arrived steaming hot, filled with chicken, rice and tomato sauce. And I was looking forward to enjoying every single moment of my quiet lunch. I was mindfully living in the present moment.

My cabernet had arrived in a stemless, trendy wine glass, so savoring my meal was in, but swirling legs and nose-diving was out. Everything was delicious though, but there was just one thing. I was only able to eat one of the peppers. And I started to feel bloated just before asking for the check.

It appeared to be a new restaurant, but gluten-free, dairy-free, and nut-free, were all common dietary labels that have been around for years. Vegetarian and vegan too. I wondered why this restaurant didn't list anything at all. A new restaurant would surely be on-trend. And this one was apparently—with their wine glass selection.

Even if it were an older restaurant, they would have updated their menu by now to keep their regular patrons coming back and new ones coming in. And no labels kind of meant no liability. It was enough to pique my curiosity, so before leaving I asked, "Have you been open long?" She said proudly, "About a year and a half."

I treated myself to an impromptu pedicure next door and then a long overdue stop at a thrift shop. But in the parking lot, when I was switching from the takeaway flip-flops into my shoes, I noticed something wasn't quite right with my knee. Making a mental note to be more careful during my workouts as I was unloading my car, my knee popped again. That couldn't be good.

At home we shared my second stuffed pepper outside sitting on the patio to hold us over until our date night dinner and again the feeling of bloatedness come over me. *Dammit.* I knew those stuffed peppers had something in them. But I didn't know if they were wheat or corn-laced.

Later at dinner, I decided to give my body a rest and scaled-down my meal with a simple grilled chicken salad. Going forward I consciously made the decision to listen to my gut.

I vowed to pay attention to those red flags with care, so bombs wouldn't go bursting into air. Those peppers gave proof throughout the night that something was still there. O' say does that outdated menu that you gave... o'er the land of the gluten-free, a home anyone can brave dangerously dining symbol-free?

Nicole Perry

Day 214: Saturday, May 5th

My husband and daughter were leaving to pick up groceries, so I asked them to please bring me back some fun gluten-free snack foods. Simple stuff like almond crackers, cauliflower crust, and some raisin toast. Mainly because when they were all eating carelessly carefree—I was feeling a little left out and lonely. Unusually, I found myself reaching for that thing called ice cream.

After coming home from the gym, I noticed my knee was acting up again. I had been very careful and babying my knees by avoiding their burpees. At my age and size, it was a blessing in disguise, to have a real reason why I couldn't do the exercise. But no matter how much it sounded like an excuse, my left knee was visibly swollen. I let out a big sigh at the thought of having to resort to wearing practical shoes on a daily basis—*for the rest of my life*. Just a few weeks previous my daughter had said to me, "You can't be fat mom if you wear high heels."

I was famished and I cooked up a box of gluten-free pasta, "accidentally" pouring all of it into my bowl. I was quick to abandon my original plan—which was to only eat half. But I kept adding more butter and parmesan in between bites. Salt and pepper too. I kept shoveling. I was eating my meal vigorously too and fully aware at every moment of what I was doing. But I forgave myself immediately. As they say, onward and upward.

We made turkey burgers for dinner with a side of corn on the cob, sautéed spinach and grape tomatoes. I do want to be mindful about how many ears I eat each year, but how many was enough to satisfy my summertime love? Where was the imaginary line between appreciation and deprivation?

Could all whole foods be the exception to my love dieting rules? And is the inability to digest corn in fact, the way to make my colon happier between colonoscopies?

Day 215: Sunday, May 6th

It was subtle, but I felt my body shift and lighten up—like almost on a cellular level. I had no idea how hard my body had worked to heal itself of toxins over these past few months, but I knew it was healing and would continue to heal with more time. My body was recovering.

What I needed was to be patient. I was on the right path, and I was sure I needed just a little more time. I made salmon for dinner with risotto and grilled brussels sprouts with a honey, garlic, and Dijon mustard dressing. The kids didn't care for the vegetable, but just like my body I was sure they would with a little more time.

Day 216: Monday, May 7th

I was prepping my house early. My deep housekeeping clean team was coming, and I was in that go, go, go mode for about an hour until I arrived at good enough.

It's amazing how fast I can move my body and how much I can get accomplished when I know my entire house is about to be cleaned from top to bottom. I showered, then meditated and they arrived in divine timing.

My day was flowing almost seamlessly. For dinner, I made pizza for everyone—including a gluten-free version for myself and we enjoyed the beautiful weather together eating outside on the deck. During our dinner conversation, I looked around and noticed that all of our pizzas looked surprisingly similar. It felt good to not look like the oddball out—for once. Theirs was a thin crust from a box and fairly small in diameter compared to delivery. Mine was made with a cauliflower crust—also thin—with my own marinara sauce and part-skim shredded mozzarella.

It didn't occur to me that the two pizzas I had put into the oven looked so similar that if you weren't watching me take one out of the box and construct the other, you might not be able to distinguish the difference. So, I asked, "Are you sure mine is the gluten-free one?"

It was my own fault. I was careless by not marking them and additionally lazy by asking my kids to bring me out a slice while they were getting theirs. Initially, my emotions were directed at them for not looking out for me, but I assured them it was my own fault. I was the careless one and it's ultimately on me. I freaked out a little on the inside and got pissed at my own stupidity. I was emotionally irrational, pacing around for a few minutes and I worked my way over to pitiful, holding back useless tears. All I could think about was how hard I had worked to take care of my body by eliminating gluten for four months, and in the blink of an eye, I screwed up.

And it wasn't even something I was enjoying on purpose. All of my efforts were not erased, but this was definitely a wake-up call to pay closer attention and care more. I am responsible for my own health. And fate is always in my own hands.

Day 217: Tuesday, May 8th

It was picture week at dance, so I was picking my daughter up from school early to magically make hair and makeup happen.

And in order to play dance hooky with her, I had to get a lot of work done first. But, before that, I had a higher priority—me.

Meditation had become essential to my routine. I was putting myself at the top of my own priority list—daily. Through my meditation practice, I was attending to myself in many ways. I was releasing stress, manicuring my nails, breathing deeply, sitting with better posture, and letting go of limiting beliefs. Pouring attention into myself at the start of each day didn't come easily at first, but as it turns out, it's a transferable skill.

Day 218: Wednesday, May 9th

At the morning mixer I attended, the only thing I could eat was the fruit, so I filled up my cup with love! The meeting was held at a location filled with outdoor inspiration and hopping back into my car I could feel the warm sun shining on my face. The energy of spring and the invitation to change was in the air.

It had been brought to my attention through sharing my new gluten-sensitive diet with a variety of people that we need to have some gluten in our bodies. But did we? In order to be tested for Celiac yeah, I get that. But did we need to have gluten in our bodies to live? And why were those people going out of their way to tell me that? Were they becoming gluten-defensive to this new phenomenon of the gluten-sensitive?

We ordered take-out pizza for an easy dinner—and I asked for extra black olives for my notably different gluten-free one.

Day 219: Thursday, May 10th

Their home fries were not gluten-free however, they did have a separate fryer for their french fries. Oh heaven! I was craving a heartier breakfast, so I ordered the fries with a one egg mushroom and parmesan cheese omelet.

For dinner, I got a little adventurous at the restaurant and ordered their creamy pesto chicken, with roasted red peppers and their gluten-free pasta. I was excited to eat something deliciously different from the usual salad with grilled chicken or even the gluten-free pizza I was used to. But when it arrived, the first thing I noticed was the color of the pasta. It was yellow—which meant it was corn-based. *Shit.*

Day 220: 198 lbs. Friday, May 11th

Courage carried me over to crystal and faith stood with me as I stepped on her. I was past the seven-month mark on Day 220 since my journey began and I was back at my original weight. But faith was still with me. Perhaps it was because I had gone over the 200-pound mark and could feel I was already on my way back down. Or it was because I was feeling and looking better. But I believe the real reason I had faith and didn't get caught up in negativity was that even though I was right back at my original weight—mentally, I was nowhere near where I had started.

Day 221: Saturday, May 12th

Struggling with carbs has happened a few times for me, but this time I wasn't just trying. I was working hard, and I was taking actionable steps constantly toward bettering my health.

I deserve to love myself and become the healthier woman that I dream of being. I can imagine that woman in my mind, and in my heart and know it's possible. I know I'm capable of becoming that woman. I was letting go of old limiting beliefs and self-sabotaging behaviors. And I was on my way to a healthier life.

Training my mind and retraining my thoughts has been challenging and it has taken time. And even though I had been accustomed to saying certain things and feeling a certain way for a number of years, I was allowing more love in. I had not loved myself 100 percent of the time during this process, but I was self-motivated, more than ever before.

ಶ ൙

Nicole Perry

Chapter 11
It's Time to Be Free

"And it is a vicious cycle indeed—when we continue to believe—that the trick still lies up someone else's sleeve."

Day 222: Sunday, May 13th

My daughter wanted to make waffles and she made mine with fresh fruit, love, and a little compassion before making everyone else's. I wasn't going to get sick from any cross-contamination, but I really did appreciate that she went out of her way to make mine first.

I had replaced using syrup a long time ago with honey and grabbed the squeeze bottle since the homemade jar my sister had given us was gone. Evenly, I spread the butter into just about every square and gave my gluten-free waffles a little drizzle. It was delicious of course, and I froze the other for the next time I was in a rush to get out the door, which usually happened at least once a week.

Everyone was being kind most of the time. Whenever my husband and kids went shopping or cooked a meal they were considerately thinking about me. In one way or another, it felt like they were all doing my love diet right along with me. It's interesting when it comes to the state of our physical or mental health—it can very quickly become a family affair.

They weren't about to let go of their pure maple syrup breakfast buddy though. It is all natural too, and it's what they love, but the amount of sugar it contains is well over 53 grams per serving. And the only thing they were measuring were sizable puddles piled onto their plates. I don't need to be a nutritionist to know that large amounts of sugar like that aren't good for the body. Especially in one sitting.

My breakfast was rational and lovely. And I planned to spend the better part of my Sunday afternoon learning about Chakras. It's something that has intrigued me for a long time, and I couldn't wait to snuggle up to my DVD player and absorb the information. But disc one was just okay, and hardly the mind-blowing experience I was hoping for. I fell flat at disc two too. I really did try to let it wash over me, but I just didn't have the patience. There's probably a chakra for that.

I do love Cliffs Notes of any kind, but I ditched the DVD idea. My personality was better suited for a getaway weekend class connecting with others in a group setting. An educational energy exchange was what I wanted. It's on my bucket list.

*Day 223: Monday, May 14*th

A different restaurant caught my eye and I pulled over to have lunch. I ordered the Buffalo chicken salad from their gluten-free menu with bleu cheese dressing. And shortly before getting the check I asked to see what options they had for dessert.

My mojo was kind of low—so I ordered their flourless chocolate cake to go. When I got home, I ate the entire piece of cake accompanied by a large glass of red wine, followed by a much-needed nap in the backyard sun.

To lift up my spirits, I cooked one of my favorite meals for dinner—pan-seared scallops with creamy mushroom risotto and asparagus—it's one of my kids' least favorites, but interestingly, my youngest had come around to the green fuzzy tipped sticks on this day much sooner than expected.

*Day 224: Tuesday, May 15*th

My vibrations were not as high as they could have been, so I went to a meeting held by one of the women's groups I belong to. I wanted to go because I knew that getting out and about would be the fastest way to pick my chin up off the floor. *Talking is an amazing antidote for any sign of depression.*

On my way back to my office I stopped for lunch and continued to talk, this time with my waitress. We traded blood pressure experiences and I was proud to tell her that I was able to lower my numbers significantly just by changing my diet. She admitted that hers was high, but that it was also hereditary. She told me that she had no choice but to take medication.

I had heard a few other people say that they had no choice too, but I wondered—was it the high blood pressure that ran in her family or—was it the food she was raised on? Could the food she was actually accustomed to eating—be the hereditary link? Was it possible for people to change their undesired history—just by tweaking those traditional recipes?

We talked very little about dressings since they are so easy to get on the side and dipping my fork into any dressing first before taking a stab at my salad was what I had been doing for years. It was one of those no brainers that stuck with me and almost went without saying. Instead, we dove headfirst into a conversation around sauces and gravies.

When I mentioned the word gravy, I could feel her energy as I watched her eyes searching her memory bank for the last time she remembered having it. Most people automatically think of special occasions like Thanksgiving or other major holidays when the subject of gravy comes up. But those complimentary juices are being served to us a lot more than we think. They are the icing on the cake to any given restaurant meal to keep us patrons coming back for more. They are the conduit to delivering two of the major hidden flavor boosters—sodium and sugar. After all, salt and sugar sell—in packaging—and in restaurants.

The very definition of gravy is not just the fat and juices that drip from cooking meat, often thickened, seasoned, and flavored. Gravy is also slang for profit or money easily obtained or received unexpectedly. Ironically, gravy is exactly the type of food that we are all being served, here, there and everywhere—deliberately. My server said she didn't eat gravy of course, but before I started my love diet—I used to think I didn't eat any gravy either.

As usual, I did the dishes before starting dinner. I poured myself a tall glass of water and thought about how my brain was stuck on *how* come I wasn't dropping any weight and I was using the very word I practically vowed not to use. It was May and spring had already sprung, which meant I couldn't blame winter anymore. But I wasn't just sitting around waiting for my body to change either. I was doing lots of things. As frustrated and impatient as I was, I had to keep in mind that I was still in the midst of—and going through—menopause.

"Push *through* the contraction Nicole," is what my doctor said to me when the art of giving birth clicked and the lightbulb grew brighter. Teaching me to push through my contractions helped me to understand unequivocally *how* to birth my baby in that moment of angst, pain, and frustration. That metaphor was so powerful to me that I filed it away until the next birth, and the next, and then the last. Those words of wisdom turned out to be words I would subconsciously live by when there was nothing left to do but be patient, be present and persevere.

I was approaching the other side of menopause or at least had high hopes that I was one of the *six-year* women and not one of the *thirteen-year or longer* ones. Every woman who has gone through it knows that it's an experience that one doesn't forget and yet—no one talks about it.

The list of ailments and symptoms is endless and at times, it felt like I had them all. Each new symptom piled on top of the previous, from the backaches that didn't lead to a cycle, to the start of a cycle that led to nowhere and disappeared into thin air. The list goes on to the hot flashes and sleepless night sweats seemingly too silly to vet, drenched in irritability and frustration is what I was.

Menopause had thousands of sucky moments for me and like any woman—I prayed for it to go away. Individually, every new symptom was tolerable, but collectively, it was a recipe for fear and uncertainty.

As blurry as it may have been up ahead in the not so far distance, I was getting a glimpse of the finish line. I believed I was coming out of the disconnect and was almost there. And yet, I wouldn't trade my experience for anything else. Not because it was almost over, but because through it all I didn't see menopause as an obstacle to overcome—but a rite of passage to live through.

Through menopause, I was becoming wiser with every absentee month that I tucked under my chastity-turned-integrity belt. I was experiencing menopause in its entirety, and it was carrying me to my next chapter. I often referred to menopause halfheartedly as metamorphosis because I was changing into something different. And there were many times I was content to wrap myself up in the cocoon of my bed and ride it out until the next day—eager for another fresh start.

My path happened to be an all-natural one, and not the chosen path for all. But choosing to have my experience in its rarest form had ultimately helped me to let go of my childbearing years, which included my youth. And my brain was slowly wrapping around the fact that I would still be a woman, but a transformed one. In and of itself, the experience of menopause has helped me to see that the physical gifts inside of me had given all that they could give. The experience of menopause had helped my mind accept that it was time.

For our family dinner, we made simple grilled chicken tenders with butter and olive oil, along with some leftover rice and fresh broccoli.

Nicole Perry

Day 225: Wednesday, May 16th

Deep inside our shopping carts is where we can hide just about anything. We can hide foods in our cabinets at home and we can eat in hiding too. But we can't hide forever. The choices we make will have to be placed on the conveyor belt for anyone to see—or eventually be exposed through our tight-fitting clothes. Sadly, the choices we make can be revealed in yet another way—emotionally suppressed for a future manifested day.

Standing in the grocery line, I was proud to place my items on the counter for all to see because they were practically judgment-free. Turkey burgers were on the menu for dinner and I picked up some fresh fruit too. Two oranges, one grapefruit, one banana bunch, two packs of grape tomatoes, one ripe avocado, a box of gluten-free crackers, and one bag of all-natural corn chips with fewer than five ingredients.

I knew everyone would appreciate the guacamole and chip surprise. My avocado dip is simple and made with nothing but all-natural ingredients. Starting with the scooped innards of the ripe avocado I added the olive oil, crushed garlic, lemon juice, a hint of crushed red-pepper flakes and a pinch of salt and pepper. It comes out great every time and it's good for you.

A fair amount of compassion is what I searched for when I saw what the woman in front of me was buying. But judgment got the better of me.

She had placed one giant Danish on the counter, along with a large bag of candy and an extra-large jumbo iced coffee. The kind that was freshly made to order and I could still see the perfect chocolate and caramel swirls through the plastic.

Instinctively, I couldn't help it. I was sneak peeking at her choices, trying not to judge her look by the cover. But it's easy to judge other people. Most of us know that. And having not walked a mile in her shoes I searched deeper for the compassion I knew I was capable of. Still, I wondered if she would ever find her way to love.

Maybe she was on her way there. Or perhaps what she was buying was not even for her. But she was not a pillar of strength or an example of good health either, so it was easy to let my mind cross the line. I couldn't help but wonder if she was holding the kind of love that could contaminate the love she already had? And was it tainted love? Then it hit me. Perhaps the path of true love was not her path to take.

I wasn't much different from that woman though because I wasn't a pillar of strength either and I wasn't a role model of good health of any kind. I had my ways of self-sabotage. *I was a binger.* I had plenty of positive moments in the public eye—and space in between my bad binging ways—and consequently, I was not completely free. But even if I was, I still had no right to judge.

Maybe I was a little bit different. I was changing with mindfulness and grabbing hold of growth through awareness. I was starting to see the light and I was turning my bad habit binges into healthier ways of snacking. Not all the time, but I was making strides. I was taking more steps forward—than I was taking backward toward awareness and self-care. I was finding myself more often than not, standing in pure eagerness to love myself more—just about every single day.

Later that night after my third glass of red wine, I made myself a small bowl of my kids' rocky road ice cream. Nope. I was, in fact, no different than that woman at the store. We both needed to feed ourselves more love.

# Nicole Perry

*Day 226: Thursday, May 17*th

I excused my daughter from school after my meeting and took her to a women's luncheon. At age 13 she was curious what it would be like and excited at the notion of swimming amongst a sea of strong women.

Scooping her up from school to take her with me was an easy decision. And I was so blessed to be able to share the empowering experience with her during these formative years. I watched her throughout the day in her little two-inch black high heels, gracefully absorbing the energy that filled the room.

Beyond myself, and the relatives in our life, she was able to observe and meet other women in her community who shared their real stories. And she got to hear firsthand how those women had overcome major obstacles and persevered to become who they are—in spite of any adversity.

Over my Arctic Char dinner, I shared some thoughts about our day with my husband. We were both amazed at how quickly she was becoming a young woman. Without a shadow of a doubt, we both agreed right then and there—that we were giving our daughter a good solid foundation for a strong and healthy outlook on herself—and life—in this 21st Century.

A healthy state of mind is essential to the human spirit. Especially in the accelerated internet world we live in. And we all know that our minds are shaped by more than what we learn from our parents, our environments, or the women we seek as role models. Our minds are shaped by our body image too. And what we see through the eyes of the world can be perceived positively or negatively.

I AM ON A LOVE DIET

When my daughter was born, I clearly understood the responsibility of raising a girl. And as she grew, the gravity of what was to come started to unfold in her early years. Weighing in at just 8 pounds and 2 ounces—she was my smallest baby.

Several months after she was born, she settled into the fifth percentile for her weight. And when we moved her to real food, our pediatricians would strongly encourage us to feed her more milk, cheese, mayonnaise, olive oil, and butter along with plenty of pasta. I remember it—like it was yesterday.

When we moved her to real food, the first time we talked about what my daughter ate at our wellness visit seemed casual, but the conversations we had grew a little more pressing with each visit. "She needs to eat more," they would tell me. "How about tortellini?" I said once. "Yes, with plenty of cheese and olive oil," was their reply. I was so confused about their suggestions that came with almost a sense of urgency. We were feeding all of our kids the same way and she looked perfectly fine. She was normal—not malnourished. She was ideal and she was healthy. And there were no other signs showing that she wasn't.

Knowing the severity of obesity in our country, I couldn't believe what they were asking me to do. My husband and I had many conversations about it and were a little shocked at each cumulative visit. Her pediatricians were thoughtfully attentive, but I thought they were looking past my daughter visually, for something that was only there in theory. I was surprised that they even brought anything up. Her placement on that chart appeared to be speaking louder to them on paper than she was as a whole person—in the flesh.

We paid closer attention, of course, but there was nothing to do. She liked eating food. There wasn't anything to change and I certainly didn't want to be *the* person in her life that caused an eating disorder—of any kind. The only thing those charts revealed to us was that 95 percent of the children her age—were bigger than she was.

In the 1970s, only 5 percent of U.S. children ages 2-19 were obese. Huh. So, since she wasn't obese today, if she were a toddler back in the '70s, she may have been on the other side of the spectrum in that 95th percentile—with the other "non-obese" kids. I make a good point.

By 2008, those numbers of obese children increased from just five percent to nearly 17 percent. And back in 2007, when my daughter was a toddler, it was frustrating that her placement in the fifth percentile on that chart was deemed inappropriate. Wouldn't the diet we were feeding her be the sought after one? *Hello!?!?!* It's like she was the last of the Mohicans. I state my case.

The question never seemed to be about if she was, in fact, underweight, but more along the lines that she wasn't in alignment with the other children her age. In 2019, the numbers of obesity in children had shockingly risen up 20 to even 30 percent. Which for me raised a huge question: Why were they looking at everyone else's body weight in the last 10 years—as the ideal or appropriate new standard?

When I was a child, I looked a lot like my daughter. And where she had placed on that chart had to have something to do with genetics. My instincts told me to keep doing what we were doing—and to not *pump her up with extra food*. It didn't feel like a healthy approach and it seemed almost irrational or even a little risky. I nodded my head in agreement at each visit and ultimately left their suggestions at the door. I trusted our pediatricians, but in this particular scenario, I trusted myself more. Shaping our daughter's mind around body image at the tender age of a toddler was already happening and I was refusing to place my trust in anything other than my own motherly instincts.

In retrospect, it was a pretty big moment in time for me as the mother of a young girl. As parents, each time we heard ourselves saying things like "finish your dinner" to any of our kids, we took a step back. We paid closer attention and armed ourselves with a passion for our family's next generation to have and consume a better healthy concept of what their body image could be. We thanked God—we left well enough alone. Because the original instructions by our daughter's pediatricians had slowly turned into mild suggestions, and finally faded into complete reflections.

Overall, our kids were not growing up on gummy worms nor were we starving them. We didn't need to change a thing. We taught our kids to listen to their doctors, but we also emphasized the importance of listening to their own bodies. Our kids all eat a diet filled with healthy family dinners and typical kid foods. But most importantly, they all like eating food, and they all stop eating when they're full.

Day 227: Friday, May 18th

Creating plenty of opportunities to take myself out to eat each week is something I love to do and the chicken parmesan with a side of broccoli sounded perfect.

It was listed on their gluten-free menu, but I asked what the multi-colored spiral pasta that it came with was made from and it was a combination of rice and corn. As tempting as it was to have it with my meal, I wanted to stick with my latest exploratory idea of removing most—if not all—processed corn from my diet. So, I ordered it and eighty-sixed the pasta. I asked them to hold the mozzarella too and to put my favorite parmesan on the side.

I've said it already but it's worth repeating. According to my doctor, parmesan cheese is an acceptable hard cheese to allow in my now highly aware, cholesterol-reducing diet. And keeping some cheese in my diet is important to me. I gave up cheese once completely. And it was not easy.

I tried living a dairy free life a few years ago and I barely lasted through day three. The idea of living my life dairy-free had come to me after a friend had told me that her nursing baby was allergic. I was one of the fortunate parents that didn't have any babies allergic to anything, but I wondered what foods our pediatricians would have suggested if my daughter had been allergic all those years ago.

My baby mama friend was in remarkable shape and had attributed all of her good health to living her life dairy-free. For years I had been trying to slim down to my first pre-baby weight. And her dairy-free perspective climbed to the top of my pre-existing, four-time post-baby condition.

After having plenty of cumulative baby weight to lose, I decided to give it a good college try. The first thing I did that day after my friend left was open the deli drawer in the fridge and zero my hungry eyes in on the brand-new, sliced deck of creamy American cheese. *Damn.*

During my first family dairy-free dinner, I had to pass the parmesan so many times to everyone else at the table—it almost felt like they were eating more of it—in spite of my decision not to. That sucked. But I got past it. Shortly thereafter, frustration kicked in again when I tried to decipher the dairy codes on each label my friend had clued me in on.

Several times I wondered whether or not conforming to a diet that was not deemed medically necessary for me was worth continuing. And if I wasn't actually allergic, where was the incentive to stick with it? While we were watching a family movie together, the black bag of white cheddar popcorn was being passed around. I gave up and snatched it.

Allowing myself a few items of exception, like that magical popcorn, would be the only way I could consider trying again to live my life *somewhat* dairy-free. I had already replaced skim milk with non-dairy almond a few years back, so maybe I could tackle dairy just like that. And it was how I was tackling processed corn.

At our date-night dinner, I ordered the gluten-free pizza crust toasted with a side of pizza sauce for dipping. And I thoroughly enjoyed having a small amount of parmesan cheese with it. I also ordered a small house salad with grilled chicken. So far so good.

Day 228: Saturday, May 19th

It had been a very busy week, we were tired, and it was raining too. There were plenty of really good excuses to cancel our Saturday night movie plans and replace it with something simpler like television and tacos—which easily transitioned into nachos. Either way, I had no desire to eat the corn tacos or chips and made myself a healthier version into a salad.

A small foundation of greens is what I started with and then layered the black beans. Next, I added a small scoop of all-natural salsa, bright green guacamole and sprinkled it with slices of black olives. Finally, I added a few scoops of the freshly cooked, taco-seasoned ground turkey with a small dollop of light sour cream. It was so freaking delicious I didn't need any dressing.

I would even take it a step further and say that it was so good, I was actually liking taco night again. A little hot sauce atop the sour cream gave it an authentic fast-food touch. Which posed the question: Why was I trying to create a healthy meal that had resembled "fast food?"

Day 229: Sunday, May 20th

I spent most of my morning writing until my husband made me a baby broccolini omelet. And it was borderline better than the tough competition of a restaurant.

Thoughtfully crafted with only the simplest of ingredients it tasted nothing like fast food. Cooking with whole foods, simple spices, and ingredients is the reason our meals are so good. And eating delicious meals was definitely playing a huge role in how I was sticking to my love diet plan.

This particular Sunday afternoon called for a simple grilled chicken family meal with sautéed brussels sprouts and some thick pan-seared, red-bliss, round potato slices. I poured plenty of olive oil while cooking and I made two easy sauces for dipping, one aioli, and a Dijon honey mustard. It was another healthy and successfully delicious family meal, but there was just one thing. We ate at two o'clock.

When eating a large family meal together so early in the afternoon I've noticed there is generally a bigger price to be paid. Sure, one of the benefits is that our bodies can digest long before going to bed, however, by the time five o'clock rolls around, we find ourselves rummaging and searching through the kitchen cabinets for many little somethings. We tend to munch our way through the rest of the night, and what's even worse than that is all the complaining we do, about what we are doing, before, during and after. We had yet to resign eating our family Sunday dinner at a reasonable time.

Day 230: Monday, May 21st

While I was eating my very healthy one egg over-easy breakfast with a slice of raisin toast and fortified side of leftover brussels sprouts in a timely manner, I sat browsing the internet.

I stopped and watched a video about a young woman in her early 20's telling her story about how she lived in a body full of excess weight as a teen. She shared her very vulnerable vlog thoughts and emotions taking us on a deep journey through what was going on in her mind back then, and how she felt about her body image today. She is one of the few to overcome the odds. It appeared she may keep her new healthy body and image too.

As a child who was born in the '60s and grew up in the '70s, I wasn't overweight as a child or as a teen. I had a fairly healthy mindset around food and body image—despite what the magazines were portraying—or the direction the packaged food industry was heading.

So, what did healthy nutrition look like in the '60s and '70s? It certainly wasn't found at the penny candy store we would go to, or in any can of spray cheese at our local supermarket. I grew up in that era of refined discovery and foods became even more defined in the '80s and '90s with better production and clever conveniences—making it even harder to look toward Julia Child for guidance, versus resorting back to Betty Crocker or giving in to Sara Lee.

In 1980 I was just thirteen years old when the controversially funny Dom Deluise movie titled "Fatso" came out. Dom's character portrayed a man who loved to eat and the well-humored messages around food spoke to both the young and old moviegoers alike.

One of the movie clips showed the cabinets in Dom's character's kitchen all chained up and padlocked nice and tight—as if that was all it would take to stop him from eating too much food. Those heavy-duty chains solidified what most were likely thinking—that it wasn't possible to achieve weight loss success—alone. The messaging was both relatable and absurd that in order to make a powerful change—we had to use force and take drastic measures. Or, if you were lucky like Dom's character, you would simply fall in love.

Watching the trailer, Dom's character didn't really look that overweight to me—compared to what we've seen since in our society. In 1980 the topic of overeating in a movie setting gave us a glimpse into the epidemic future of our country. But as far as movies go, it was good material for comedy.

Unless you were struggling with your weight of course. Then standing in public all those years ago to get your ticket might send you into a tailwind of mental frustration, anguish, or virtual embarrassment.

When I was growing up there were a few people in my life who were considerably overweight. And as a teen I watched and absorbed unhealthy perceptions around food and body image unfold. In my life and on the movie screen. Wasn't it inevitable? That once I became an adult, I too would find myself searching for solutions to get myself back on the right track—just like Dom and his fictitious feud with his fat? My mind was consciously developing while I listened and learned—and subconsciously,

I witnessed the adaptation of food addictions in the people around me who I loved.

Back in the day, the messages we received were similar to what we see today. And now, we're conveniently provided with illustrations of the new and improved or fast and easy, carefully executed by the seemingly skinnier and virtually healthy. When you sprinkle decades of mixed messaging and add to it the unavoidable act of aging, the fairly healthy body image I once had changed dramatically. It was an easy recipe for obesity.

Like many, the people in my life struggling with their weight bought into the diet and weight loss industry, as would I—eventually. That industry that continues to hold the fictional key to what we think will magically help us succeed. *And it is a vicious cycle indeed—when we continue to believe—that the trick still lies up someone else's sleeve.* Ironically, we remarkably buy into and consume unrealistic thoughts of idealism—and we pay for it all, eagerly and voluntarily.

It would be foolish to insinuate that any of us are victims of such marketable circumstances and that we are somehow unwilling participants that have been roped into any such commercialism. We're not quite brainwashed, but ultimately, we're all under the influence of some subliminal messaging whether it plays a lead role in a movie or is one of the extras in any other scene. With decades of knowledge tucked under our belts, we are still being spoken to from both sides of the mouth. Be healthy—but drive thru. Oh, and by the way, now you need to take this.

Sitting in my kitchen I took my mouse from videos back over to analytic searching and quickly discovered that out of the 327 million Americans, there are an estimated 160 million that are in fact obese—or are already on the path to getting there by being significantly overweight. America was ahead of all the other countries. Of course we were winning.

Day 231: Tuesday, May 22nd

There's an average of 125 calories in one five-ounce glass of wine and most pours in restaurants are six to seven, which can then bump those calories up from 150 to 175.

A realistic pour at home can generally exceed seven ounces, which can stretch that glass into the 200 range, easily. But sometimes, whether or not the calories are in fact, empty or wasted—having a glass of wine is an easy way to unwind. And sometimes after a long day, an extra unnecessary glass of wine is actually necessary.

Relaxing with a glass of wine before and during dinner is commonplace in our home, and it's not unusual to continue after. On this particular day, I seemed to be on autopilot though, and too much "relaxing" isn't good. Automatically, I was pouring myself another glass of wine after dinner, but I stopped and stood there staring at the glass. Almost examining it. Something was different. And I was seeing that glass from a different angle or perhaps through a new lens.

It wasn't about whether I was seeing the glass half-full or half-empty. Something had changed. Just like when I had seen that pizza crust with lust. I couldn't put my finger on it, but very carefully—and with intention—I watched myself pour that wine back into the bottle in slow motion as though I were watching from somewhere up above.

I AM ON A LOVE DIET

Day 232: Wednesday, May 23rd

Running and shouting from one person to the next I pleaded and begged as quickly as I could. There were far too many people that needed help. No matter how hard I tried, I couldn't help them all. I was only one person. And then I woke up.

The dream I found myself immersed in came out of nowhere and was completely unexpected. I was a little afraid of what I might find, but I took a quick peek inside my interpreted dreams analysis book. Dreams are very interesting and can tell you a lot if you look deep enough, but they can also be very confusing. In this particular dream, all of the people around me that needed help were dying.

As much as I hoped the dream was an exaggeration, I knew there was a hidden meaning. It could have been an underlying message that something in me had already died, or that something else was about to arrive. But I wasn't sure. And as scary and overwhelming as the dream was, I knew there was a message I needed to hear. Probably more than one. Anyway, it was highly unusual to wake up that way, and I found myself neither wanting to explore it—nor able to ignore it.

Day 233: Thursday, May 24th

Thirty-two years ago, on this date I was walking down the aisle at the age of eighteen for the first time. It was a very young age to be getting married and if I had the chance to do it all over again, I would consider the more fun and less commitment option like getting a couple of roommates. If we all knew then what we know now right?

When I think back, I don't remember too many people in my life encouraging college, but then again, I was an extremely willful and independent young woman. If there was ever a real wish to be made, I wish I could go back in time, and convince myself to listen to all advice. But mostly to sift through it before making any permanent decisions about my life.

This date in my family also marks the day my paternal grandfather passed away. It was several years earlier that he had lost one of his legs from the knee down due to diabetes. The memories I have as a kid are still clear of him washing his stump out in the open. It was what we called it back then. Today the politically correct term has evolved into having a residual limb. And the amputations due to diabetes since the '80s have also evolved significantly. One article I read said that following a diabetic amputation, up to 50 percent of people will die within two years.

I searched my memory for the emotions that filled the living room back then and what I remember most was that there was practically no animosity. I'm guessing it was due to the fact that my Pépère was grateful to still have his life.

Gratitude is what I remember, and maybe a few silly jokes to lighten the mood. I am definitely grateful that I don't have diabetes and fairly certain that diabetes won't get passed down to my children. Grateful and confident, but hopeful too.

Day 234: Friday, May 25th

Luckily, I was listening. My mind didn't have to shout at me at all. I knew I needed to dial it back. Before I did anything I took a hot shower. *And I gave myself permission to take a mental health day.*

It was a gift really. I was consumed with emotions, so I accomplished only what I had to. I chose to step away and take a break from the outside world—*for just one day.* I allowed myself to take some time to get quiet, breathe and listen. I was mourning something. And I wasn't exactly sure what, but I knew something was going on with me since I had paid little to no attention to what I was eating for two days. Respecting my emotions is one thing, but what I was doing was mindlessly eating emotionally, and subsequently, disrespecting my body.

Depression is something that can feel like a heavy burden or an anchor, maintaining a firm hold to keep us from moving forward. And guess what? We are human—and human beings have to move. We have to move our minds—and keep them moving in a forward and positive direction.

Sometimes, with all of the hats that I wear or roles that I play, I feel like I'm holding that anchor in my hands or the weight of the world is invisibly hanging around on my shoulders. But like anything in life, we can choose to see the negative or positive. And I am finally able to see the positive in my own moments of anxiety and depression.

It is just a feeling. And that feeling of weights, anchors or worlds, can automatically feel lighter or be lifted completely, simply by putting my feelings into perspective. It is important to feel—and I am capable of moving through those feelings in a healthy way—with some help. And sometimes I have to help myself by giving myself permission to take a mental health day.

The positive has come full circle for me and is crystal clear now that I've chosen to see it. When I feel any hint or sign of anxiety or depression kicking in, I recognize it for what it is. *It is a built-in, beautiful, internal mental clock that wakes me up and tells me—it's time to feed myself more love.*

That dream I had was just a dream, but it stuck with me like a powerful movie. Through my journaling, I had been dissecting my history and doing a significant amount of memory diving. I was taking a lot in and as much as I knew that brushing over my past wasn't an incentive to propel me into my future, it was important to acknowledge my history and see it for what it was. I could have been mourning my past, but whatever was happening, I was able to instantly dial down the feeling of depression when I surrendered to that built-in beautiful internal mental clock that was speaking to me.

Day 235: 197 lbs. Saturday, May 26th

Eating down the house is what we do sometimes. We take inventory and make do with what we have. It's such a great opportunity to take stock and get creative, which can either cause frustration or encourage a sense of gratitude.

Basically, we force the kids to be grateful—and they get frustrated. But dropping hundreds of dollars at each pay cycle on large grocery shops was the routine I wanted to get away from. Because like many people, we can tend to stock up on a lot of junk, filling our freezer with frivolous foods. We don't even have that much room and I know darn well that the buck doesn't ever stop there. We always forget something or run out of milk.

We can get carried away with those several smaller shops in between too. There are so many incidentals not on our lists that when I take a closer look at my checkbook, that large shop and all the little shops add up to something just shy of insanity. We only have a family of six to feed—not sixty.

The intention is always for the bigger food shop to last two weeks and it rarely, if ever, does. Purchasing all the extra processed food was not lasting either. And it wasn't feeding our family love.

However, buying the ingredients for the meals we actually want to make was the one thing that was starting to organically make sense to me. We still had a significant amount of mind shifting to do in our family but focusing our attention on a few meals every couple of days could be a much smaller hit to our wallet at month's end. And bring more seasonal vegetables in.

Food has gotten so physically and financially refined that it has become cheaper to purchase the enriched, hydrogenated, bleached, modified, and extracted. We needed to become more mindful by pushing our carts into the produce section and pull ourselves away from the packaged direction.

Somehow, we slipped back into reaching for the faster and easier, which is why putting on the brakes by eating down the house would help us recalculate or reroute. Life happens.

Day 236: 196.5 lbs. Sunday, May 27th

"Would you like butter?" was her standard question. And I said no thank you to the extra saturated and cholesterol, presumably dyed with yellow number five.

I'm sure that movie popcorn was hydrogenated, saturated or both, because it took several hours until my body finally felt normal again. It was an eight-dollar lunch, that 848-calorie bucket that I ate. And it sat in my stomach like a dead weight.

This time for dinner we made a variety of healthy choices like turkey burgers, grilled zucchini, and sweet potatoes to please most at our table. Along with the moderately unhealthy sausage and white buns. *Baby steps.*

Day 237: Monday, May 28th

I had given in to that bottomless bucket of temptation many times—and just like giving in to that popcorn—I still get the urge to go down the easier dieting road—in search for something "out there" that I think will magically cure my "in here." Especially when I see someone dramatically lose 70 pounds in a matter of a few short months.

Just as eating a giant bottomless bucket of movie popcorn that isn't love—I also have to keep reminding myself that going on another diet wouldn't be feeding myself love either. *It has to come from within. And until I find that burning desire to love myself all day and every day—no diet in the world will ever work for me—and I'll never be free.*

Day 238: Tuesday, May 29th

For no particular reason, I had a plain bowl of fruit for breakfast. I wasn't giving up on carbs by any means or punishing myself from the unnecessary indulgences I had engaged in. But I just thought I would start my day simple—without any extra calories.

It had taken an enormous amount of effort over these past few exploratory months to work each new little habit into my day while simultaneously removing the bad. And the idea to start my day out with something as simple as some fruit came naturally. I was relearning how to love myself in a new kind of way.

Learning to look in the mirror and love myself exactly as I am was what I was doing too. My eyes, my hair, my nails, my skin. Even the fat that still lies here within. Every flaw and feature, every curve and fine line. The body I was blessed with, gifted and assigned.

Day 239: Wednesday, May 30th

The majority of my morning was spent at a coffee shop and then after dropping my son off for an appointment—I took myself out to lunch. My eyes gravitated toward the veggie burger on their gluten-free menu and my non-vegetarian waitress swore by it.

I ordered the bunless beauty and interestingly it was green and strangely soft, like a pillow. It was amazing and quite possibly the best veggie burger I had ever had. It was beyond delicious and anyone who even came close to my table would have ordered it too—simply based on the yummy noises coming from my core. The coleslaw was equally satisfying, and I intentionally ate half of the meal, just so I could eat it again as a snack later in the day.

My husband and I met at a restaurant downtown near the water and I ordered the grilled salmon for dinner. It was served with a balsamic glaze, but it sounded like it fell under my "gravy" category and I remembered reading that some balsamic dressings may be loaded with too much sodium.

On the contrary, the bottle of balsamic I had at home only had 12 percent of the daily recommended allowance. I guess it could use more investigating as to what a glaze consisted of. But still, my daily blood pressure had already been compromised and I didn't want to risk getting it on the side. I had to decide. So, I traded one evil for another—the bleu cheese dressing.

Standing in my kitchen later that night, I ate slice after delicious slice of the kids' American cheese. I knew that it wasn't good for my cholesterol, but it continues to remain one of the most precious indulgences for me. It wasn't part of my new dairy reducing plan, but I was eating it anyway. I had been feeding myself dairy for years, and evidently, my body was craving it.

It was an easy decision to make when I had decided to reduce my own cholesterol through the food that I eat or didn't eat—and I was still determined. I want to heal my body naturally and it was taking time. Our bodies crave what we feed it and I had been feeding my body animal fats like cheese, milk, yogurt, butter, eggs, pork, shrimp, burgers and "gravy" for years.

I want to be the one to get my cholesterol in check, but I also want to do it in a way that doesn't mentally make me feel deprived or shock my body. Shocking my body isn't love. It's just mean. I want to heal myself in an achievable way and find that balance of how much animal fat is okay for my body to consume in one day.

In retrospect, reducing one's cholesterol numbers in three months or even six hardly seemed realistic. Eating that cheese in my kitchen was what my body needed. I wasn't removing all dairy or animal fats. I was slowly weaning myself off by figuring out what my body can handle without sending my numbers out of whack. It might take up to a year to figure out that balance, and I was still on a mission to finding it.

I AM ON A LOVE DIET

Day 240: Thursday, May 31ˢᵗ

I grabbed an apple and a handful of nuts for the road after eating breakfast and while my hair was processing, I flipped through some photos on my phone. Coming across a very unflattering recent picture of myself I realized I still had a long way to go. I've got rolls—I count 'em.

The younger days have come and gone for me, along with being carded, construction worker whistling, and the good old-fashioned car honk followed by "Hey babe, I'll be back to pick you up later!" If a flattering look comes my way, it's generally from a man 20 years my senior and likely because I'm the youngest—or perhaps the only woman in the room. These days I'll take what I can get.

Becoming a member of the aging society is all fairly new to me, and I read that one of the saddest things in the world to see is an aging woman start to disappear, especially after reaching the seasoned age of 50. Aging, unlike dieting, is completely out of our control, and I wondered, if I stayed at my current size, was I on an even faster path toward that so-called invisibility paradox?

So far, not that much had changed for me. Well, if I don't count menopause, stretch marks, wrinkles, gray hair, and weight gain. And I was long past measuring up to the younger, prettier, and skinnier twenty-year-old's. And even their thirty and forty-year-old elders. But was I in an even worse position by being an aging woman over 50, who is also heavy? Was being heavy *and* old a double whammy? I was certainly not ready to disappear though and vanish into thin air. And I was definitely not ready to be left alone to any corner rotting chair.

In my community, I am still somewhat relevant, but I have no idea how long that will last, or when the real fading will begin. Perhaps the so-called invisibility factor is evidence that we do live in a society that doesn't honor or respect the aging person in general. But even still, I know plenty of older women who command attention. And they are not just celebrities, but women within my community that seem to invite and attract respect without even trying. I hope to become one of them, sooner and later.

It is inevitable—that one day I will look in the mirror and see a 100-year-old woman looking back at me—108 if I'm lucky. But if becoming invisible is, in fact, inescapable then I hope it takes a really long time for the insensitivity to permeate under my skin, and I'm oblivious to any of the imaginary tiny violins.

Beyond being desirable to my husband and needed by my children, I believe that in order to stay relevant and remain visible against the prevailing disposition of our society—the desire has to come from within. If I matter to myself, I will matter—period. And the old phrase "treat others how you want to be treated" has never been more prevalent.

If I value my elders, I too will be a valued elder. If I am interested in others, people will find me interesting. If I continue to seek independence, I'm less likely to become dependent. If I don't want to fall into the so-called senior society trap—or be habitually dismissed, unquestionably, I have to be the one that comes from a place of worthiness.

We wrapped up our date night early and while my husband was searching for just the right amount of romance, action, and comedy, I did a little searching of my own for inspirational aging women and found many to admire.

Although, I wasn't sure I could ever go to that place where people do just the right amount—to smooth out, tighten and erase. In my particular case, I don't think it will help me be in a better position of visible space. I was leaning more toward the actors or celebrities who appeared to be embracing each year with just enough elegance, wisdom, and grace.

Day 241: 196.5 lbs. Friday, June 1st

It was an understatement for sure to say that I was proud of myself for how I was taking charge of my own health over the past eight months.

Even through the binging hiccups—because they were becoming fewer and farther in between. When our waitress came over to take our lunch order, I sat with my friend tall in my chair spilling with pride. I mentioned to our server that I was a little high maintenance and removed a few things from a salad on their menu and added a few other things to it. The friend I was with was a mentor for sure and just happened to be about 20 years my senior. She was also practically half my size and when it was her turn to order she said with a great big smile and a little bit of a giggle, "I'll have the same salad, but I'd like to have it exactly as it appears on your menu."

A tinge of humiliation set in. I felt laughed at and my face turned beet red. I was embarrassed and I felt ashamed that I had gotten to a place where I couldn't even order a salad as it appeared on the menu. What I really felt was stupid. As if my requests were pitiful and pointless.

Then I felt ridiculous for feeling proud about how far I had come, since clearly there were no visible signs that I had done much of anything to the people I knew. I still looked fat. Then I got pissed and angry for openly labeling myself again as a high maintenance person and wished I hadn't placed my order first.

Lots of emotions came over me in that one single moment and I felt guilty—for wishing she was invisible. But then I thought about a few weeks earlier when I had lunch at the same restaurant with a different friend and mentor. That friend loved what I had ordered. She was openly impressed and ordered the exact same thing. On that particular day, I felt good about my choices when I left, and I wanted to clone her.

The two different lunches with two different ladies at the same cafe brought up completely different feelings and emotions for me. At each lunch, I had arrived in great spirits, proud of myself and practically high on life. I admired and respected both women too. Clearly, there was more I needed to do, to reposition my good disposition.

One lunch had left me feeling elated and accepted, while the other left me feeling deflated and rejected. Still, the one common denominator in both scenarios was me. I was loving myself and my body, but I was still allowing outside energy influence the good energy in me.

Chapter 12
Putting My Mindset Where My Mouth Is

"And coincidentally, I was learning how to change my mindset—while I was changing it."

Day 242: Saturday, June 2nd

There's something about this particular salad that I can't seem to replicate. It's ginormous and delicious. The oil and red-wine vinegar blend always comes on the side and the roasted red peppers are seasoned to perfection—the Italian way. Directly on top, front and center, is an abundance of thickly shredded mozzarella cheese. The salad is like a gift, bound up so tightly with plastic that it seems to double in size when we unwrap it.

My daughter and I stopped to pick up two of them before heading over to my mother's house for the afternoon. We settled into the kitchen and enjoyed our salads with a full-bodied red blend followed by watermelon and grapes for dessert that were already on display when we arrived. Gingerly, I popped a piece of the perfectly cut square fruit into my mouth followed by several more while we chatted.

We moved our conversation over to my mother's closet and I tried on a ton of clothes for the remainder of the afternoon. My daughter sat quietly on the bed in the near distance on her phone providing rational opinions when needed and threw us an occasional smile while watching the dynamic duo in action.

Squeezing my body into one outfit after another had introduced so many ridiculous topics and limitless laughter that we could hardly contain ourselves. But the laughter coming from me was merely a hollow mask hiding how painfully embarrassed I was about the shape of my body.

Bloated and gassy was how I was starting to feel while I was showing off the variety of constricting fashions. And on the ride home, I asked my daughter to do a quick search for me, curious if there were any side effects from eating watermelon. She began with… Does watermelon make you bloated? Then she moved on to become gassy, retain water, fart, burp, pee, gain weight, increase your blood sugar, until finally she typed—give you diarrhea.

I had experienced most of those things after eating our lunch, so I made the decision, at the very minimum, to temporarily eliminate watermelon from my love diet—and to no longer eat heaping amounts of it.

Day 243: Sunday, June 3rd

While my husband was fixin' to cook our family meal, I sat at the island nibbling on a few cashews, which quickly led me to eat the remainder of the bag. There was no sense in leaving hardly a handful.

He stepped outside to cook the chicken on the grill with some sweet potatoes and large tomatoes and I stayed in the kitchen to make the salad. We didn't seem to have any traditional ingredients in the house, so I did my best with what we had.

First, I threw together the last of the spring mix, baby kale, and arugula onto our plates. I tossed in craisins and pumpkin seeds along with a little leftover broccoli I found in the fridge. Finally, I topped off our salads with some savory parmesan shredded from the block. They not only looked like they were made by a clever chef, but also as if they came from a fancy restaurant—served just shy of the gourmet dressing.

I was completely stuffed after eating our family dinner around three o'clock. And it was only about an hour later that I noticed my daughter getting ready to bake a cake in the kitchen. She loves baking so she was sort of becoming our own personal connoisseur. She had picked out the boxed cake mix in her small protest against the gluten-free pancake mix that my husband was going to buy because she said it was too "gritty." But my husband was also protesting and drew his line in the sand at purchasing duplicate loaves of bread and pasta to accommodate my new gluten-free life. During their shop together she worked her magic and asked for something completely different, cake. Of course, he said yes.

It's not my intention to take over the entire house with my specific dietary needs and because I appreciated all of their advocacy—individually and collectively—I wanted to help by compromising in any way that I could. I made a great suggestion to take the gluten-free muffin mix that everyone loved—and combine that with the *gritty* pancake mix to dilute it—adding to it some fresh blueberries. It isn't rocket science and it was a creative idea sprinkled with a dash of patience.

It's fun to experiment. And I wanted to help create a great signature family pancake recipe that we could all enjoy without having to purchase and make separate mixes and batches. I knew my suggestion was fantastic, but I was the only one who was the least bit enthusiastic.

Day 244: Monday, June 4th

My day began with a quiet meditation and the desire to look for my yoga mat came out of the blue. I ran with it, hopping onto the floor for just a few minutes. Whenever I did yoga, I felt empowered, flexible, and healthy—whether I did it for five to ten minutes—or I vanished into a mindful fifty.

Calculating a specific amount of time to exercise each day or week was quite possibly boxing myself into a very unnecessary motionless corner. The pressure I put on myself was stifling. In my mind, if I wasn't able to exercise for a significant amount of time—I would automatically think—why bother trying.

Not measuring up or keeping up would usually introduce subtle feelings of paralysis. Shortly thereafter, making the commitment to bring back exercise, brought on an abnormal feeling of claustrophobia that would start to present itself. I would quickly waiver from my original goal, which in hindsight was never very realistic to begin with. And was more along the lines of desperately optimistic. So when the idea came to me at that moment to spend just a few minutes of my time hopping onto my matt, it opened up my eyes to the possibility that the amount of time I dedicated to moving my body each day was not nearly as important as the act itself. Regular and notable intervals would surely find their way in overtime.

Day 245: Tuesday, June 5th

[Deep sigh.] I was in shock when I heard the news about Kate Spade. I didn't even own a single product from her line. But I did know who she was. Whatever Kate was going through—I wondered if she was also experiencing the extra challenging layer of menopause.

The news brought me straight back to when I first heard about Robin Williams. And beyond the feeling of disbelief, again I felt sad, confused, and frustrated. It's always extremely sad and unsettling to hear about anyone dying. Obviously, I didn't know Robin or Kate, but what I felt was completely unhinged—my heart left swaying in the wind.

When I was just ten years old, I remember when I heard about Freddie Prinze who died by suicide. He was only 22. At that age I thought—how could anyone so cute not want to live. I wished I could have told Freddie with my ten-year-old crush of love that anyone who knew him wanted and needed him to stick around for a really long time—no matter what. If *I* only had known him, I thought. But I was just a little girl.

Celebrities are the ones we're made aware of. They are the faces we recognize, but the reality is, for every celebrity that dies by suicide, there are thousands of people that die by suicide right along with them. According to the American Foundation for Suicide Prevention, suicide is the 10th leading cause of death in the United States. And in the year 2017, there were 47,173 recorded Americans who died by suicide, along with 1,400,000 estimated suicide attempts. In my opinion, anyone who has thoughts about suicide needs more love and attention—period.

The bottom line is—fear, anxiety, and depression can affect any gender or race. It does not discriminate and without question can contaminate. And reaching out can immediately lighten the weight.

National Suicide Prevention Lifeline

"Reaching out does not define me as a weak person. It only defines a moment in my existence when I needed strength."

<u>One does not have to be in crisis to call or connect</u>.

Text CONNECT to:
741741
Massachusetts State-Wide Samaritan's Helpline:
877-870-HOPE (4673)
National Suicide Prevention Line:
800-273-TALK (8255)

I have learned to live with anxiety and depression myself. *And living with anxiety and depression takes practice.* Through my experience, I finally found it so much easier to sit with—and nestle into those moments and emotions that persist, than try to resist. Because within chaos and/or confusion—clarity can't help but emerge. *And like anything else in life, learning to navigate my own emotional path takes practice.* I no longer suffer from anxiety or depression—I simply figured out a way to manage it.

My life is not perfect by any means and there are still many messy moments that I wish I could erase. I'm sure there will be more. But I decided a long time ago that I do want to feel. I want to experience all emotions—not just the good ones.

Feeling sad or down is something no human being can avoid. And we have to learn how to manage every emotion. It's just not possible to prevent every sucky emotion from seeping in—or escape every shitty moment in life. And I attribute being able to manage my emotions by simply seeking support whenever I need it, which is like placing my own oxygen mask on first.

A brand-new therapist or coach is always refreshing to me and I have seen countless over the years. I am human and far from perfect. I only know what I know. And there's a shit-ton of things that I don't know. *But there is one thing I do know—reaching out to talk can lead to self-love magnified. And the number of people who are eagerly awaiting to lend an ear or provide a shoulder to lean on—is practically limitless.*

I for one always appreciate a kind soul that is willing and able—to cup their hands and hold them out for me—just so I can simply get a leg up. Whether I surrender to blind faith by listening to a new voice, or I talk to someone I trust, I keep talking and listening—until my heart, mind, and soul adjust.

The fact of the matter is—it is humanly possible to reprogram negative thought patterns with rational ways of forward thinking—with some help. *Reaching out does not define me as a weak person. It only defines a moment in my existence when I needed strength.* And I am living proof that a person can change negative thought patterns. I just happen to be one of the lucky ones that was gifted a second chance. And I forgive myself.

Day 246: Wednesday, June 6th

When I arrived at the restaurant to meet a friend for lunch, I was starving. The funny thing was, even though she was just a friend, I was more passionate about talking than I was about eating.

Day 247: Thursday, June 7th

Desire comes from within, but the idea I had been working on for so long—was no longer working. It was a great concept, but I kept getting stuck and hung up. I was getting so lost in the details that the direction I was heading in—was pulling me away from my original intention, which ultimately was my truth.

After I jump-started my brain with a cup of oatmeal and a simple black coffee, my lovely new friend and I got straight to work strategizing. I salvaged what I could and broke the mold by recycling my old idea. Almost effortlessly, new and fresh ideas began to flourish.

Just up the street a short distance away I arrived at the luncheon I had organized. The staff was extremely accommodate-ing to a few of my requests and had gone above and beyond what I could have expected. Practically everything was placed lovingly on the side with the exception of the guacamole and the grilled chicken. It was gorgeous. My mouth was salivating at the sight of the beautiful piece of art that was placed in front of me. It was interesting and it was delicious. Once again—the dressing went untouched.

I AM ON A LOVE DIET

Day 248: Friday, June 8th

Spending the day at the spa is something I wish I could do more often, but I am still very grateful that I can afford to pamper myself every now and again with a few gift cards.

Quietly, I sat alone in my thick, solid-white cotton robe and slippers, while peeling an orange cutie with grace and intention. Even if it were for just a millisecond, I gifted each person I came in contact with a gentle smile that reflected automagically back to me. With a heightened level of appreciation, I let each moment of peace and serenity wash over me and thought about how it would feel if I simply allowed the abundance of gratitude spill over into my daily life—into my meals—into me.

The subtle scent of the tiny cup of cucumber water was refreshing and then cleansing when I tasted it. I felt nothing less than blessed as dignity and respect ignited my every step. I was highly in tune to each of our five senses and how powerful they are collectively—but also amplified individually. Consciously, I didn't take a single one of them for granted.

In the center of the room, water flowed against a colossal stone, gently dripping soft and soothing sounds for the listeners. I absorbed everything I could feel and see and resided in complete awareness while waiting to be called for my facial. I thought about the most powerful sense of all—the human touch.

Pure and blissful was how I felt as my spa day came to a close and my husband was meeting me for dinner in their lovely garden bar outside where we shared a grilled artichoke appetizer and a Spanish alioli sauce served to us on a rustic wooden board. We took turns sipping from a cold bowl of refreshing gluten-free gazpacho before I ordered the grilled chicken iceberg wedge salad for my main course—without the bacon.

I described how peaceful my experience was and how my only expectation throughout the entire day was to cherish every single moment. And then we heard the news about Anthony Bourdain.

It's a new day and people are getting more creative with cries for help. What can I say? I wish he could have found the love deep within his core—and let that love soar.

Day 249: Saturday, June 9th

Thankfully, we were scheduled for the early show and my daughter's call time was at 9:30 in the morning. I woke up early, had coffee with peanut butter on toast, and began the process of ballet hair with a sense of calm and ease. It was her eighth year of dancing and my thirteenth year of living vicariously through her.

Watching my daughter gracefully grow into a young woman was nothing shy of miraculous. And this year's recital would be filled with more memorable moments to capture. She was old enough now to do her own makeup and was far better at it than I. So, when she was ready, I dropped her off and drove back to the house to finish getting ready myself.

One by one we hopped into my car to leave and just as I sat behind the wheel I said, "Oh shoot, I forgot to do my meditation." I was fairly certain that I would get back on track in the morning and just as I was letting the thought go, I heard my mother-in-law from the backseat say, "Me too." It completely caught me by surprise and I was a little excited at the notion that we had a new common interest beyond parenting so I said, "I didn't know that you meditate?" to which she replied, "Oh, I thought you said you forgot to take your medication."

I AM ON A LOVE DIET

At intermission, we were all pretty much hungry so at the concession table, I reached past the chocolate bars and candy to buy a few bags of plain chips, knowing they had the least amount of ingredients. They were chemical-free, and it was just a little snack to hold some of us over. I found everyone and started to pass the small bags around to anyone who was hungry and noticed my mother already eating from a dirty bag of Doritos.

I couldn't help myself. I looked directly into her eyes, pointed at the bag and wisely whispered, *"That's not love."* Without skipping a wiseass beat or peeling her irritated hungry eyes away from mine—she crunched up what was left of the bag—and shoved it into the arms of my forty-five-year-old baby brother and smiled.

It was nearly two o'clock in the afternoon by the time the recital had come to an end. We quickly took pictures, and spontaneously agreed to meet back at the house. On our way, we stopped at the store to pick up some pizza and salad for everyone, and without realizing it, they had stopped too. Of course, they did. We were all famished.

We should have communicated after the show about each of us planning to pick up food. But no one was thinking clearly, except for where our next meal would come from and how quickly we would get it. Perhaps organizing a lovely breakfast for everyone at the house prior to the recital would have been a better idea. Back at the house, we placed the mish-mash mound of cravings onto the island counter and all dug in.

Nicole Perry

Day 250: Sunday, June 10th

Eating while standing is something I still do. I have every intention of sitting down to enjoy my meal, but sometimes I don't make it to the chair.

When I was placing my one egg-over-easy onto my gluten-free buttery toast and added a little hot sauce it happened again. I was just gonna take one bite and poof—it was gone.

Living consciously inside my so-called new *lifestyle, my life* was really not *all* that different. Just like eating while standing, I still do a lot of the same things I used to do. I still attend the same family functions, the people in my life are the same, and I'm still the same person. I haven't changed my *entire* lifestyle. I've just *redesigned a part of my life*. In fact, it's only the concession I choose that's different, and the food on my plate that has changed.

Before creating my love diet, trying to teach myself how to live an *entirely* new lifestyle was virtually a mission impossible. Like trying to teach an old dog a really hard new trick—without having the skill set. The thought of having to change *everything* scared me straight into doing nothing. Half-heartedly, I bought into every other so-called "life-changing" easier thing.

Some people can take huge leaps of faith regardless of any circumstances and embrace drastic change, which likely stems from being forced into that fight or flight mode. But I had never experienced any real danger. My internal battles were small and inconspicuous in comparison. And no matter how frustrating becoming a heavier person was, my mind and my body had adjusted and adapted to the new normal. Sure, I was sick of dieting, I was sick of feeling sick, and I was desperate, *but my life*

I AM ON A LOVE DIET

wasn't intolerable. The size I became was manageable—and I had gotten comfortable.

In my mind, instinctively changing my *entire lifestyle* meant I would have to deny myself and miss out on *all* of the simple pleasures in life, while everyone else was still enjoying them—without me. To even consider changing what I was doing—*all at once*—didn't feel possible. It was daunting and I imagined it would feel just like trying to quit smoking while still living in a house full of smokers.

Crouched love snuck up on me over time and, as the years shrunk by, I was loving myself less and less. My body's craving for more love grew stronger and louder, screaming at me in the tone of high blood pressure and bad cholesterol numbers. My organs were begging me to stop the insanity of what I was doing. And I had spent a few good solid years ignoring the clues.

Reversing the damage, slowly overtime was the only way. I had to change. But my body needed me to do it slowly and get uncomfortable. I hadn't lost any significant amount of weight yet, but I was finally listening to my body and my body was starting to show signs of gratitude. I found my mission possible. And it all began with my heart.

My mindset was in a completely different place than it was exactly one year ago. And sticking with my love diet, my mind and body would both be in an entirely new place in one year from now. *My entire lifestyle wasn't different*—but my life *is* better. *Amen to that.*

My daughter and I settled into our Flashdance chick flick, taking only a short break for her to get something fun from the ice cream truck. The movie is and always will be one of my favorite inspirations.

I let the creative dancing seep into my mind along with the desire to push beyond my own limitations. Each of the dancers exuded sheer will and I studied their every move—as though I could somehow be their understudy. The movie took my mind far away from the heaviness that I still carried—peacefully into the arms of determination.

Day 251: 197.5 lbs. Monday, June 11th

Standing naked in front of my all-but-full-length mirror and saying I love you to myself with sheer unadulterated honesty wasn't easy. It took the concept of saying *I love you* into my own eyes to an entirely new level. But I did it. No matter how pretentious it seemed, I immediately looked for the positive.

While it took a tremendous amount of compassion, dignity was the first thing I found in my olive-colored and now un-taut skin. My body held 50 years of wisdom and was riddled with rivers of stretch marks—a price I was willing to pay during my child-bearing years. And then I saw it. My body had changed. To the left of my jelly roll that I have in common with millions of other women, and just before the dimples of cellulite that sprinkled the lower half of my body like stars to the sky, what was once a pair—was now barely there. One of my fat folds had all but disappeared.

I never did take any measurements at the beginning of my love diet or before starting the gym workouts. But I guess it didn't matter. I was only going to the gym once a week and progress was actually happening. Seeing that fat fold all but gone was the greatest visual reward I could have ever asked for. The change might seem small to some, but I gave myself a giant pat on the back with a smile.

Gleaming with pride and time on my side, I took a moment to organize my spices while waiting for my toast. It's amazing how much one tiny piece of progress can lift one's spirits. The positive energy I exuded spilled over into my lunch and afternoon with many more satisfying moments of simplistic gratification—*turned up on high.*

Day 252: Tuesday, June 12th

The fight I had with my daughter while I was placing the chicken on the grill outside for dinner didn't matter. She was working on her opinion skills along with her teenage notions and later kindly apologized.

Ironically, I was learning how to raise my kids—while I was raising them. *And coincidentally, I was learning how to change my mindset—while I was changing it.*

Day 253: Wednesday, June 13th

"In your own home" were the words my heart clung to and had been longing to hear. I had been thinking about trying this new video workout program and privacy had climbed up higher on my list of precedence. *My exercise regime was greatly in need of a shift* and there was a free in-person trial session I could attend to get a taste of what the program would be like. It was not that hard to squeeze the one class into my calendar since it was only once, and the unlimited workouts would be conveniently accessible online.

At my fingertips, I would have the extra support of a built-in local group coach. It was practically perfect. No longer would I have to race out the door, be embarrassed in public about my limitations, or feel so self-conscious that I was instinctively overcompensating for being the oldest and the most out-of-shape person in the room. She also came with a nutritional background which was the bonus that made it a no-brainer. Obviously, I signed up.

Fundamentally, the accountability would still be on me. It's great to feel strong and be able to say that I did something by myself, but the truth is, most of the time I need help. Help feels good! And to know that someone else had my back was exactly what I needed to level up.

Day 254: Thursday, June 14th

My brother and I were meeting for lunch and I ordered one of my favorite summer treats—steamers. A pound was the perfect appetizer to satisfy my craving and I had their gluten-free cheese pizza for my main entre.

I know, I was far from being a saint. But treating myself while staying within the realm of my love diet was—in my mind—perfectly acceptable. And I hardly ate half of it. A typical burger with fries is what my brother ordered and if my husband were with us, I'm sure he would have had the same.

Neither my husband nor brother ate like that every day, but the truth was—what they chose to eat was none of my business. I can care. And sure, I can talk about my love diet with my loved ones, even lovingly lead by example, but no matter how much love we have for someone else—the desire to care about our own health and well-being has to come from within. It just has to.

The reality is—there wasn't anything that anyone could have said or done to make me see that most of the food I was feeding myself—wasn't love. I had to see it for myself. What I discovered is that I actually do care—more than I was leading myself—or anyone else to believe.

It took a long time for me to figure that out, but I did. And no matter how much effort I put into loving myself more—it still doesn't make it any easier to continually watch the people I love eat meals that are blatantly unhealthy. No matter how inconsistent or intermittent, I know firsthand how painful it can be, to grow up watching someone you love sabotage their only body—and slowly kill themselves with food.

Day 255: Friday, June 15th

The easiest gift I can give to myself and my loved ones—is to simply feed myself love. Eating my homemade gluten-free muffin in the car, I drove to that free workout session I was invited to. It was a little tricky to find, but it was my first time, and I wasn't about to give up. Pulling in and out of a few parking lots and spaces, I was officially late. The other gal was too and thankfully, it was really not a big deal.

After signing the disclosure, I put my latest treasure down. A water bottle that had a center core holder thingy that you could put a couple of pieces of fruit into that help flavor it. It was the perfect invention for anyone who was the least bit water challenged. Setting my fresh and clean pear water down, I walked into the wall-to-wall green turf full of equipment, ready, willing and kind of capable.

When she started talking about her videos that we would be able to follow online, I got a little excited about how we were combining education and muscle building in the privacy of our own homes. In my head, I was imagining myself doing the workouts, but I Freudian slipped that I couldn't wait to watch them. And the only thing they heard me say was the word *watch* and giggled at my suspect ploy at enthusiasm.

Rushing home to change, I barely had any extra time to spare. The trial session was great, but it did consume most of my morning. Thankfully, the new program would be online, saving me tons of my precious time.

Arriving at my lunch meeting, I ordered the chicken parmesan. I said, "Hold the hoagie please but I'll keep the side of gluten-free fries." I had earned it.

Day 256: 196.5 lbs. Saturday, June 16th

Like fruit flies to summer, my acne was back. Not in full force but just enough to make me wonder if it was something I ate or if my heckling hormones were just poking fun at me again. My husband insisted it was neither. He said it had to be bacteria-based.

A potential bacterial infection was not on my short-list of self-diagnosis, but the power of suggestion can be strong, and it got the better of me. Without delay, I washed all my makeup brushes with antibacterial soap and made the easy decision to do it more often. Washing my brushes was a really good idea. I was taking better care of my skin too. But deep down I knew that the returning acne had to be a sure-fire sign that my health was still a work in progress.

When I look at the facts, in less than eight months I had been undiagnosed with Grave's, told I was inches away from having Hashimoto's and being spoken to in the same manner as diabetic patients. Whether the signs of acne were visually valid, or the recent results were inconclusive, being slapped across the face over and over with a variety of issues—was concerning at the very least.

It was interesting that each of the challenges I was facing were all stemming from my immune system and I was becoming less of a stranger to the topic as I aged. When I look back into my past, the psoriasis that appeared in my twenties and the rosacea I had learned to live with were issues that I shouldn't have been so quick to dismiss as simple signs of aging.

Ironically, research shows that autoimmune issues are more prevalent in women and are becoming notoriously widespread. In this day and age, it seems we are practically expected to have one, and considered almost alien if we don't.

Clicking through social media, I happened upon a photo of Kelly Clarkson. The accompanying article said that she had attributed a recent 40-pound weight loss to discovering that she had an autoimmune disorder and had no choice but to change her diet. For a millisecond, I wished I had no choice and that I could simulate whatever disorder she had, just so I could fast forward to a 40-pound weight loss too. But it wasn't a real wish. No matter how many close encounters I had, I certainly didn't want to own any of it.

I was envious about her weight loss after reading the article. But I was grateful too, because I was already doing some of the very same things she was doing. Like buying mostly organic and eating gluten-free. I was pretty sure that I was right behind her and would soon have a significant weight loss too. All I needed was a little more time under my belt. Well, actually, I needed a lot more time.

What I found intriguing; she was also incorporating non-GMO foods free from pesticides and following a diet low in lectins. The non-GMO foods were slowly working their way into my life too—just like the organic was—but learning more about eating a diet lectin-free was new on my radar. It is interesting and I would definitely consider it, but everything I decide to do—has to not only be healthy and easy—it has to be sustainable for me.

I also have to remember that my love diet isn't a fad that will come and go, or someone else's diet either. It's something personal that I'm creating from scratch—for myself—at my own pace. I'm not going to do anything just because it sounds good, or because someone else is doing it. What I'm creating is my own forever diet. And I need to be careful and only introduce a change when I'm ready. And if it will work for me—for the rest of my life. Especially at my age. Because introducing too many new tricks at one time can very well send me straight into overwhelm mode. Aka, quitting.

Clearly, I am at the top of my own priority list, but just like they say—patience is a virtue. I'm depending on myself to be rational. I'll do what I need to do. Slowly and steadily. The easier and better way; by incorporating and reducing one thing at a time until I can get the hang of it. And equally important—to see if it's even worth hanging on to.

My husband and I ate at the same restaurant we typically go to and were getting tired of their menu. We were stuck and mutually agreed to search for another place to make our new regular.

Day 257: 197.5 lbs. Sunday, June 17th

Each year we like to kick off our summer with an awesome family tradition. And growing up in New England made having clam boils easy. What I love the most is that almost everything is thrown into the same large pot which makes even the hot dogs, sausage, and potatoes taste just like the ocean. *Yum.*

Undeniably, what makes any tradition special, are the memories created, not just eating certain foods. And with this tradition, we like talking about our summer as we drive down to the fish market and park the car on what seems to be a somewhat dangerous cliff. We love admiring where we live and cautiously take in the ocean view thousands of feet below, getting out of the car carefully and occasionally snapping a photo.

We love the powerfully contagious energy we receive from the moment we step foot inside the shack. The small red building looking like it was somebody's home once upon a long time ago. On display across the way are delicious spicy quahogs we love along with the local clam chowdah. But as we took in the inventory, I quickly realized we had to make a few adjustments and compromises this year to our family summer tradition.

The quahogs were not gluten-free, and I was avoiding sodium-rich soups, so we passed on both of those. The kids didn't really care all that much and really they were just happy to be there. My husband was being very understanding too, about how my love diet was superseding everything now. But as usual, like powerful magnets, the Maine lobstah bin pulled us in.

Since learning about cholesterol and that shrimp was higher in it, I assumed lobster was too. But what I actually found was that there are only 72 milligrams of cholesterol in one 3.5 oz. portion of Maine lobster with approximately 98 calories. Shrimp, on the other hand, has about the same calories in one 3 oz. portion, but they have more than double the cholesterol with a whopping 180 milligrams.

They say that the current recommended going rate of cholesterol for the average person to consume is 300 milligrams, and only two hundred if you are at risk for heart disease. Now that I have been made aware that my cholesterol numbers were out of whack, obviously, I want to be sure I consume plenty of foods that will help me increase my healthy HDL—and avoid the saturated and trans fats that are, in fact, the dangerous fats.

My head continued to spin around whether or not shrimp was okay for me to eat on a regular basis. For every article I found that said eating shrimp can be dangerous to anyone working to reduce their numbers, I found another one that said the good cholesterol found in shrimp cancels out the bad. And some articles were proudly claiming that eating shrimp in moderation is perfectly acceptable.

Frankly, the word moderation itself brings out the bitch in me. There's nothing concrete about it and it has become such a wavering red flag that sends me steaming with frustration every time it pops up. Too many questions were going unanswered in my head.

What the heck did shrimp moderation look like any-way? Would eating thirty-six, eighteen to twenty-four count standard shrimp cocktail at any given holiday party put a cork in my heart? Or are we talking two to three little cute tail-on or tail-offs with a fancy restaurant meal each week be okay? The farther I fell down the winding rabbit hole of information confirmed what I already know. It was best for me to keep little miss shrimp on the barbie back burner temporarily. Just like they say—when in doubt, leave her out.

Everyone was okay with slimming down our clam boil though and letting go of the extras. Including that pricy Maine lobstah. We did quite a bit of adjusting, but still, we had plenty of steamers, corn on the cob, baked beauties, and salad. It was all delicious and more than good enough to get the summer going.

I AM ON A LOVE DIET

When you get right down to it, each little individual moment leading up to the event is what keeps our tradition alive and strong. And the clams. None of the flavors meshed together like they've done in the past and our skinnier clam boil was not the same. But nonetheless, it was definitely less of a mess.

Aside from our abbreviated clam boil, the tradition that I want to pass down the most to my kids and grandkids above all other traditions is to respectfully make sure they feed themselves love.

Day 258: Monday, June 18th

It was time to let go of my original idea to combine my OB-GYN and Primary Care Physician. I really did think it was a good idea to blend them into one—especially for someone like me—who had not been to see a doctor for quite some time.

I didn't think it was a genius plan, but I did think it was clever. I admired myself, for coming up with the idea that would get my butt into an appointment. I was saving precious time as well as energy—and it worked for a few visits. Little did I know that I would discover a lot more than I had bargained for. And evidently, I needed more specialists. So just like any other idea that no longer serves me, it was time to let it go. The world we live in is a little more complex than it was a hundred years ago.

Our bodies aren't much different, but in this day and age, we know more about the body. And although there is a bit more poking and prodding, it is smarter to have more eyes and ears—at our fingertips. It was time to temporarily stop some of the self-diagnosis and get advice from real professionals. So, I enlisted a new PCP! And made an appointment with a dermatologist too.

For a quick breakfast, I had some granola with fresh fruit and when lunch rolled around, I had a basic salad. I tossed in some broccoli, olives, tomatoes, and homemade honey mustard dressing and followed my salad with two gluten-free cookies for dessert. There was one thing I noticed though, after breakfast and throughout lunch my attitude was turning. And I wondered if I was experiencing the late change-of-season blues.

Day 259: Tuesday, June 19th

Crying was all I felt like doing when I woke up and while I sat braiding my daughter's hair for field day, I wondered again if it was menopause getting in the way of my positive energetic path.

It was also very frustrating how long it was taking for my body to adjust to my new eating style. Two hundred and fifty-nine days long. I was still going up and down the same two pounds and having my weight yo-yo was one thing, but my mind was swaying back and forth from grateful and hopeful to cynical and doubtful.

It would be so much easier to live without the extra fifty pounds of weight that I unwittingly lugged around. And I'm sure it would help me mentally—if my body was healthier physically. The sun was shining but my spirits were a little on the grey side. I know that my thoughts create my own reality, but I couldn't help but need another spark of results or a glimpse of something positive to help shift my emotions.

I was doing all the right things by spending more and more time every day on me. I was meditating, being mindful, gardening, exercising even, and still the real solid change I was hoping for wasn't happening fast enough. And then I had a tiny lightbulb moment. *The one thing I could control—was the here and now.* And there it was. The other positive I needed to cling to.

I could do another one of the in-home workouts—inside the privacy of my own home. Energetically, I gravitated towards the concept and it couldn't have come at a better time. Look out candid camera! Here I come!

Day 260: Wednesday, June 20th

This day marked the second consecutive in-home workout. Third if I count the tryout. I was feeling pretty good about the accomplishment. Way to go me!

I made a bowl of fruit with almond milk drizzled with a little honey for a quick breakfast and skipped the granola entirely. I was having a fair amount of writers' block, but I was ready to hunker down into a quiet home office day and hoped I would finally break the chain.

Day 261: Thursday, June 21st

Talking about my book with my daughter, I said, "Don't worry, I have plenty of fat photos if I need them for before and after's." Simultaneously, we both caught my belittling words as she gave me a quick look of disappointment as if she were the parent.

Barely sipping my coffee, I hardly touched my eggs or potatoes. And the pear I ate on the way to my meeting in the car almost squirted juice all over my silk blouse while I was driving. The words that had slipped off my tongue were still dangling in the air. The very attitude goes against what I practically preach, and I couldn't believe I had said—what I said—out loud.

Changing our thoughts isn't something that comes easily for most and I was no different. The thoughts I had spoken were more than words. So, I forgave myself for the juvenile jab and continued focusing on letting the positive new thoughts crush the old and to keep doing what I was doing—until the positive was strong enough to hold.

I had some more fruit around ten o'clock and when lunch rolled around, I found myself ordering the same salad I had the week before with chicken, guacamole, salsa, and sour cream. This time adding shredded cheddar. I only ate half of my meal at lunch and enjoyed round two around three. The dressing still went untouched.

Day 262: Friday, June 22nd

It's funny how old mindsets can stick with us. Like "waste-not, want-not". Limiting beliefs can strongly override and shove aside a new positive vibe.

I made two slices of gluten-free toast and turned them into tuna melts with a side of broccoli, avocado and a few almonds for lunch. It was too much food though. For some reason, I was overcompensating from the modest breakfast. It was all good and healthy, but I was beyond stuffed. And the only reason I kept eating was because I didn't want it to go to waste.

We had pizza again for dinner, mine gluten-free, and I only had two slices. However, I did have four gluten-free cookies for dessert. And then, just before ten o'clock while watching a movie I snacked on some gluten-free crackers, avocado, salsa, and olives. That's one of the things that alcohol does. It lowers our inhibitions and lets the old and tired mindset from the past crush the positive affirmations that I worked so hard for.

Chapter 13
What's in My Gut Could Help My Butt

"I had to keep shifting so it would come naturally, and my mind would be strong enough mentally—before my body could let go physically."

Day 263: Saturday, June 23rd

There are plenty of theories claiming that everything starts with the gut and I was developing a greater understanding of the concept. After all—we are what we eat.

I wanted to learn more and found an article that said our gut can be affected by other things beyond what we eat—things like anxiety and depression. So, I kept reading.

Then the article said that *the* anxiety and depression that does, in fact, affect our gut, can, in turn, be the root cause of acne. Huh. The feelings I had with anxiety and depression weren't there every day, but they did pop up often enough to make me wonder if the depression I was experiencing—was from the acne that was a considerable source of anxiety for me.

Having a moderate amount of acne routinely reside on my face was not easy to live with. It's frustrating. Our face is the first thing people see. And over these past few years—having acne—has undeniably taken its toll on my self-esteem. I know a lot of people can sympathize and some can even relate. My only saving grace—was knowing nothing ever stays the same.

No matter how ingrained into the brain or heart-carved into any tree—the simple fact of knowing that nothing truly ever lasts forever was the positive affirmation that I clung to. And I held onto that power card tight in my back pocket—spackling my way day after day.

Most of us know that the skin is the largest organ we have, but learning about how the skin, the brain, and the gut all intertwine—was pure knowledge divine. Although, I did have to admit the new theory added a little layer to my frustration. Just when I thought I was inching closer to some kind of finish line—another twist around the human body was defined. The only question I had left—what the heck did I do with the information.

Since eliminating gluten from my diet, my skin was looking much better. I was having many aha moments every time I looked in the mirror. But just a few weeks after a simple day in the spa—which was really just a whole lot of napping wrapped around one lovely facial—I noticed that the acne was starting to come back.

It was kind of crazy to think about. Not that the acne on my face could be from what was going on inside my gut, but that what was happening in my gut could possibly be influenced by what was going through my mind. Crazy, but possible. I knew I had a lot of thinking to do. To figure out what thoughts I could be feeding my mind that were gut-friendly—but ultimately skin-safe.

My husband was starving, and we were stuck in traffic. Not a good combination for anyone. And when we arrived at the restaurant, he rushed his order off the menu and impatiently waited for it to arrive. Inevitably he was turning our simple date night dinner into something similar to an urgent food challenge reward about to be received on an episode of Survivor.

We used to order our meals with our drinks when the kids were little because time was always of the essence. But did he really need to resort to such hurriedness when our kids weren't even little anymore, or even with us? Couldn't he have just eaten something, like say, I don't know, perhaps a meal, around lunchtime. I wished he wouldn't risk putting his body through that—never mind me.

The salad I ordered was beautiful and I was in no rush to wolf it down. It had baby spinach, bleu cheese crumbles, and berries. I swapped out the walnuts for almonds and added grilled chicken. Our server described their balsamic glaze that it came with as unbelievably delicious, but when it arrived it looked more like a strange light brown glue-like paste. I was so glad I had asked for it on the side. Humbly, I requested their bleu cheese dressing instead.

Dipping my fork into the dressing first I got in a delicious measured taste with each and every bite. My salad was very good, but something was different. I generally take half home and this time—I was able to eat the entire thing.

When I discovered that I was an emotional binge eater it was a huge revelation for me. And now that I've had some time to let it resonate, I can't seem to let any thoughts or acts dissipate. No matter how significant a binge or how meager any act is—being honest with myself is crucial—and my eyes were opened wise. Whether the binging is conscious or disguised—it wouldn't be smart of me to ignore any of the signs.

Binging is subjective too. Only the binger can know what is considered a binge. And no matter how much dismissive support I receive from anyone else in response to one of my binging confessions—I can't take any binge lightly. Only I can know if the act itself is, in fact, a binge. And beyond the quality or quantity of food—what's equally important is that I recognize the emotions that can send me recklessly into abandoning all principles set forth from within.

Living in a heightened state of awareness of course is helping me embrace how susceptible I am to this eating disorder. After all, most habits don't change overnight. And this was a disorder that I had acquired over several years, which I only truly discovered a few months ago.

Change takes time. And deep down in my heart what I wanted more than anything in the world was to change. I am ready to recover. And I was beginning with *observing* whether or not the food I chose to eat was in fact, an actual binge—or would lead me to one. I was learning how to manage my behavior. And then I remembered again: *Awareness IS the change.*

Later that night I had two slices of gluten-free toast with peanut butter and followed that with a small ramekin of granola and almonds while watching TV. I was okay with what I ate because it wasn't too late. My body was craving food, I was eating in moderation, and more importantly—I was not emotionally eating. I am recognizing what I am doing, complimenting myself when I do well, and finally, forgiving myself if I don't.

I AM ON A LOVE DIET

Day 264: Sunday, June 24th

My daughter and I were attending a baby shower in the early afternoon, so I ate a simple but solid meal before we left. Two eggs over easy with olive oil, a side of broccoli, and a cup of berries with almond milk.

The brunch was at a lovely restaurant and they initially served coffee, fresh fruit, cheese and the only thing I couldn't eat so far were the crackers. The mimosa I had was heavy on the orange juice, but I let that go as we settled into our table. The main course was individually plated. Each one was served with stacks of pancakes, scrambled eggs, mini pulled pork sandwiches, bacon, and a deeply pigmented saffron rice.

Everywhere I go I tell the staff about my meager dietary gluten-free restriction along with how mindful I am about watching my sodium, but for some reason, chefs seem to misinterpret what I say to my server and think I need my food to be bland. I don't have a dietary spice restriction. I love to get creative and use a variety of spices—almost religiously. I just need to figure out a way to convey that to the magicians in the kitchen.

Discreetly, I mentioned my gluten-free needs to our server, completely forgetting about the low sodium piece. I was later handed a special plate with only the eggs, bunless pork, and saffron rice that was moderately sprinkled with whole corn. Everything was really good, and it appeared that forgetting to mention the low sodium piece did the trick.

There's such a subtle difference between overeating and binging and I don't deliberately try to do either. But sometimes it just happens. And since I had been somewhat limited with my entree—I overcompensated by eating more than enough dessert.

The two desserts they served were both gluten-free and I began with the flan and excitedly I moved on to the Portuguese rice pudding. After devouring every delicious bite of each, I sat there feeling completely stuffed, and guilty. Still, I could have eaten another pudding or flan in its entirety—with only a hint of encouragement.

There was nothing emotional happening with me, so this was undoubtedly an example of overeating. The concept of only eating until we feel 80 percent full popped into my mind because I was well beyond it. Perhaps the theory was just what I needed to start paying closer attention. And having a healthy gauge to measure could easily be added to my existing love diet list. But what the heck did eating until we feel 80 percent full feel like? The only percent I was skilled at, was nearly zero, or anything over a hundred.

Then I read a short blog about a woman who wasn't sure about the 80 percent rule either. And what she did was eat slower during her meals to see if that would help her figure it out. Very unironically, it did. A little more than three quarters into each meal she felt *the tinge* and it clicked. She said it wasn't that hard to do so I tried it. I ate slower for just one meal to see if I felt the same tinge and I did. Evidently, eating slower is key. Or perhaps listening to what my body is telling me is what will actually open the damn door.

I made homemade pesto for dinner with fresh basil leaves, olive oil, parmesan cheese, pine nuts, salt and pepper. I placed the pesto on top of my raw zucchini noodles for myself along with some cherry tomatoes and we all enjoyed some haddock with butter and a simple side of rice. I tossed frozen broccoli in the microwave for an easy additional side for the kids too, just in case.

Together, my husband and I watched a movie and I poured myself another glass of red wine along with a small ramekin of granola and nuts, this time adding raisins to the mix. I opened up my personalized love diet list and added the 80 percent rule to my healthy love diet plan. *God, I am loving my diet!*

<u>*My Love Diet*</u>:

1) *Feed Myself Love*
    a. *Is Love on My Plate, In My Bowl, In My Cup?*
2) *Minimize Sodium*
    a. *Remove High Sodium Caesar Salad*
    b. *Remove or Reduce Soups, Dressings, Sauces, Gravies and Dips.*
3) *Reduce Animal Fats*
    a. *Red Meat, Pork, Shrimp, Yogurt and Soft Cheeses*
4) *Be Mindful of Carbs*
    a. *Remove or Reduce to Size of Fist*
5) *Let go of Pizza*
6) *Remove Deli Meat*
    a. *Including Bacon, Sausage, Linguica, etc.*
7) *Live Gluten-Free*
8) *Exercise Any Amount—Three Times a Week*
9) *LOVE My Body as It Is Today*
10) *Eat Slower. Listen for the 80 Percent Tinge.*

Day 265: Monday, June 25th

The last day of school had arrived, it was a half-day, and my two youngest asked if they could stay home.

When I was growing up it wasn't customary to ask your parents if you could actually skip school—we just did it. And it was usually on a whim, which obviously came on a sunny day of a test. At first, I selfishly hesitated to give up my last few hours of peace, but then I said okay and embraced the generational skipping school shift. It felt kind of good giving in to their menial request, but then it was official—school was out for the summer.

The energy in my home was anxiously relentless and I could hardly focus on anything. So instead of wallowing in frustration—I escaped into a meditation. I got hit with a great virtual snow globe idea to shake things up. It was bound to settle all our vibrations and bring them into a state of equilibrium. Plus, I was getting in some exercise.

Moving around as much of our outdoor furniture as I possibly could by myself, I created just enough noise to pique their curiosity. Then I insisted they help with the heavy lifting. The beauty of it was, moving things around together required teamwork. It's the same furniture we put out each year by the same sets of hands, but gaining a fresh new perspective was what we all needed.

Nudging the energy back into my corner, I flashed a few of my parental metaphors at each opportunity. Physically moving the outdoor furniture helped us mentally move our minds and it carried our conversations back into cohesion. It was just like being handed a fresh new salad that I've seen a hundred thousand times. Our back yard and summer were looking delicious again.

I AM ON A LOVE DIET

Day 266: Tuesday, June 26th

Introducing a new coach into my life who's also equipped with a background in nutrition was a really smart thing to do. Following her lead, I was already excited about not having to worry so much about animal fats—for the most part.

With her assistance, of course, I was sure that reintroducing a few simple items would be fine. Like the occasional yogurt for breakfast and for a snack once in a while along with some cottage-cheese every now and then. It seemed reasonable. And I could also check to see if adding a little light sour cream to a healthy omelette with black beans and salsa would be okay.

Beans felt tricky though. And since I wasn't sure if they were a protein, fat or carb I did a quick search. They were low in fat, mainly a carbohydrate and a good source of protein. I had always remembered that beans were the staple for vegetarians, so I assumed they were mostly protein above everything else. Which was interesting that they were a combination.

You would think I would know since I did embrace that diet once in my twenties. But I was a cheap vegetarian. And it was by happenstance. I didn't eat a lot of beans. I just couldn't afford to buy meat. My diet consisted of three main staples: cigarettes, white zinfandel, and ramen noodles. Listed in order of precedence of course.

The brilliant vegetarian idea came to me officially one day when I decided to live my life up a notch and put back the beef and chicken-flavored ramen, exchanging it for the more sensitive oriental kind. As an independent twenty-ish-year-old woman it was a shiny light-bulb moment for me. And from that moment on I was proud to call myself *a vegetarian!*

Spending as little of my social time as possible to research how to live a healthy vegetarian lifestyle, I was an unhealthy one. In between waitressing, clubbing and my fortified port wine wheat thin meals, reading labels was the only thing I did and avoided the simple ingredients I had been raised with; beef, chicken, and of course, the other white meat.

I think I did allow some seafood in, but still, I was mainly ridding my body of meat and I did it the best way I knew how. By eating plenty of eggs, cheese, crackers, and of course, Raman noodles. I allowed myself to only eat anything without eyes, and for some strange reason—it seemed rational to eat what an animal had eliminated.

It was very likely that I had consumed a fair amount of cholesterol clinging to that status I had claimed. And I did it for almost two years. Until one day when my husband and I were dating and he invited me to his company cookout in Charlotte, North Carolina.

The smell of the meat on the grill ate away at my homesick aura and brought back years of memories to the forefront of my weakened taste buds. Salivating beyond my expectations, I finally gave in after eating several bags of chips at the lame attempt to push my craving deep down inside.

Blatantly eating an entire burger was something I couldn't bring myself to do, so I rationalized and ate my first hot-dignity-free-dog in almost two years. Camouflaging my frankfurter in the lesser evil of the bun I smothered it in an abundance of ketchup, mustard and relish and never looked back.

Someday, I might become a vegetarian again. But if I were so inclined I would strive to be the real kind. The type of person that suddenly unleashes an abundance of compassion from deep within for all living creatures and the planet in which we all

I AM ON A LOVE DIET

benefit. And by the flip of a switch choose to live life with more intention and meaning—effortlessly and organically.

I don't know if that will ever happen for me. And for the time being, I placed some black beans onto my salad and then added artichoke hearts, diced Roma tomatoes, a carefully sliced hard-boiled egg, a few slivers of avocado and a dollop of light sour cream. Even though I hadn't had the sour cream conversation with my new coach—yet.

I had to leave early to attend a board meeting and didn't have much time to make a large family meal. Turkey burgers were an easy go-to, so I made mine with a gluten-free bread-bun, lettuce, and tomato. Smothering it in ketchup and mustard too.

When I got home, I poured myself a glass of wine and sat on the deck outside with my family before calling it a night. It was such a good idea to focus on bettering my sleep habits. I was getting to bed by a reasonable time, which was usually by eight to nine o'clock. I was even letting go of reading in bed along with that very unnecessary last-minute, sleep-sucking phone-flipping.

What I was doing was getting into the new habit of simply climbing into bed and exercising gratitude while falling asleep. Honoring my body's need for proper rest was pure love and I was starting to give myself a good foundation every night.

Day 267: Wednesday, June 27th

Living in the present moment was something that was beginning to come naturally. It felt so good to reside in almost complete awareness—most of the time.

The first thing I did was make a cup of black coffee and do some dishes. Next, I refreshed the pitcher of water on the counter with sliced lemons and left it on our island as a visual reminder to drink more. Effortlessly, I moved on to writing, followed by breakfast, a meditation, a dance workout and then showering.

Loving myself through a variety of ways is what I want to do every day. And that is why I gave myself plenty of time to do all that I did—before leaving the house by 9:30 am. No matter what my schedule looked like, exercising a medley of self-care rituals is what I was committed to do daily.

Before walking out the door I grabbed an apple to leave in the car, just in case I wasn't able to get lunch right away after my interview.

Day 268: 196 lbs. Thursday, June 28th

Mindfully standing at the kitchen sink I could feel the cool breeze coming in through the window while I was washing the dishes. And just as I was thinking of a wicked cool idea the wind blew increasingly. In that moment I felt like I was channeling one of The Witches of Eastwick.

I was only down about two pounds and was having some normal moments of doubt, but somehow, I knew that everything I was doing had to be working. And I hung in there with hope on my side, which had arrived in the form of a coach.

She was introducing me to some best practices like how to measure portions. And the way I was proportioning my food was weigh-off. I was excited to learn more about the latest and greatest tricks and she helped me to use my own fist as a visual guide for the one protein *and the two—not one—preferably green vegetables* at each meal. I thought that our fist was the visual for carbs too, *but what I learned was that it's actually our cupped hand.*

Through the help of my new coach, each discussion gave me more power cards to put in my back pocket. She also taught me that I needed to include a healthy fat with each meal. And she was right. I was feeling fuller, longer. My body was craving more greens, and I wasn't as hungry in between meals. I didn't have the need to bring celery with me anymore or beat myself up with carrot sticks. The body craves what we feed it—and evidently fat is the new phat!

Day 269: 196.5 lbs. Friday, June 29th

The first half of the year had gone by in what seemed like the blink of an eye. And I still had the desire to take in more and absorb everything like a sponge. Learning, mistaking, deciding, loving.

Tossing the zucchini spirals into the saucepan first I added olive oil, spices, and two scrambled eggs into the mix. I had heard that zucchini spirals were a great way to trick our mind into thinking we are eating pasta, but I love zucchini so much it wasn't really much of a trick. Adding a splash of water into the pan in lieu of milk, I covered the dish to be sure my makeshift omelette was cooked all the way through.

Wondering if sour cream had any nutritional value what-so-ever, I did a quick search. It turned out that two tablespoons of sour cream had half the calories of a single tablespoon of mayo and had less saturated fat than a 12-ounce glass of two percent reduced-fat milk. Sour cream also made the shortlist of fatty foods with healthy benefits. It was last on the list, but it made the list. I placed my gluten-free buttery toast onto my plate next to the omelette topped with salsa and light sour cream.

When I finally remembered later in the day to ask my new coach if it was okay to have a little sour cream once or twice a week her response was interesting. She suggested yogurt instead.

Day 270: Saturday, June 30th

I believe that manifesting what we want is possible. Even if it's simply seasonal. Our main floor central air conditioner had kicked the bucket and as my daughter and I were working our way to the register, several were magically stacked up by the grocery line neatly and conveniently as tall as me.

It was incredibly accommodating, we needed one, and it was dirt cheap. Even if it wasn't technically the correct BTU's for our space, to me it was good enough and as they say, one of those no-brainers. My daughter, however, was mortified at my excitement for the bonus find.

Somehow, the very thought of my lifting it to get a price check was beyond embarrassing. She became almost shockingly insistent—shushing and pleading with me not to do it as our line got shorter. The more she insisted—the more I was taken aback. I never realized how uncool drawing attention to yourself was for a pre-teen these days. Even secondary attention.

In my eyes, it was pretty funny though—to do that back and forth verbal dance and see a different side of her. Through the purchase, I couldn't hold back the giggle that bubbled up through my voice any longer and it peppered every rational word I said.

Chicken marinade in ranch dressing was on the menu for dinner with asparagus and sweet potatoes on the side. Whilst I was preparing another delicious and simple family dinner, I explained to my daughter how she would come to appreciate that small air conditioner we bought in a matter of a few minutes.

Later that night, sitting by the fire, the kids were eating toasted marshmallows and I gave myself permission to have one for old time's sake. Interestingly enough, it tasted equally as good as it did bad. I must be half-way there.

Day 271: Sunday, July 1st

A veggie omelette drizzled in healthy olive oil fat was how my day began and later for a snack, I had some cottage cheese with honey. For lunch, I wanted to make a protein shake, and it was the perfect opportunity to experiment.

I was out of protein powder, but I can get pretty creative in the kitchen so I thought I would whip up my own concoction. Beginning with some almond milk I added a splash of orange juice, some frozen strawberries and a half banana. It was hardly tasty or refreshing—even after adding cinnamon and cocoa. But Rome wasn't built in a day so I figured I could work on it more over the summer. Or at least be sure not to run out of powder.

The conversation I was having with my Mom began with pecans and quickly shifted. My mother said, "I know—I need to diet *and* exercise." So immediately I said, "No you don't. Not at first. Just do what I'm doing Mom and start with one thing until you nail it and gain some confidence." But I don't think she heard me because she was adamant about not wanting to buy a bunch of stuff. So, I said, "All you have to do is start feeding yourself love Mom. And what I mean by that is just start paying attention to what you are feeding yourself. Is it a lot or not enough? Are you depriving yourself of nutrition—or are you over-indulging in something else? My point is to just start by feeding your body love and play with that for a few days—or even weeks—until you feel like you can tackle the next thing. Then when you are ready to introduce something tangible or let go of something that you've always wanted to eliminate; it will be easier to do. Not only because you want to—but because you are building a foundation for yourself and you'll be ready." Then I said, "Are you happy with your current size? Do you want to gain weight or let go?" She said she would like to let go of about fifteen pounds, so I said, "Well you need a plan, right?" Then she said it again, "Yeah I know—I need to diet and exercise."

Our conversation was all via text and she added that she hated the word diet. I texted, "I hate the word hate." Then I wrote, "Just keep in mind the #1 rule is to feed yourself love. And when you are ready, add something as your #2 rule that you want to pay attention to—just like I did. Whether you eliminate, introduce, or reduce, pick something for that number two spot that is really important to you and that you want to accomplish above and beyond anything else. I chose to focus on reducing my sodium first because I went to the doctor my blood pressure was unusually high. Pick something that you know you can do, and that you actually want to do. All you have to do is make it realistic and achievable." Then she said it. "But Nicki, you have only lost like two pounds and you have been doing your love diet since October."

There it was. The statement stung my face, but I held my grace. I said, "I may not have lost forty-five pounds Mom—but I certainly have not gained it back either—along with an extra ten." I added, "It's taking my body some time to adjust to letting go of the Copper IUD and remember—they did find bacteria on it at the lab too. My body is getting used to the fact that I am eating more cleanly and my positive state of mind would never be where it is today had I not started my love diet. I am human. I do still binge eat while standing in my kitchen and drink a little more wine than I should at times. But my habits are changing. And it takes time for real change to happen and for it to be sustainable. I love myself far more now than I ever have before my love diet—and even at the beginning of it."

It appeared I had just given myself the mini pep talk that I needed to hear. Then I texted her my most up-to-date personal love diet list. Immediately she texted, "What no shrimp!" I said, "No Mom. This is *my* love diet and I am sharing it with you so you can see it as an example. You have to create your own love diet so that it will work for you, your body, your age, and your life. I'm not eating shrimp for a good reason. I need to get my cholesterol in check. If you want to let go of that fifteen pounds, it starts with recognizing what is no longer serving *you*—not me. And acknowledging what it is you want to do—or not do. But also forgiving yourself for how you got to where you are in the first place. You don't need to go on a diet Mom. *You just need to pay attention to your diet.*"

After all that texting I was exhausted as I'm sure she was too. Switching gears, I made all of us stuffed gluten-free mushrooms, haddock and yes—garlic mashed potatoes in the middle of summer for dinner.

Day 272: Monday, July 2nd

I had already invested ten days and it didn't appear that anything had changed. Inside or out. But I read that it was best to give a probiotic up to thirty days to work its magic.

Some people experience positive results in just one day and initially, my husband did too. But even though it didn't last, he read enough about it to believe it was still a positive addition to his faithful daily supplemental routine. And I was convinced too. I hadn't experienced any routines that stuck with me over the years, but I was willing to give it a try since it wasn't, in fact, a diet. *It was a compliment to my love diet, and I also agreed it was a good idea to be more pro than anti.*

As a family, we do try to avoid antibiotics as much as we can, but sometimes there's just no escaping it. In January, I had to take it. Antibiotics seem to kill everything, but it didn't kill the acne on my face, so it must not have been bacterial. Which sort of led me in the direction of what I had originally self-diagnosed. The acne had to be hormonal or worse, auto-immune.

With all of the buts lining up, I couldn't ignore my gut. And it made the decision to keep taking the probiotic easy. To see if cleaning my gut flora—would help my facial aura.

Day 273: 199 lbs. Tuesday, July 3rd

There was still a degree of resistance in me. Like accepting that the number of carbs recommended is actually the size of my cupped hand and not my fist. And it makes me cringe to think about the hundreds of plates or even thousands of heaping bowls of pasta I had made myself over the years, not to mention what I'd been served and consumed in any given restaurant.

Half-heartedly, I picked the smallest of the baked potatoes and only took one half, slicing it lengthwise to make it look bigger on my plate and placed it next to my turkey burger. I was being diligent about portioning out realistic amounts of carbs at each meal, but the number of carbs we are supposed to eat was not easy to wrap my brain around nor my stretched-out stomach. Regardless, later I found myself in a bit of a binge.

It was a healthier binge, but clearly what I had eaten at dinner was likely not enough carbs, protein, fat—or something, because what I did notice during that moment of weakness was that there were no signs of emotions involved.

Nonetheless, I really don't want to binge eat at all. I want to eat like a healthy-slash-normal person. I want to let go of the extra body fat that I have accumulated and have been carrying around with me over these last six-ish years. What I want is the simple act of feeding myself nutrition—*to be easier.*

Making the decision to not binge eat while standing in my kitchen unless it was healthy food was a good decisive shift. But I was not quite there yet. *I had to keep shifting so it would come naturally, and my mind would be strong enough mentally—before my body could let go physically.*

Day 274: Wednesday, July 4th

We were excited about enjoying the holiday, which was also my son Duke's birthday. With a full day planned, we began it with a morning at the beach.

We used to bring a ridiculous amount of food with us years ago each time we went, and the activity became less about being together as a family surrounded by beautiful scenery—and more about what was inside the outdoor pantry. So we made a simple decision to each eat a good solid meal before we left. We only live a mile or two away, so packing up and leaving early if someone was hungry was never a big deal. Even when our youngest was only about two—the one thing we agreed to stop bringing was food.

Our plan after the beach was to serve a light lunch and I grilled up everything fast and easy on the stove top. My husband's eyes grew wide, thrilled at the notion of being able to enjoy sausage again when he saw me take the chicken version out of the fridge. The product was good enough and free from nitrates and GMOs. The hotdogs were kosher too.

When I was prepping the side salad, both of our mothers had called and texted unexpectedly. They each wanted to stop by and give our son his birthday gifts, so of course, we invited them to join us for lunch.

In my eyes, the eight hotdogs, four sausages, side salad, and the cake I picked up for dessert was plenty of food for the six of us—and still suitable for the additional two. But as soon as my mother walked into the kitchen, I could feel her eyes skimming across the island, thinking to herself that I definitely was not serving enough food.

When I was growing up my mother would always have an abundance, serving everything in elegant dishes, silverware and pressed cloth napkins that I helped iron. She has the ability to stretch any meal to accommodate a variety of taste buds, levels of hunger and any unexpected drop-ins. Perhaps there was always plenty of food because she was usually hosting a party or holiday gathering, but nonetheless, it is instinctual for her to have more than enough—and stretch any meal into the following week. My husband's mother has a different approach, but still has it down to a science. There is the perfect amount of food for a few to enjoy seconds—and rarely if anything is leftover.

In our home, we try to incorporate a little from both sides. And on this particular occasion, our intention was to stick with the original plan to serve a light lunch—since six of us were leaving for an early "day of" birthday dinner too. I didn't think it was necessary to pull out any more food. Not until I asked the question, "Who wants sausage?"

Day 275: Thursday, July 5th

Everyone that walked by me wanted to taste the peach I was slicing so I shared it. And I thought for sure someone would want the last of it—so I left it. But the one sliver just sat there stuck to the pit. I finally took it. The only one willing to get their hands sticky in the slightest bit.

Scooping some Greek yogurt into a bowl I added the peach to it along with some cinnamon, honey, and a few pecans. Almonds are my usual go-to nut, but pecans are good for you too, which makes for another delicious and healthy alternative. And I was discovering that having diversity was key for me to continue eating healthy.

I'm sure I was just trading one evil for another, but I swapped out the feta cheese for bleu cheese crumbles for my date night salmon salad dinner. And I also swapped the balsamic dressing out for the bleu cheese. *Again, baby steps.*

Day 276: Friday, July 6th

It was already almost ten o'clock, so I headed up the stairs to meditate before the rest of the day slipped away. Then I took the concept of binging to another level. I opened up my guided meditation by Deepak-Oprah and one meditation led to several.

I hadn't worked out the entire week, so I hopped onto my yoga mat for a little stretching in between meditations listening and absorbing. It felt really good to combine their wisdom and meditative music into my yoga practice. It was a great morning filled with self-care and bringing myself back to center was just what I needed.

I was feeling menopausal again and emotional. Living through insurmountable uncertainty was not easy and it can be especially frustrating when the heaviness that we women feel is no longer followed by the satisfying release of a fresh clean start. In my experience, by the time I realize I am in the midst of a ghost cycle, well, the endless ride seems to start all over again. It is such a balancing act that very often feels like my life is a circus.

After lunch, I gave myself permission to enjoy a small gluten-free brownie to satisfy my chocolate craving with a small glass of red wine that quickly turned into two.

Day 277: Saturday, July 7th

While the kids settled into their vacation mode, I settled into a level of frustration. This time around my kitchen. No one was doing nearly as much as I thought they would—with or without a dishwasher.

It is interesting how the people in my home can avoid the kitchen seemingly without having any anxiety or guilt over it. Inevitably, I am the one who cleans it. But this time I went on strike. No matter how much it went against my core—I did no more.

Deliberately, I took the last egg to make myself breakfast. I scrambled it into the pan quickly and added the leftover vegetable medley from the fridge and yes—I left the mess. I had an additional side of yogurt sprinkled with blueberries, pecans, and cinnamon and did my very best to pretend that my kitchen was in fact clean. And just before heading to the groomer, I grabbed another Greek yogurt snack and didn't look back.

Lucy was trimmed and revealed the skinny little muscular thing that she is underneath all that fur. She is pretty healthy, but during the summer she gets so much exercise that we have to increase the amount of food we feed her a little bit, and in the winter, we feed her a little less. We assess the seasons and change our dogs' diets when necessary. *What a concept; Pay attention to my body and adjust it accordingly.*

My husband made salmon for dinner along with some rice, but for a family of six, one cup hardly sufficed. And the vegetable side was the afterthought that arrived, a little too late to make it to the plate.

Day 278: Sunday, July 8th

It felt like I was taking only one step forward and then two steps back. My stomach not only felt bloated—it looked bloated. I was eating emotionally again or should I say *menopausally*. I was a bit of a mess, which of course, led me to feel a little anxious, stressed, worried, and depressed.

What I've noticed is that whenever I am emotional, I tend to fall back into the old nail-biting habit too. For me, it's a way to exert the energy of what is going on in my mind and get it out. Nail-biting is not something I like to admit, but it is what it is and the act itself can actually help relieve anxiety for me.

It's a physical outlet that happens automatically when I'm working, driving, and even watching movies. It happens when I fall deep into my thoughts or have intense conversations. If I am not paying attention, I can take it too far. And I am fully aware that it can resemble the likes of cutting.

Wearing fake nails is a great way for me to avoid nail-biting, but it is also a way of living on the surface and avoiding my emotions. I love the glam for sure, and when my nails look nice, there's less of a temptation to grab a small hangnail and let 'er rip. The fake nails are indeed a great trick.

But I made the decision to not cover up my nails anymore. Because I was just covering up my emotions. I am such a visual. And seeing the status of my fingernails and cuticles was helping me to be highly in tune and aware. What I wanted to do was to address my nails as part of my healing process—not hide them. And boy my nails were a wreck. Seeing my nails in their rawest form was what I needed to see, because it was crystal clear to me—that I was not loving myself nearly enough.

Albeit my hormones had kicked back in, it was a beautiful day. I did my best to get back on track and loved myself with some easy gardening, reading, and writing. I had some yogurt for breakfast, ate some fruit for a snack and made myself deviled eggs on a bed of greens for lunch. And everyone was chipping in before and after dinner again.

Our attempt at a sliced turkey breast stir-fry dinner was okay and luckily cumin goes with ginger, because I was cooking without my glasses again.

Day 279: Monday, July 9th

Flipping through the internet I came across a quick video of Oprah saying she usually gains eight to fifteen pounds during the holiday season—and that for the first time ever, she had stayed the same. We were six months away from the holidays, but with almost 100 days left of my love diet to go, it was interesting to think about.

Perhaps it was the same thing that was happening to me. At this stage of the game, maybe my body needed to stay the same

I AM ON A LOVE DIET

before my mindset could completely change. It might take more than a year for me to let the weight go and I woke up realizing that my body was used to storing all of this fat. For a long time!

Yes, I had made many efforts over the years, but they were mostly faint. And placing my head in the sand in the dieting industry land—was the heaviest price to pay. Like the perfect storm, the person I had physically become was not just because of one single thing. It was a combination that eventually made this fat lady sing.

The environment and manufacturers have both played their part, but ultimately the majority of the roles were played by me. I needed to be the one to see. To sift through the noise and listen. Because I wasn't just stuck where I was at with my fat. I woke up thinking about the alcohol I was drinking.

Eliminating wine altogether would not be a realistic goal though. It's not what I wanted to do. But I wanted to cut out the extras. Was there still time to cut back on my consumption of wine? And if Jesus could turn water into wine, could this child of God turn her wine into water?

Day 280: Tuesday, July 10th

My routine was way out of whack. I didn't have breakfast until almost ten o'clock in the morning and completely skipped over lunch. By mid-afternoon, I was starving and made some more deviled eggs. But I only ate one. I had to leave unexpectedly to go and pick up my son.

In the car on the way home, we both laughed a little about how we would look back at his ruse, pretending to walk to work for weeks. He was embarrassed that he didn't plan very well for the transition. And secretly, I hoped he wouldn't ever keep secrets from me about his health.

Day 281: Wednesday, July 11th

At breakfast, I had a really simple but delicious yogurt with one of my youngest son's unsweetened applesauce school snacks. I could only imagine what it's like to be an eleven-year-old and I was a far cry from being a teenager too. But I could relate if I thought about it hard enough.

Love is what I give to my kids, and I want to feed love to the little girl who lives inside my heart too. She has been longing for the tenderness of self-care for years and I imagine myself holding her hand, telling her with confidence that everything will be okay. And that she has nothing to fear, we are strong, and together we only have everything to gain.

My day blissfully continued until taco night. The stand-up shells were stale, but luckily the kids found a fresh pack of soft shells tucked in the back of the pantry. We settled for leftover tomato sauce in lieu of salsa and were all underwhelmed by the leftover rice. Chopping the romaine lettuce with some hesitation it practically went untouched after learning about the recent E. coli outbreak in the news. We topped everything off with the new yogurt that replaced our sour cream and through our taco meal gratitude was hardly anywhere to be found.

Day 282: Thursday, July 12th

Sitting at a picnic table outside, I pulled out my laptop while my son went in for an interview. It wasn't easy for me to focus surrounded by so much nature and the fact that our vacation was fast approaching—but I did try.

Failing at the first attempt to link my wi-fi—I let myself wander over to text. My Mom was chiming in and letting me know that she was trying my love diet concept and had been loving herself more through awareness since our conversation. I was so proud of her—for trying—and doing. And after I sent some encouraging thoughts it suddenly occurred to me. She may have been waiting all this time for my body to change—to see if this path was worth her time to give it a try.

Day 283: Friday, July 13th

We spent the entire morning packing the car but first I enjoyed a few moments of peace sitting in my shade garden drinking my coffee.

While I was writing, I looked up briefly from my phone and saw a cute little grey bunny hopping towards the safety of the fence. It didn't seem worried at all about our three dogs relentlessly chasing her. I followed her fluffy white tail as it bounced across the lawn like a song and I thought to myself how I was on a similar mission—to get to a safer place and to let nothing stand in my way from achieving that freedom.

છે ✑

Nicole Perry

Chapter 14
Ignorance IS Bliss

"I had barely touched the surface of that sugar challenge—and already it was a huge wake-up call."

Day 284: Saturday, July 14th

No scale here. Of course, it would be a silly thing to do. Bring a scale to a campground—on our vacation—and weigh myself in the woods. As much as I like to embrace that OCD of mine, the thought never did cross my mind, which is interesting to think about. That it was not at all absurd to have a daily routine of weighing myself at home—just because it wasn't in the dirt.

I contemplated again, what it would be like to let it go and wondered if I could ever live my life free from it. That crystal scale that almost never gives me what I want, which is just a few daily glimpses of hope or a sneak peek into a skinnier future. I know there are some people that do let it go—but I'm sure those people don't have any real issues with their weight or a single pound of fat to lose. And I'm pretty certain at this point in my life that ditching my scale isn't how I will lose weight—let alone keep it off.

In a way, I was giving my power away to that scale. But only some of it. My scale was a symbol of love and for me letting go of it was like saying I didn't care. I do care and I wasn't at a place where I could let it go, yet. I wasn't just looking for a magic number anymore. What I was more attached to—was measuring my progress.

Either way, if I did try to let it go, I'd be placing the power elsewhere—in its absence—and I want to be the one holding the power—with or without it. Someday I may figure out how to let my crystal scale go and still care. Perhaps the better way to live is only weighing in at the doctor's office or when I feel a major change happening in my body. Or is it? *Perhaps the only way one is able to let go of their scale—regardless of size—is by facing our emotions—not by ditching a seemingly inanimate object.*

And there we were. Like scraping the spindle across the vinyl—vrrrpp. Boom. We arrived at our Cape Cod camping vacation. Every summer for almost ten years we plop ourselves into the woods—nestled in a sea of pine trees. We relocate ourselves to a destination well known—in the middle of nowhere.

With only the sun, the sky and the earth to comfort us—the only glamping going on was a blown-up mattress, swimsuit with matching coverup, and a layer of concealer. The mascara—completely optional. Although, I did bring some falsies the year I lost all of my eyelashes when I got caught up in the lash extension trend. It was kind of funny gluing them into place sitting at our picnic table in a sort of what not to do kind of way.

Purposefully, we strip away most of the comforts of home and layer on a little simplicity and humility. No beds, no kitchen, no couch or television. We are unplugged with just a couple of tents we stake to the ground, claimed on a small piece of land, not too far and away from our own. And just close enough—to call our little sweet home away from home.

Well, we do still have our phones. But does anyone—go anywhere—without their phones anymore? Technically yes, we are still plugged in, but we are mostly *dialed in*—to each other. And we ration our batteries for priorities like catching up on the latest episode of Big Brother. The kids all save most of their juice for staying connected with their friends on social media and as for me—I save most of my power to write. After all, a writer still whits in the woods.

Kicking off our family vacation, I looked through the cooler we brought filled with just enough of the typical stuff to get us through a few meals before a second grocery round in P-town. I whipped together some chili for lunch on the portable outside grill beginning with the standard olive oil, chopped onion, and diced green peppers. We kept it lean by adding ground turkey, and of course some essential spices conveniently stolen from our kitchen at home like basil, parsley, paprika, cumin, salt and pepper. For the beans, I added cans of black, navy, and kidney along with one large can of crushed tomatoes. Our camping chili 101 turned out to be pretty darn good and was really not that far from what I would have made at home.

It felt so good to take a midday nap on day one and it felt even better to do it again just chillin' at the beach in the sun. Occasionally, we looked out at the beautiful ocean together and

I AM ON A LOVE DIET

admired the confident and impressive glutes in the young Brazilian bronzed bikini butts that walked on by and I wondered if I would ever be able to go back to those days of almost being one of them again.

The seals were bobbing their heads in and out of the water and my eyes yearned for every glimpse of their silky puppy-like whiskery faces. The ocean was beautiful, and I noticed an older fit man off in the far distance swimming in his shiny black wetsuit. If I had to place my bet, I would have easily guessed that he was 65, or even 70. I continued to watch the elder man like he was the star behind my documentary lens. And then he walked out of the ocean onto the beach—grabbed a surfboard—and went back out. Wow.

Thoughts of guilt, what-if's, and maybe I could do that too immediately filled my head as I watched the man. The thoughts eventually evaporated though as we walked back to our exertion-less campsite. Grilling up the new nitrate-less chicken sausage for dinner I reheated a few baked potatoes for the grill that I had microwaved at home and served a house salad with avocado, pear infused vinegar and olive oil for the dressing. Finally, we all enjoyed some fresh blueberries for a fun dessert, along with the gluten-free brownies we brought from home.

Day 285: Sunday, July 15th

Eating breakfast together as a family is something we hardly ever do at home, so cooking it up while camping was kind of nice. Eggs were on the menu along with some turkey bacon to try. I toasted some gluten-free raisin bread for myself and english muffins for everyone else. We always bring a couple of nostalgic cans of baked beans too, but I knew it was hardly healthy, so this year I chose to pass.

Each sunny day was more than an opportunity to enjoy a beautiful day at the beach and I insisted everyone wait for me. It was at least a one-mile hike round trip, or more, depending on where we decided to sit. And I knew it was the only exercise I was gonna get.

Later we stopped to get the good old-fashioned American emergency peanut butter and jelly staple from the grocery store. It jogged my memory of visiting my Great Gramma who lived just one house over from my Grandmother. My mother and aunts would send bunches of us over to her house, assumingly to get a moment of peace. We were little, somewhere in the range of two and six-years-old, and I can still see my Great Grandmother sitting in her kitchen chair—each pointy corner of her Cat-eye black glasses embellished with a hint of fake bling.

It was a time when locking the house wasn't necessary and we made ourselves at home from the moment we surged through the door. In my memory—as Bob as my witness—I led the Rugrat crew and volunteered to climb up onto her kitchen counter and rummage through her cabinets to find the infamous peanut butter and jelly she claimed to have. Fluffernutter if we were lucky.

She hardly moved a muscle as I thoroughly searched for the good crackers trying my best not to disrupt her Mother Hubbard cupboard. I thought she must have been at least ninety, but she was definitely a twentieth-century Great Grandmother watching a slew of unruly kids in the early '70s. Yeah, peanut butter and jelly is still a good staple to have around.

I AM ON A LOVE DIET

Day 286: Monday, July 16th

My vacation had barely begun when I opened my phone and the first thing I noticed was that I had been invited to take on a sugar challenge by my new coach.

It was the best kind of challenge. All I had to do was read labels and be mindful. I was curious and it seemed simple enough. Introducing more love into my life was something I wanted to do every day not just on Mondays or the days that might be convenient. So yeah, I wanted to keep loving myself on my vacation. Plus, I was already staying clear from most sweets by eating gluten-free anyway. I figured this would be a piece of cake.

Bananas are undeniably a whole food, but they are fruit—so obviously they have some sugar. I practically eat them every day, so it was the first thing I searched for using a small amount of my precious phone battery power for. Right away I found that one medium banana was loaded with 14 grams of sugar. *Damn.* But it was still a whole food and an all-natural one, so I wasn't sure how much it really counted. It's a really good question.

Watching my daily intake of sodium and animal fats to gain control of my blood pressure and cholesterol was something I was already doing, so it made perfect sense to dig a little deeper and investigate how much sugar was actually considered normal. According to the American Heart Association, the recommended daily amount of sugar for a woman to take in was less than 20 grams. *Shit.* I had been reaching two-thirds of my daily quota by kicking off just about every day with a freaking fourteen-gram banana at breakfast. And sometimes I had it as a snack*!*

Panic shot through my fingertips as I searched some more. This time, I opened the cooler and grabbed the honey. Inside one tablespoon it also listed 14 grams. I grew even more agitated sitting starchily at our poignant picnic table. I counted out the small handful of blueberries I had just recklessly tossed into the pool of honey that sat on top of my yogurt. My convenient camping breakfast was becoming my nemesis.

As calmly as I could, I guestimated the amount of sugar I was about to eat and started a pitiful paper napkin journal just on the other side of our scrabble scores. It added up to be a lot of sugar leaving very little wiggle room for the rest of the day. After back-tracking a few meals—I put down the pen.

It was what it was. And what I needed to do was to gain back control as soon as possible. The least I could do moving forward at the very minimum was decide not to eat any bananas the same day I had honey. Done! My body was happier from the changes and shifts that I had already made, but this latest discovery about sugar was huge. My scribbled notes were the writing on the wall that I was bound to see—eventually. *And without a shadow of a doubt, what I had just discovered about sugar, could actually be the reason why I wasn't losing any weight, why dieting had become so difficult for me as I aged, and why I kept quitting. Ho-ly Shit.* Evidently, I was far more sugar challenged than I realized.

Never did I imagine that I was consuming too much sugar of all things, not to mention my heart was taking another big hit. And it was a hard hit to take. Like the time when I was about twelve, freely running backward in the park—bursting with enthusiasm and laughter. And just at the exact moment when I turned myself around—my face smacked into a tree.

I was okay of course. And I will be okay. But I did feel like I had just smacked into a wall. *I had barely touched the surface of that sugar challenge—and already it was a huge wake-up call.*

I continued counting with my kosher camping hotdog and makeshift gluten-free bread-bun exception at lunch topped with mustard, relish, and a line of ketchup. It was crystal clear that everything I was eating was laced with sugar and I was kicking off each day with about 30 grams. Brewing over my own ignorance, I destroyed all evidence of the cheap condiment narcotic and licked up every ounce of it.

I was in shock and a little freaked out about how the heck I would be able to reduce sugar at all, but I still forged forward. Writing in my throwaway journal at dinner I noted my bunless turkey burger with half baked potato and avocado salad. After a long day of self-diagnosed sugar dependence, the only good news I clung to was that the glass of wine I just drank only had about 1.5 grams—so I grabbed the box and poured myself another.

Could I claim that I knew exactly how many calories, carbs or fats were appropriate to take in on a daily basis for a woman my age with my unique body type? No. And maybe I didn't need to. I am smart though and like most people, I knew that 38 grams of sugar in one can of soda was not good.

I also knew that sugar definitely turned into carbs. Or was it vice versa? And carbs most certainly turned into fat. I think. What I did do at the start of my day was pass on the helping of nostalgic baked beans in a can. And I'm glad I did, because when I read the label I found out that in just one small half-cup there were twelve grams of sugar. I'm not even sure if the noted 550 percent of sodium or the 29 grams of carbohydrates mattered anymore.

Learning what the heck the average amount of sugar is actually appropriate for a typical woman to take in on a daily basis regardless of our age or size was mind-blowing to me. And if I didn't know what the daily recommended number was, I wondered how many other women didn't know what it was either. That sugar challenge was literally a game-changer for me, but also a huge blessing in disguise. I knew this was a pivotal moment in my love diet, and still, I couldn't help but wonder, why was I just learning about how ambiguous sugar was. And then it occurred to me. I must not have been anywhere near ready to hold that power—until now.

Day 287: Tuesday, July 17th

The sugar saga continued, but I had to dig even deeper. Armed with the daily guide for a woman was not enough to equip me and my family. I had to search for what the daily recommended amount was for men and children and the numbers continued to bewilder.

For men it was a whopping 36 grams and it was more annoying to discover than it was surprising. But men burn it off much faster, so it made sense. After all, men are hunters and women are gatherers. But children are dependent, and their daily recommended allowance was the most alarming at 17 grams.

The thought of what my children were potentially consuming right here in my own home was scary. *But having this new information about sugar was powerful—and I was so grateful to be in the know.* Discovering the dangers of sugar was just the beginning and for the sake of my kids' futures, I had to inform them about the simple daily recommended guide.

Standing there in their skinny little, burning-it-off-as- we-speak bodies, they rolled their eyes at the sense of urgency in my voice. It was reasonable for them to think I was overreacting, after all, they are kids. So initially being dismissive was normal. But as their mother, it was just as natural for me to want to protect them. *I knew it was crucial to educate my kids about the gravity of sugar being downright seductive, dangerously addictive, and deceit-fully cumulative.*

There was no going back. I couldn't unlearn the information and I didn't want to. It was eye-opening that I never knew what the amount of sugar recommended for the average woman was, and what I was literally consuming. I had wasted years of my life engaging in countless diets and in all that time, I was completely oblivious to the real dangers of sugar.

Sure, sugar is talked about a lot. But all of the diets I had participated in were only suggesting me to remove obvious sugars like cakes and cookies. I honestly don't remember a single diet informing me about what the daily recommended guide was for a woman—or her child.

I am smart. And maybe I didn't read deep enough into the intricacies of those diets. But they never really kept my attention long enough either. And suddenly I felt paranoid. Like there was some kind of conspiracy going on in the world to keep ordinary people like myself in the dark. Although it does make perfect sense. For them to have the need to lead me to believe—that only through them could real success be achieved. And I would forever be at the mercy of a diet. Let's face it—it all comes down to money. *The industry needed me to keep investing mine and I was their ideal client. A middle-aged, overweight, desperate woman, with a next generation of malleable children.*

Limiting my sugars throughout the entire day on my own to less than 20 grams was not easy, but I had to keep trying. Continuing to love myself, I counted four grams in one slice of gluten-free raisin toast I had for breakfast, which I ate, with real butter, along with two eggs, some zucchini, and avocado and at lunch, I noted 11 grams. I didn't have any snacks throughout the entire day and at dinner, I counted a total of eight. For the entire day of being extremely aware, and working diligently to reduce my own consumption, my total sugars for the day added up to 23 grams. That was not easy!!!

The information I held was still pure power. I was no longer ignorant about sugar or at the mercy of anyone else. Limiting the amount of sugar going forward, that I was willing to allow into my now sacred body, would easily make the cut into my love diet list.

<u>My Love Diet</u>:
1) Feed Myself Love
    a. Is Love on My Plate, In My Bowl, In My Cup?
2) Minimize Sodium
    a. Remove High Sodium Caesar Salad
    b. Remove or Reduce Soups, Dressings, Sauces, Gravies and Dips.
3) Reduce Animal Fats
    a. Red Meat, Pork, Shrimp, Yogurt and Soft Cheeses
4) Be Mindful of Carbs
    a. Remove or Reduce to Size of Fist
5) Let go of Pizza
6) Remove Deli Meat
    a. Including Bacon, Sausage, Linguica, etc.
7) Live Gluten-Free
8) Exercise Any Amount—Three Times a Week
9) LOVE My Body as It Is Today
10) Eat Slower. Listen for the 80 Percent Tinge
11) Prioritize Meditation Daily
12) Reduce Sugar to Less Than 20 Grams Per Day.

Day 288: Wednesday, July 18th

It wasn't easy to physically or mentally continue but I kept on keeping on. I had my one slice of gluten-free bread with butter, a slice of turkey bacon, and two scrambled eggs for breakfast. And just before leaving for the beach, I grabbed a quick snack.

When I held the squeezable honey jar over my yogurt, I hesitated for what seemed like an entire minute before finally adding just a drop into it. I was sticking with my decision to no longer, carelessly, pour heaping tablespoons of honey into any of my meals, but I wondered—would plain yogurt be palatable without the sweet luxury. And would I eventually get used to it?

Carefully being mindful about how much honey I was willing to allow myself was a good thing, but I was so pissed at myself for forgetting about the blueberries and tossing them into my yogurt—again. Yes I realize that blueberries are a superfood and we've all been taught that we need to eat two to three servings of fruit each day. *But fruit has sugar.* And maybe what they have been recommending all these years was wrong. Perhaps it's supposed to be more along the lines of two to three berries—or bites.

Limiting how many blueberries I eat is a good idea—I think. For now anyway. And vowing not to have honey the same day as a banana too. But frankly, I don't even want to eat bananas anymore. At least until I can figure this out. Or get a hold of my figure.

Once I actually acquire a fit body, it may not even matter. Because what I had learned throughout my dieting years, versus what I was witnessing in the real world were conflicting to the average unfit person—or non-nutritionist like myself. Bananas are the perfect whole food example of why proper nutrition can be so confusing.

Years ago, I was hanging out with another mom in my hood on a playdate with our kids and she mentioned how she loved bananas. Without giving it a second thought, she said she ate bananas every day and sometimes had two. She had a kick-ass rocking hard-body and I'm sure she still does. I certainly knew that eating bananas back then or even today wasn't going to magically give me a body like hers, but I was listening. And it was interesting. She was the ideal person to look up to with such a healthy body image. She was managing her weight extremely well and sustaining it.

I have never personally experienced a fit body to the degree of my neighbor, and if I had, I probably wouldn't think twice about eating bananas either. But I don't have a kick-ass rocking hard-body.

Each time I tried to follow those diet removing banana rules the memory of that mom stood out in my mind. It just never made any sense to me why I had to remove a whole food like a simple banana. Removing bananas from my diet at any time didn't seem smart, but after learning about their sugar content, my theory shifted. And now, I get so pissed at myself for all the times I ate them.

For the time being, I was happy to remove bananas. Until I know or learn better. After all these years, I wish I had known the real reason why so many diets wanted me to cut the bananas out. I wish I had known about the 20-gram gauge for a woman. *I wish I had known about sugar.*

The funny thing is—which is really not very funny at all—we all know when someone has an addiction to food. And it's also clear when we see someone with a positive, healthy body

I AM ON A LOVE DIET

image. It's either an amazing triumph—or a struggling disease. Whether we eat carelessly and tolerate the eyes of judgment in public, or we hide how we really eat alone in the privacy of our own home—what the world sees is our size. And size matters.

Size matters to me when I see the mannequin in the window sporting a fabulous outfit that I want to own in P-town, but when I try it on—I am too embarrassed to come out. And too disappointed in myself to discuss. Size matters when the jeans don't zip and only three bottoms in my closet seem to fit. Size continues to matter when I receive a meal smaller than my eyes had hoped for—and that my stomach is quite capable of holding much more. It was only 11:30 in the morning and I had already reached nine grams of sugar. My body was still crying—feed me, Seymour.

At the beach, I heard a woman in the distance with two toddlers talking with a friend. She asked the kids about what they wanted to order for lunch and wanted to know specifically what their favorite was—a hamburger with fries or a cheeseburger. Her mind notably elsewhere. She was clearly obese and while she maneuvered through the wading water, my heart reached out to her.

But whether the compassion I held for her was misplaced energy or not—I'll never know. Because for all I knew she was happy with her size. She did, after all, bravely plop down to sit in the water with those kids, which was something I couldn't even imagine doing. And whether she was happy or not, I still felt her pain. And I knew I didn't want to keep living in the body shape that I had—that could potentially lead me to a body shaped like hers.

Watching her scared me. I knew the issues with my weight paled in comparison, but then again, I was nowhere near skinny either. I knew that. I have eyes and dressing room mirrors. I was just skinnier than her. So, I saved some of that compassion for myself. I didn't have the courage to sit on the land or even in the water like she did. The thought of getting back up again was far too embarrassing for me. But then again, I didn't have to. My kids were older and that one summer I stuck to the safety net of my beach chair—turned into several.

Charting out all of the cumulative years of roller-coaster dieting was not just about my lack of willpower though. The size I had become was the result of many things. And I can see clearly now that I no longer want to remain a prisoner inside my own body—stuck deep in the cells of sodium, cholesterol, gluten, and now sugar.

The information I was accumulating was powerful. I was finally beginning to create a fresh new mindset and nowhere near comfortable anymore. I was on the path to feeding my mind and body better fuel to keep progressing, shifting, and yes, changing. *Real change will happen. It has to.* And I believe it will. Because I was determined. I had come way too far to accept that my current size was as good as it was ever gonna get.

Someday I hope to have grandchildren and I want to be able to move with them—with pride—at home and at the beach. Standing, walking, sitting, crawling and maybe even stop, drop and rolling around on the floor with them. *In the end, the will to change my size must be strong, but the desire to care and love myself has to be stronger.*

By two o'clock I was already at 20 grams—and forgiving myself for getting there.

Day 289: Thursday, July 19th

Continuing to go through life pretending I was content or ignoring my health by rationalizing was something I didn't want to do anymore. And what I was doing every day since my love diet had begun—was mentally free myself from that absurdity. I want to be further away from the debts of obesity not fall deeper into it. I want to break free from the misery and be significantly healthy. And because I was taking better care of myself—it was starting to spill over into my family.

Plopping ourselves back into civilization at the local grocer, I took great pride in being the person in my family that was open enough to discover the information about sugar. Within minutes of arriving at the store, we were all counting sugars, one-upping one another at each opportunity. It was crazy cool and fun for me. I was not only translating the information that I learned, but I was acting on it, they were listening, and it was turning into the game we all wanted to win.

Day 290: Friday, July 20th

The phrase waste-not want-not lingered in the air of my awareness again. I wasn't brought up in the Depression but still, I was raised by a community who was and the urge to not be wasteful is strong and comes naturally.

My daughter had offered up the last few bites of her baked potato, but I said no thank you. There is only one gram of sugar in one small potato and the two bites she offered me were barely less than. But still, I was full. And it felt good to respect my body by not consuming the tiniest extra bite—just because. Although, root vegetables didn't concern me hardly as much as the banana did.

Even a medium carrot only has three grams of sugar. And enjoying a few condiments I thought would be okay too while I embraced this newest addition of reducing sugar to my love diet. As long as I paid close attention to the quantities of course. If I wanted to treat myself with honey, there are only about four to five grams of sugar in one *teaspoon* depending on the brand. And if I wanted to adorn my turkey burger with my favorite childhood ketchup condiment, there were only about four grams in one single tablespoon. With an average of fourteen grams of sugar in one medium banana—they were loaded.

As I took the time to start adding all of the sugars up from breakfast, lunch, dinner, snacks, condiments, any extra bites, and even wine, it was accumulating to a ridiculous number that was well exceeding the daily recommendation. But I was completely on board about continuing to practice reducing sugar, because inevitably it would lead me toward positive results. And frankly, it would be nice to simply put on a pair of pantyhose again without feeling like I'm about to give myself a hernia.

Reducing my sugars was the carrot and the stick. I felt like I had found a real fountain of youth and my mind was already envisioning getting my cute little skinnier body back. And oh, the dresses I would love to fit back into again! It would feel great to wear some of my old power dresses and even the almost new Mrs. Cleaver green holiday taffeta one that I bought at a thrift shop without trying it on. When I attempted to put it on at home, sadly I was about five pounds away from slipping into it, and ten pounds away from zipping it.

So far, I was kind of reducing my sugar radically, which was sort of forcing my body to hold onto every ounce of fluid in me. In just four days I was sporting a new set of cankles. But on this 290th day, I have to say, I was fueled by the excitement of seeing how quickly, or slowly my body would adjust to living even more cleanly.

Skinnier does equate to more wrinkles, but the feelings of empowerment were magnified the more educated I became and in control of my own mind and body. *When I am healthier—I am better mentally. And when my mind is in good shape—it makes me want to be more fit.* I would take healthy and wrinkly over the latter any day. And most of my wrinkles are camouflaged by tattoos anyway.

My coach also told me in a private message that letting go of most sugars would help clear up my skin. And she encouraged me to continue reducing all unnecessary sugars that appear in almost everything. Boxed, canned and bagged. Natural, refined, and yes, organic. It was good to pay attention to every place they hide, remove most of them, and count the consumable gems.

Day 291: Saturday, July 21st

That's what you do when you have acne. You sit at your campsite and layer on concealer and foundation at the start of the day. It may have left me wide open to judgment from passersby, but if I'm perceived as some kind of glamper, that's okay by me. Concealing my acne keeps my mental health in check and gives me confidence. Plus, we were leaving.

As I sat alone at our picnic table reading my book and drinking my last cup of shitty coffee in the wee hours of the morning I took in the last moments of peace. Daddy longlegs were everywhere, multiplying by the minute almost. Delicately, one walked over my phone with me into the next page of my book. And another crawled across the glasses on my face as I quickly jumped and quietly flicked.

Still, I was not ready to leave the simpler camping life deduced down to one small dirted area. Giving away the last stick of butter to our momentary neighbors, we had one last breakfast on the grill, a hike to the beach, packed our bags, and we were gone.

Day 292: Sunday, July 22nd

Our vacation had come to an end and coming off of the vacation fringe I sat at our morning shade garden and soaked in what was left of the afternoon sun.

It had been nine days of not weighing in and almost six days of eating as cleanly as I could. Our resources had been limited, but I was so proud of myself for embracing the new challenge, through eating mostly outdoor grilled food.

I took ownership of what I chose to put on my plate—and into my mouth. And I ate as much salad as possible without getting sick of it. I felt better already, and I couldn't wait to see how I would continue to feel as the next few weeks and months unfolded.

Watching something scoot under the wheel barrel I absorbed the energy within my own backyard and shifted out of our vacation mode. A tremendous amount of peace washed over me. We were home and I was ready to take everything I had just learned about sugar and knew to be true into my everyday life.

Day 293: Monday, July 23rd

Settling in at home I acknowledged that something was very different. My mindset had shifted just a little bit more in a positive direction—again. The Wellfleet flea area market blanket turned tablecloth helped me to see our backyard as our own little oasis. And I want to stop and smell the roses more often and observe the beauty around me—not just what's going on with me.

Our yard was full of perennial gardens that were mostly in full bloom when we arrived back home. From our white, yellow, and peach daylilies, to the original daisy starter garden we created, to the most recent shade garden addition. All of the work to be done physically as well as metaphorically going forward seemed hardly the task—and daunting, all at the same time.

Day 294: Tuesday, July 24th

The simple act of having my blood pressure checked brings me so much joy now. I look forward to the results—because I was the one bringing my numbers back to where they needed to be.

When she walked into the room, the first thing I noticed was she looked at least 20 years my senior. Then she said she had already done two yoga sessions before making her rounds, so when she wasn't looking, I rolled my eyes at her question about whether or not I exercised. I knew what I needed to do. But my new primary care physician could see clearly that I hadn't done much of anything legitimate—on a regular basis—for quite a few years. She was also half my size and exuded the strength of an ox. I would have been willing to bet against myself that in a pinch she could have easily taken me.

Sitting in her exam room, I smiled tossing my new knowledge of sugar and invisible hair into the air. I was starting to acquire more information about nutrition than the average person and my doctor wholeheartedly agreed with me, easily adding "Sugar is the root cause of most disease." What she said made perfect sense and I shared her disdain for sugar, wittingly adding, "I can't believe how much it's in almost everything." She replied almost with a big fat 'duh', "It's because it's addicting."

She was smart but underwhelmed with my new-found discovery and gave me a look of disappointment when my so-called new and improved blood pressure numbers revealed 120 over 100. I was so embarrassed. Immediately, I confessed and said it must have been because of the salt I was adding back onto my plate at the picnic table. Hardly showing any compassion for all that I was learning and had accomplished, she threw me another look, this time it was a *you look smart, why aren't you acting that way* vibe. And I didn't want to pick up the shameful reality she was putting down.

Insisting that I do something, she said, "You need to work up a puff. Not any of that leisurely walking and talking stuff." And evidently the local gym and in-home workouts I mentioned barely impressed her. I guess there still was hardly any progress showing on my outside. Then she said to not eat anything white. I totally get the white flour, and of course, white sugar, but it was the "nothing" that caught me by surprise. I should have liked her because she was healthy and smart, but I didn't fully understand the no white rice or white potatoes part.

I didn't care to look at their non-crystal doctor-office scale after receiving the deflated blood pressure results. Their numbers were always higher than mine. The day was also half over, and I was full of clothes and jewelry, which I'm sure equated to at least two or three pounds. Mid-day also meant I had breakfast and lunch so, right there, was another two or three more. Four to five pounds makes a big difference in my book. And when I think about it, I almost want to fast for my next appointment and take the earliest slot I can, just to see what their scale really has to say. At three o'clock in the afternoon, this patient was plumb out of patience but just before I left, we checked my blood pressure one more time and it came down to 120 over 86. A day late and a dollar short.

Day 295: Wednesday, July 25th

My tiny and fit primary care physician was right though. Moving my body on a regular basis was essential to my mission. Whatever I chose to do didn't matter. I just needed to choose something and stick with it. But exercising was already starting to work its way back into my life because I had joined a gym, which led me to the latest in-home workout training thing.

Then something amazing happened. I came across a new dancing thing on Facebook. As skeptical as I was about giving my debit card information into the hands of the internet land, I did it. It was a real program and I jumped in. Before, during, and after the new dance workout—I kept thinking to myself—*OMG this is perfect for me.*

My entire morning was amazing. I spent the first two hours totally on me. Loving my dogs with coffee, then dancing, showering, meditating, and breakfast. I did it all before the first child got up. Then I watched a quick video trailer.

I couldn't tell you exactly how the heck I was steered in the direction of the video, but it was entitled Eating Animals. And OMG it was shocking. It actually enticed the omnivore in me to skip completely over vegetarianism and head straight to the world of vegans! But I couldn't help but wonder how the heck a mother in a house full of meat eaters could become a vegetarian. Was it even possible?

Back to "nothing white," I then watched another short video. This time it was a vegetarian actress. She was showing what she liked to cook for her kids and husband—in her amazingly skinny and healthy little body. And the meal she was preparing had the very white rice that my primary care physician had just told me to stay away from. Therein lies more of that confusion.

Day 296: Thursday, July 26th

Measuring my progress is why I step on my crystal scale each day, but I hadn't weighed in since before we left for our camping vacation. At this point, I was serious about thinking about trying to let it go. I have to admit that there were at least three to four moments when I had been tempted but just stared at crystal in a show-down. And I let it go. I do want to measure my progress, but I also want to pay attention to how I look as a whole person too, not just consider myself another size or number. And weighing myself might not be serving me anymore.

Now that I have been on a journey of introducing more self-care and self-love long enough, I don't think the green light to eat whatever I want will reappear if I don't know what my number is. I care too much about my body and my health now to resort back to betraying my soul like that. And having said all of that, I still need to be mindful of the old habit—if I am able to set my crystal scale free. After all, history is the greatest predictor.

Lying on the floor with my feet in the air, I noticed the swelling had gone down and my cankles were turning back into ankles. I smiled at the small but glorious progress and wondered if it were from the almost two weeks of reducing sugars, the two days of dancing—or both.

I AM ON A LOVE DIET

Originally, I thought the dance program I found online was one of those *too good to be true* kind of things. But it was real. And it is easy and fun. I felt good about myself and I wasn't dreading it. It was in the privacy of my own home and I could take my enthusiasm to whatever level I wanted to take it. I loved it. And it felt like a workout I wouldn't ever get bored from.

My team meeting was on the schedule and I had a quick green chocolate shake for breakfast. It was low in calories and sugar. And the words "green" and "chocolate" sounded like an amazing combination suggested by my new coach. Adding one scoop of the powerful powder to my shake would give me all the greens I needed to eat, in one shot, right at the start of my day.

Again, it was another no-brainer. But as open-minded as I was trying to be, it looked and smelled a little like dried manure. I do love to have an easy shake once in a while, but after following the directions it tasted a little like the shit it probably was, and I knew I would have to tweak it quite a bit.

Canceling my afternoon appointment, I ate some carrot and celery sticks for a total of almost four grams of sugar. And then at lunch, I made a simple salad with leafy greens, bleu cheese crumbles, olive oil, diced sweet potato, cucumbers, black beans, and a little salt and pepper. *Sweet mother of Jesus it was good!*

Day 297: Friday, July 27th

My new routine was to blast the music and dance in the privacy of my bedroom, but everyone was still sleeping. Thankfully, dancing can be done anywhere. *Obstacle schmobstacle.* I stuck with my plan, put on slower music, and danced sort of modernly—alone in my kitchen. Perhaps another missed calling.

I followed my routine with a meditation and then got ready to go. Before driving to my hair appointment, I added some of my own protein powder to my green chocolate shake mix and it came out pretty good. My entire fast and easy breakfast came out to be 110 calories and less than two grams of sugar. Nice!

At the restaurant on our date night, I switched up my meal quite a bit. Check this out. First, I asked them to remove the candied pecans. They're usually not gluten-free and loaded with sugar. Easy-peasy. I also asked them to hold the sautéed onions and the craisins. Check. I swapped out the feta for bleu cheese and since I removed so many things from the salmon salad, I asked for a side of asparagus. Done. It was beyond delicious. Frustrating only to me though—because I am still so salmon challenged at home.

Two healthy-sized glasses of chardonnay went down easily prior to—and with my meal. It had to be upwards of two grams of sugar per glass. And when she encouragingly asked if I wanted another, my shoulders physically shrunk with shame. Guiltily, I said yes. Complete awareness is still a good thing.

Day 298: Saturday, July 28th

Some things in life are truly embarrassing. Like that time when I walked into that tree as a twelve-year-old little girl. And it was avoidable too—had I caught a clue. As an adult, events can be even more embarrassing. Like the time when my husband and I were running in races together and I decided to sign up for a half marathon—alone.

I was totally fine to do it without him and finishing the race was not the embarrassing part. What was embarrassing was when I finally did get to the end, everyone had all but gone home and the finish line was practically non-existent. I did do it. And yes, I did finish, but embarrassment was still the stronger emogi that came to me crossing the imaginary line, not pride. But why?

To diminish my own humility, I selflessly joked a little and told my friends that I came in tenth—*giant pause*—to last. Giving myself even more bonus points I would further go on to highlight all of the people I had beat who quit—or even left via ambulance.

All jokes aside, I would never "quit-shame" anyone for real, because we all have our own journey to experience. And to sign up for any half or whole marathon, triathlon, 5k or 10k is taking a giant leap in a positive direction. I was proud of myself for doing it. I was just a little more embarrassed that I struggled with it.

My husband and I no longer run together in races and I only ran a few short times after that at home and we found a new common pastime. Writing in accompanied silence.

Casually writing together in our backyard, a new embarrassing moment took the stage. I got up to get another cup of coffee and my chair broke. More specifically, two slats cracked in half, more significantly, under my ass.

It was so embarrassing that my mind immediately raced to the time when we bought three new teak folding chairs on sale for the outside. Straight out of the box my husband sat in one and came crashing to the ground. Yes, it was vital for me to remind him of that day. And we were tired of breaking chairs together separately. Of course, the Nantucket red broken chair became his, and I gave him a slat off my newly claimed Adirondack.

Day 299: Sunday, July 29th

Skipping my dance workout for a second day was something that I didn't want to do. But I did want to have a quiet morning to write and it was calling me more.

We had a traditional family reunion summer cookout to attend and I made an avocado dip and a sweet potato one with zucchini and celery sticks. I also brought along a simple salad with cucumbers, bleu cheese, walnuts, and olive oil. And I made some deviled eggs too. I wasn't sure what everyone else would bring so I was sure to make plenty of food that I knew would be question-free.

Steering the conversation toward sugar everyone guessed at my question about what the daily recommended allowance was. I had no idea what it was just a few short weeks ago, so I don't know why I was so surprised that no one else could guess it either. One person said eight, another guessed twelve, then six.

In my mind, women struggle more than men with our weight. I think most of us anyway. And surprisingly, none of the women that I asked knew about the daily sugar recommendation. Like me, they also didn't know how many grams of sugar they were consuming on a daily basis.

It was a thought-provoking subject that led everyone to give their advice on how much we are supposed to exercise while the bowl of Doritos got passed. When I searched later, the statistics actually show that it's 3 out of 4 men or 73.7%, versus 2 out of 3 women or 66.9% that are in fact, obese.

Day 300: Monday, July 30th

For the first time in almost six years, I had not gained any weight at my wellness visit. Now there's a positive worth revealing—and remembering. I hadn't lost weight either, but I did lose some blood pressure points that were very notably back on track.

So far, what I had proudly gained were two clean ovaries, a clear mammogram, a clean colon, and a uterus on the mend.

Day 301: Tuesday, July 31st

There was hardly any food in the house, so I had a simple protein shake for breakfast with a slice of toast and peanut butter.

Later that night at the networking event there wasn't much that I could eat, or should I say that I wanted to eat. I'm loving my diet so much now that it's getting easier to see what foods are better for my body. I did try a delicious gluten-free lobster and cucumber boat, but I shied away from the mozzarella and grape tomato sticks. I was avoiding the soft cheese, but more importantly the little app sticks were so long I was afraid to poke the back of my throat. Maybe they forgot to test them.

Day 302: Wednesday, August 1st

For the first two to three hours of my day, I spent the morning on me. My dance workout was becoming religious. I made myself a shake and some toast before showering and left for the radio station for a recording.

For lunch, I stopped and had myself a cauliflower pizza with a glass of wine followed by a grocery shop. I was so excited at how much food I purchased for only $218 for our family of six that I posted a pic on Facebook. Our day ended at our new favorite farm-to-table restaurant for our anniversary dinner.

Later my daughter Greenleigh said excitedly, "There are almost too many snack options." While my son Duke was happily making himself an organic, non-GMO, yogurt with some gluten-free granola. I thought it was interesting how everyone was beginning to see clearly that eating healthy was the better way to be.

Day 303: Thursday, August 2nd

Beginning at six o'clock in the morning, I did everything from coffee to dishes, to dance and meditation, to having my protein shake and doing the bills, to taking care of the dogs and making my bed. All before 8:30 am—while every kid was still "sleeping."

Coming back home from my meeting to have a quick lunch, I went upstairs to my bedroom to close the door and work in solid uninterrupted peace and quiet. When I finally emerged around six o'clock to start cooking, I was bombarded with questions about what was for dinner and why was it taking so long. Yep. Summer. I took a deep breath, made a plate for myself, and took it outside to eat in peace where they all followed me.

Day 304: Friday, August 3rd

There is no secret. *We all have to exercise—regularly.* But—and it's a big butt—the act of exercising had slowly become the obstacle in front of me that I constantly found myself trying not to climb over. And evidently, 80 percent of the population was not exercising regularly—right along with me.

Like most of my accomplices, I found plenty of excuses why I couldn't get to it. A knee issue, no time, other people to take care of first, no money, work, hangnail, you name it. When it came to exercise; where there was no will, there was definitely no way. And according to a quick and simple internet search, 20 percent of the people who exercised regularly were generally between the ages of 18 and 24. We could probably walk into a well-populated fresh and trendy hot new restaurant on any given Friday night and confirm the math just by taking a simple quick look around. Nowadays, younger people are generally more fit.

Ironically, when we reach the age of 25 is when our prefrontal cortex is fully developed. It's the rational part of our brain that responds to good judgment and awareness for long-term consequences. It's also when the complex decision-making and planning skills come in. And it's the part of our brain that links personality, the will to live, and how we moderate social behavior and what can play a huge role in our brains' development are in fact, our experiences, or lack thereof.

Realistically, the window of opportunity to decide which exercise we want to incorporate regularly into our lives—lies in our 24-year-old hands. And for most people, that year goes by in the blink of an eye.

Had I known those statistics at the age of 18 or 24 I'm not sure I would have done anything differently. But it is interesting to know that just when that rational part of our brain kicks in, 80 percent of us have already kicked out the exercise thing.

In many cases, it takes something very dramatic for someone to wake up. Like finally being tired of wasting another minute on any stupid diet, reaching a certain birthday milestone, or being handed some unfavorable results and it took all three of those things for me to kick it into gear. Making the decision to treat my body with a higher level of respect clearly came from the act of aging itself, not from my fully developed prefrontal cortex.

Nicole Perry

Now that I am fully aware, and my body continues to age—I am on a mission with ambition—as if my desire had been set on fire. At age 50, I care more than I ever have before about this one body of mine and I look for every bitty source of fountain of youth that I can find. Dancing every day was something I looked forward to and it had routinely worked its way into my days, and my life. My body was changing for the better and so was my mindset. Not at light speed to convince my new doctor, but I was changing in a way like never before. When I'm dancing it doesn't even feel like I'm exercising, and I no longer care about how much I sweat or pay any mind to the hot flashes I get. Whether just before taking a shower in my workout clothes, or I'm dancing in my kitchen in front of the stove, I am finally having fun moving my body.

℘ ℘

Chapter 15
What Do I Want?

"What I want is to have so much love for myself, that sticking to the guidelines that I have created—is easier than breaking them."

Day 305: Saturday, August 4th

Two frozen strawberries are what I tossed into my green chocolate protein shake for breakfast. I was skipping my dance workout, but still—I was starting my day out on the right foot.

We were spending most of the day driving to New York for a college tour and I knew a good protein shake would hold me over. I didn't bring a single snack with me—just a cup of black coffee for the road. Interestingly—it was the first time I didn't think twice about when or where my next meal would come from. And it was the first time in ages I didn't accumulate any anxiety over it.

A few hours into the drive my son and husband both needed a bathroom stop so we pulled over to my favorite coffee shop. I still hadn't worked up an appetite so all I asked for was a simple black coffee. When I came out of the bathroom, both of them were standing in line scanning the menu enthusiastically with their eyes. I took a look too, but I passed. Everything they were offering included a gluten-filled something.

Just as my husband was about to pay for my coffee and their extremely unhealthy late breakfasts I chuckled at the individually wrapped gluten-free brownie I saw conveniently placed by the register. The words "gluten-free" were highlighted, front and center.

Obviously, it was full of chemicals, but I was curious and picked one up. Flipping over the perfectly portioned two-inch delightful looking square dark chocolate the first thing I checked to see was how many sugars were in it. And there it was. Thirty-four grams. It was a magnificent moment for me. I smiled with confidence at the cashier and said *no thank you* as I put it back.

Before I started that sugar challenge, I might have gladly eaten it. Well, probably not. Due to the paragraph of chemicals. But it was getting easier for me to see sugar *and* let it go—now that I know. I felt jacked, I was no longer ignorant, and I didn't even need the coffee. Organically I was caring about myself even more.

In my opinion, the number of grams listed on the label is practically useless—without knowing how much sugar is actually appropriate for someone to take in on a daily basis. And it didn't take long to see that I had graduated from that particular fast-food restaurant, with enormous pride. From deep inside, I smiled again when I told my husband that I could no longer eat there. And the one positive I found as we were walking back to the car—I could still enjoy their delicious black coffee anytime I wanted to.

The podcast clip I was submitting for a potential broadcasting award this time was from a show I did on suicide prevention. The subject came up on the ride and I said to my husband, "I didn't want to die all those years ago—I was only 16. That one afternoon had spiraled out of control just from simply feeling what many teens feel—a little invisible."

Whether we are kids or adults, it is quite a journey to find our own place of individual human balance in this great big world. And I was finally finding that balance for myself. I can see it happening in my kids too. Even when they disappear into their rooms to claim some distance or a little independence, they still have the desire to be seen and heard.

Young adults and teens especially are in a constant mode of discovering who they are at their core—along with who they want to be. And they hold tight to that urge to be different—even though the acorn doesn't ever fall very far from the tree. The truth is, I shook my own tree all those years ago, and I almost destroyed it. Today, I feel pretty darn grateful to be able to watch each of my acorns turn into beautiful trees—planted all around me.

Day 306: Sunday, August 5th

Cleaning my youngest son's room to get ready for back to school, we found a miniature tin still sealed with shortbread cookies in it from his Christmas stocking the year before. Listed under sugar it said eight grams in a single three-cookie serving. And I was excited by actually discovering a cookie with low sugar for the kids. Yay me!

Elated by the bonus find, we unsealed the container together and gave the cookies a try. I closed my eyes and savored the flavor until a few bites were already in and I said, "Oh shit!" quickly tossing the rest of my cookie back into the aluminum. It wasn't gluten-free.

Constantly, I ask myself the question: What do I want? My most recent answer: *What I want is to have so much love for myself, that sticking to the guidelines that I have created—is easier than breaking them.* Just like the way I threw that cookie back into the aluminum tin.

Day 307: Monday, August 6th

When I discovered the actual amount of sugar that I was taking in—I was mortified. I knew I wasn't eating doughnut holes or mini candy bars every day—not even before my love diet. But after all these years of working so hard to eat cleaner and thinking I was eating healthier I didn't even think twice about the amount of sugar that was hiding in my food.

Straight out of the gate that seemingly little simple sugar challenge was staggering, and I was disgusted. Not at the quantities of sugar that I found, but more because the sugar that I was finding—*was in everything that I was eating.* And then when I came full circle to learn exactly how many grams of sugar a woman is supposed to take in on a daily basis—it was the icing on the cake. Counting every little one, two, and three grams of sugar throughout each day was adding up quickly, and it was mind-boggling to think that my body might have acquired an addiction to it.

Although I was already showing signs of better health by removing most sugar, abstaining from sugar completely might lead to withdrawal, deeper cravings, and yes, quite possibly—binging. If I wasn't eating doughnut holes and candy bars before my love diet, I might just resort to them now, especially if I tried to cut myself off from sugar completely.

Stripping my body 100 percent from anything that I had been feeding it for years was not a good idea. No wonder I kept quitting diets! They were all designed to remove sugar—all at once. It clearly wasn't realistic, and it isn't a short or long-term solution. I love myself. And weaning myself off over time—in my opinion—was the only way to reduce the majority of sugar from my body—and my mind.

Uncontroversially, sugar affects the brain in the same way that drugs do. And we have so much compassion for those who struggle with any addiction to drugs that we support weaning them off in safe environments—usually under the supervision of medical doctors and psychiatric care. To insist anyone, remove sugar all at once from their diet, could practically be considered inhumane.

I don't know much about the brain, but I'm a fast study, so I educated myself. The first thing that came up in my quick little brain search was that little thing we've all learned about at one time or another—dopamine.

What I read and finally understood was that dopamine acts as an informant. Apparently, it's a chemical released by our nerve cells that sends signals to other nerve cells, teaching our brains to want to repeat pleasurable experiences. And our brains build up tolerances, aka desires, to those pleasurable behaviors—whatever they happen to be. Humph.

Our bodies are so smart. And it just so happens that sugar is extremely susceptible to increasing our dopamine levels—*just like drugs*. The brain evidently has several dopamine pathways too, so it's a lot to think about. But let's face it—dopamine is a buzzword. It's been tossed around so much over the years it seems to have lost most of its power. Like that sad little shrunken birthday party balloon found three days later behind the couch. *Oh yeah, there's that dopamine.*

My life is complicated enough, and I need simplicity. I also love myself dearly and I knew that there was no way I was going to put my body through any sugar-removing shock-therapy. That's just torture. And dopamine is a messenger. So, I want to increase it—not kill it. So, to keep it simple I figured all I needed to do was stay focused on reducing my sugar, while simultaneously increasing my dopamine levels in healthier ways. Like listening to music, eating plenty of protein, meditating, and yes, exercising.

All of the decisions I had made and worked on over these last 307 days were paramount to preparing a good foundation for me to actually be able to take on that sugar challenge. *Can I get a Hallelujah!* Come to think of it, had I been introduced to that sugar challenge on Day 1, or even on Day 90—I'm not sure if I would have been ready. And removing all sugars, just like all carbs or all dairy—all at once—*was not realistic for me. What was realistic and achievable—was to keep introducing or reducing—one thing at a time until I nailed it.*

Day 308: Tuesday, August 7th

While my first cup of coffee was brewing, I washed a few dishes then took my phone out to the shade garden to write. My routine continued with a meditation, followed by a dance workout, shower, and breakfast. After making another cup of coffee I was finally ready to head into my home office around ten o'clock.

I was beginning to understand the real significance of putting myself first every day—in every way. Not just around food. I didn't just get it. I was living it. My desires had flipped. And I was refusing to step one foot into my office—until I got several of my "me hours" in first. And those "me hours" were starting to take me well into the late morning.

The first time I mentioned my new routine and concept about my *me hours* to a woman I knew in passing, I got the most unbelievable look. Maybe it was shock or perhaps it was fear. But in the seconds I looked into her eyes, I could feel that she wished she could do the same, if the box she had put herself in wasn't so deep. And climbing out on her own now or asking for help may not have been a visible or practical option either.

But why should opening an email or sending one come before loving myself at the start of each new day? Why should checking into social media immediately upon waking—come before meditation, exercise, or even feeding my body nutrition? *What was it about me—that made me believe—that my personal morning routine had to begin with other people?*

When I first started taking this journey and writing this book, I shared how 20-minutes of yoga followed by 20-minutes of meditation, or vice versa, was like a thorn in my side. I was open about how I constantly had to shift and keep working at putting myself first and clearly, I struggled with it. Now, my morning routine of pouring energy into myself has organically grown to nearly three to four times the size of what I was trying so desperately to force myself to do. *And that was only ten months ago.*

The thorn had indeed shifted—to be anything preventing me from loving myself first. Putting myself above everything and everyone else was the key to my mental health. Of course, I knew that doing things like meditating and exercising was *what I had to do* in order to feed myself more love. *But now it's what I want to do.* When I wake up in the morning, I want to spend my morning with me and fill up my cup first. Whether I start with coffee, nature, writing, meditation, dance, breakfast, or even all of the above—what matters to me is my love.

Day 309: Wednesday, August 8th

We all want what we want yesterday. And I was working hard each and every day so that I can have what I want today, and tomorrow. And what I want is to have a fit body—inside and out. Right now and in my future. I want to walk up the stairs alone when I'm over 100 in heels—without holding the railing. They might be one-inch kitten heels but still.

My virtual dancing coach said if I want to have a fit body, *I* have to be the one to move it. No one else can move my butt for me. I was becoming a believer—while I was doing it. I had about two weeks of incorporating dance almost daily into my routine and I was starting to look forward to it.

I'm sure the way I move my body now will look a little differently than when I'm older. I may not be able to dance the same way as I do now or clean out the garage with the same amount of vigor, but I will be doing something. Whether it's dancing, yoga, or moving plants and light furniture—*when I'm lucky enough to spend a few of my end-of-life years living in an assisted living facility, I want to be the one moving my own body.*

Day 310: Thursday, August 9th

Perhaps dairy wasn't the devil after all. And gluten might not be the beast society portrayed it to be either. The cruel monster I likely needed to run far away from—was sugar.

When I first became gluten-free a few people had mentioned to me that it may help my skin and right at the beginning, I had a great incentive to stick with it. By becoming gluten-free I was avoiding a variety of baked good temptations too—which was already helping to reduce a lot of the sugar hidden in my diet. So living an almost gluten-free life was a really great place to start. And now that I was becoming more aware and paying closer attention to where the sugar lies, it was starting to show in my face—and I was beginning to seal my own fate.

Doing what works for me I know is the key to longevity. And the simple act of incorporating a variety of music to my dance workouts was helping me shake it up—a lot. Everything I was doing was working. So far so good. But I couldn't help but wonder would surrendering to what works for me continue to work?

I'm a Sagittarius and I can tend to get bored easily with routine. So, I asked myself the question about what I want again, but in more detail. Would I be able to continue this path, for the rest of my life? Was eating gluten-free, reducing sugar, and dancing all sustainable? A really good answer popped up into my head; *Our bodies crave what we feed it.*

My husband and I took ourselves to our new favorite farm-to-table restaurant for dinner and it was delicious. Salmon, risotto, and a few complimentary lobster lettuce cups. *Delish!*

Day 311: Friday, August 10th

Out of pure curiosity, I took a leap of faith and tried on some clothes I hadn't worn in a really long time. I was feeling good about how I was feeding my body. And I thought for sure I would be elated by something, since I had been dancing for a few weeks.

I would have taken a tight zipper close or at least one almost closing. But the clothes that I thought would close didn't even come close. It felt like nothing had changed. To say that I was disappointed was an understatement. I was crushed. But I had an appointment at the dermatologist to look forward to. So, I surrendered to one of my typical go-to outfits.

I was excited to talk about my skin and to receive some real professional insight, advice, and solutions about anything and everything. When I arrived the two nurses asked me the standard question, "So what brought you in today?" Naturally, I mentioned everything I could think of. Opening up the floodgates to let it all flow comes pretty easily to me. Must be from all that therapy. I was happy to share and talk about the one thing I was an expert on, me.

When the doctor came in and asked the same question, I repeated a similar song and dance. But I had forgotten to mention one important thing that I originally revealed to the nurses. And it didn't dawn on me until I was clicking the button to open my car door. It was like once I put the information out into the air the first time—mentally it felt like some of the issues were

I AM ON A LOVE DIET

addressed and even resolved. Huh. Sort of like when I used to say that I was going to start exercising and eating healthier.

At this appointment, I mentioned to the nurse and assistant the importance of addressing the bumps that appeared on two of my fingers. When the doctor came in, I completely forgot about it. Even though the assistants were typing away all of the information I had shared the first time, they didn't fill in the gaps for me either. That's so extra.

I was getting so frustrated with myself each time I kept repeating the pattern. What I really needed to do was stop being an entertainer at each appointment and become more of a manager. The changes that were happening in my knuckles were probably attributed to aging or some kind of early onset of arthritis, but I was doing my best to not self-diagnose. And discussing my issues at the time of a preventative visit—does not a hypochondriac make. Everything is important. And I think the rational solution for me going forward is to bring a shortlist to every visit—that way no bump ever goes unturned.

Day 312: Saturday, August 11th

Another baby shower was on our calendar for my daughter and me to attend and of course, I wondered what they would serve. There were plenty of pancakes and bacon, and luckily for me, they had eggs.

My love diet list was getting long, but it was actually easy to follow. I hardly ever had the need to look at the list. It was easy to remember because every diet rule I was creating for myself was coming from a place of love. Every choice I was making—and what notably landed onto each of my plates—generally led the discussion toward the human diet wherever I went too. Of course it did. At our table, we got into a great conversation about the powerful information I learned about sugar. I couldn't help but share it with the people I love.

Next on our agenda was my daughter's simple birthday sleepover. I picked up the usual pizza, popcorn, and cake but "forgot" to buy the soda. Oopsies. I did, however, give the girls unlimited access to my awesome homemade soda water maker as a quick alternative. We usually get a regular cake, but this year my daughter insisted on having the old-fashioned ice cream kind. Which didn't matter to me since I wasn't going to eat it anyway and ironically, the cake melted.

Regardless of how small her party was, it was her birthday, so we readily threw good money after bad and ran out to pick up another one. Hardly any of the party food was on my love diet list, but I wasn't really craving ice cream or pizza, so it wasn't a big deal. The popcorn, however, was a different story. During the course of the evening, I found myself eating that popcorn in heaping amounts like there was no tomorrow.

The good news was that I was being mindful and stopped. And the other good news—the actual ratio of bringing good food into our home vs. junk had shifted. What used to be 40/60 had changed to more like 85/15. And it started with taking back the grocery shopping and budget around it.

My son Reece even said he was glad that they still got to eat some of the fun junk food they love, but he appreciated learning about healthier organic options and also lower-in-sugar ones through my many findings. Gratitude was finding its way back into our house on a regular basis. I was purchasing less food and more often. So much so, that we hardly ever needed the fridge in the garage. The so-called second icebox that had melted the cake.

Day 313: Sunday, August 12th

We waited for the last of the sleepover pickups to wrap up and enjoyed a lazy day hanging out, lounging around watching movies. My routine was thrown off a bit, but I still got in some writing, and a dance workout too.

Day 314: Monday, August 13th

My dance routine was becoming my daily dose of medication. And when any feelings of depression set in—the one thing I always know——the feelings always go. I believe I have accepted the emotion for what it is, and it helps to know deep down in my core that it will pass. One of my favorite quotes is the one about how nothing lasts forever. And I like to hear those words as a positive.

What helps me get through to the other side—is to pour my attention into doing things that I love. Dancing lifts me up and it was keeping the feelings of depression in check and at bay and with every new day—peace is always waiting there for me, readily available. All I have to do is decide to embrace it.

Day 315: Tuesday, August 14th

Purposefully, I trimmed down my servings of fruit each day down to one to two berries. It wasn't easy to do, but I was eating smarter and not willing to sacrifice most of my daily grams of sugar—all in one place.

I also deduced the banana portion I chose to toss into my protein shakes from one half down to one quarter. I know it may seem extreme, especially since bananas are a whole food, but for me, I felt like I was just being highly aware and diligent. And I knew I was bound to shrink in size by every little bit of sugar reducing I tried.

The curiosity was building each time I walked into the bathroom and saw crystal just sitting there. It's not a crystal ball I know, but I would look over at her and wonder if I felt light enough and worthy of a check. It had been about a month, but I was still trying to wait until the end of my journaling journal experiment on Day 365.

Instead of stepping on it, which I may or may not have been disappointed by, I looked in the mirror and studied my body. Without any clothes on I did see a slight difference. My body was changing oh so subtly and some of my body fat looked like it may have been turning ever so slightly into muscle.

One pound of muscle weighs exactly the same as one pound of fat. But I have learned that muscle actually takes up less space than fat. And I found a great visual for that. One tangerine equates to one pound of muscle, while one pound of fat is roughly the size of a grapefruit. Ahh grapefruit. I do like to eat them, but only on occasion. *A grapefruit diet is not realistic. A love diet is personal.*

Day 316: Wednesday, August 15th

Self-care can look like a few things for me and currently it comes in the form of meditation and dance. My new rituals do continue to shift but I absolutely love how they generally take up at least two hours or more, each morning.

Working from my home office can be a challenge for someone like me who has that infamous undiagnosed ADD. A simple thought that pops into my head can send me darting out of my chair and diving into a drawer, closet, or dryer. Needless to say, it has become imperative for me to work on my self-care early in the day, to be sure that caring for my own body and mental health doesn't get overlooked once, twice, or three times for this lady.

Building my "me" time into my day first was such a smart thing for me to do. And refusing to step one foot in my office until at least ten o'clock felt good to turn my end-of-day from four o'clock to five.

Fridays are practically becoming an entire "me" day as well as the occasional Saturday morning. I needed to because I was adding more writing into the mix. My me time was transitioning to more family time too. The more I pour time, aka love, into my self-care regime, the more I wanted to have more of it. Living life doesn't mean I have to grind my fingers to the bone—just because I work from home.

Watching an Oprah video, she said, "If you are not in the driver's seat of your own life—your life will drive you." It gave me the confirmation that I was indeed on the right road. I love starting each day with a huge focus and awareness on self-care, peace, and love. I know I have a purpose to motivate and lead. But I was also meant to live and breathe, dream and achieve. Albeit I was moving at a snail's pace, I was the driving force behind my own life.

During my mid-month grocery shop, I wanted to get only the bare necessities to feed my family of six. I was curious to see if our bill could land below $300 and it did with $40 to spare.

The groceries would last about two weeks and we'd only have to replenish a few small items like milk and fresh vegetables. The thing that was most impressive was that I hardly got any packaged pantry or frozen food at all. About 95 percent of everything I put in my cart was pretty darn healthy including mostly proteins, veggies, brown rice, and potatoes.

Walking toward the checkout aisle I passed some granola bars that used to be one of my favorites. And just for kicks I turned one over to read the sugar content. This one only had five grams, which was better than most seemingly gluten-free granola bars and snacks that pretended to be healthy.

The brand I was holding had a low sugar content and it was almost all whole food inside. It's not a bad thing if it's an occasional thing. You know, once in a long while. But I was eating them almost daily—thinking I was eating my way to healthy. Until I discovered the recommended daily amount of sugar that is appropriate. Once again, the nutritional numbers on the back are practically useless.

Day 317: Thursday, August 16th

Beginning with a great meeting, an awesome interview, and a lunch connect, my day was filled with amazing energy and ended with a boat cruise in the harbor.

I offered to be the one in charge of the food of course. It does make good sense for the people who have sensitivities or allergies to be the ones taking care of it. I placed the vegetables, olives, cheese and gluten-free crackers front and center and put a small basket of regular crackers in the back for a back-up.

My catering skills always come in handy for events such as these and when I mentioned to one of the guests that the gluten-free choices were on the main platter, and the non-gluten-free food was placed in a separate basket in the back, she was surprised because most people give the sensitive food an almost forgotten after-thought and I had switched the bait. It made perfect sense to me though and it's something we could all be doing more of. Place the dangerous food in a separate location in the back and even add a scarlet letter.

Day 318: Friday, August 17th

My youngest son Duke and I drove to Hyannis to look at a pre-owned car. I had purchased a few cars by myself in my life. Even in my twenties and I thrived on the feeling of accomplishment. Especially the way society deemed the act almost unachievable for a woman. I would turn the tables even further by beginning the conversation about anything but color.

It was so insulting to me as a woman, when the sales guy started our relationship that way. By asking me about the smallest detail of what color I was looking for felt so demeaning and sexist like we were standing smack in the middle of the fifties. There were so many other things to take into consideration that were more important like can my stroller fit in the back and how many radio stations can I set. Color was practically last on my list and hardly the driving force behind any decision I made. My focus was more about functionality and mileage. As if the only thing we women care about is the freaking color of the car or that it matched our purse. *Geesh.*

I wanted to purchase a car based equally on function as well as color and style. And the car I found online had a great big fat sold sticker on it when we arrived. Ironically, I had just led a mini-mastermind meeting with an exercise about manifesting what we want. And there I was, test-driving something else that I could care less about.

Nonetheless, it was still an action step leading me closer to where I wanted to be. And what was now more importantly at the top of my short list—was finding a vehicle with really good energy.

Day 319: Saturday, August 18th

Listening to the soft drops of rain sprinkle onto the umbrella on our deck brought me straight back to the recent days of when we were camping. Our little family vacation where I had learned a lot about where the sugar lied.

I went back into the house to make myself a simple breakfast and together my son and I examined the cereal box. It did only have one gram of sugar, however, looking further at the milk I noticed that it contained 12 grams per serving. What the heck? *At 50 years old, I had absolutely no idea that there was sugar—lurking inside dairy.*

Lactose was something I knew nothing about. But in the simplest of terms, what I learned was that it's the sugar that naturally occurs in the milk's process that gives it the sweet taste. And people that have a lactose intolerance don't have enough lactase, which is the enzyme our bodies use to break down the lactose in order to absorb it.

Furthermore, I learned that lactase helps turn lactose into two things: glucose and galactose. It's common knowledge on the web. And one of the funny things was that the difference between glucose and galactose is that one sits on the right side of the molecule while the other sits on the left. Holy converting compound cat-woman, even on a cellular level we've got a left, and right wing*!*

I AM ON A LOVE DIET

But here's the thing. For the body, glucose is the primary source of energy, and in fact, is the sole energy source for the brain. No pussy-footing around. It's important. And if our bodies in fact need glucose to survive, we have to be absolutely sure to have plenty of naturally occurring sugars clinging to the masses of our asses.

But where do we find good sources of glucose besides dairy? And how stupid does it sound to ask if a restaurant has a galactose special or ask for a little glucose on the side. Once again, my good friend carbohydrate flew into view. Glucose is of course found in bread, pasta, potatoes, rice, vegetables and fruit as well as fish, meat, cheese, and peanut butter proteins along with fats like butter, dressings, olive oil, and avocado.

Aside from the fruit and dressings, the listed sources were good news to me. Luckily, my love diet consisted of all those things. And it was a good lesson for me to learn about how sweet the body can be. I didn't need to live my life lactose-free because I wasn't intolerant. So I took a raincheck on mastering the proper dose of lactose. And as it turned out, all I had to do was continue reducing processed food. Overall, I was grateful to pay closer attention—to the human body and its broader spectrum.

Peacefully, I took a nice deep breath and continued finishing the remainder of my cereal with almond milk outside. The cool breeze had finally broken the heat wave and brought a smile to my face. I was planning a special afternoon celebrating my daughter's and mother's birthdays. And later, we went out for our traditional family "day-of" birthday dinner.

While everyone dove into the complimentary sourdough rolls, I ordered the gluten-free pizza crust with some marinara sauce for dipping. We all ordered pizza for our main course, and once again, mine was made from their gluten-free crust. It was another nice night, but I was more than full. And once again, before we even left the restaurant I was already beyond bloated.

What the heck did I just feed my body? I did my best to count up everything I ate, on the proprietary napkin this time, and the approximate number of sugars that were hiding in my food. Both pizza and tomato sauces had lots of sugar, as did the cheese, and the crust. I didn't eat all of my appetizer, but I did eat almost all of my entire single serving size pizza.

In one sitting, I think it was safe to say that I had consumed over 20 grams of sugar. Everything I ate was processed and surely whatever levels of sugar I had in my body had spiked. No wonder I felt bloated. Processed sugar was literally making me fat.

Day 320: Sunday, August 19th

It had been about four to five years since I took the time to help my husband out by giving his closet a thorough cleaning. And it was the perfect rainy day to tackle the task. But was it really a gift—to do it for him?

Don't we all need to go through and clean out our own stuff? I had gone through so much over these past eight months and it was clear as day to me—that I was the one who needed to do my own re-org. By cleaning up my mind, with my body, and through my spirit.

Day 321: Monday, August 20th

My closet was clean.

And the reason I cleaned it was because I care. Beyond my body, I want to care about every aspect of my life. And the simple act of cleaning my closet feels good. Any closet is the perfect place to put the stuff I can't seem to let go of. Or hide the things I don't want other people to see. But it feels good to look at what's really going on and take in the inventory. Especially at the precise moment when it's easier to close the door and walk away.

My clothes weren't falling off, but they were fitting better. Especially after accepting that sugar challenge. And exercising was part of it too. During my workouts I was reaching beyond 15 minutes and even dancing up to 45. Mentally and physically, subtle changes were happening.

I was still using my mirror instead of stepping onto my scale, but piece by piece, every little action step I took was making a difference and filtering through, each time I took the time and cared.

Day 322: Tuesday, August 21st

When I first began my journey, I couldn't even think about wasting any of my precious time trying to meditate or do yoga. My instinct was to pour my attention into my business and family. I was always directing my energy into where I thought it "should" be.

Somewhere I read that it's critical to have a routine each morning at the start of the day. But all the complaining I did about exercise, meditating or anything else in my life that needed my attention was in fact, what was keeping me stuck.

As luck would have it, there wasn't ever very much leftover energy, and it became even easier to avoid me. The escape is always temporary though because reality eventually will show up. And through this mindful journey, it finally clicked for me. I made the decision to start my day with me and to use the time in my one life more wisely.

Day 323: Wednesday, August 22nd

The mirror had been my only measuring tool since our summer vacation, and I hadn't given in to my scale yet. The temptation was still there because crystal was still there. But with each passing thought that showed up, I let it go. I swore I was down at least eight to ten pounds, but I was embracing the why's behind my thoughts and asking myself; did I really needed to see the number?

Dancing was my new thing and it was something I was finally sticking with. It had been almost a month of letting go of most sugar and I was so sure my body was adjusting from working out too. Each time I saw the scale, I looked into the mirror to find some love instead.

I was eating and being smarter, not working harder. And working smarter helped open up my afternoon to take the kids back-to-school shopping.

Day 324: Thursday, August 23rd

It is interesting how that table had turned. I was pouring more attention into me and everything else in my life was falling into place energetically.

At my morning meeting, I introduced a new twist, and everyone loved it. Driving to the radio station, I felt like I was literally floating on cloud nine.

I AM ON A LOVE DIET

Chapter 16
Embracing My Why

"And I was curious to see how my body would react, and how I would feel without a perpetual medicinal mask."

Day 325: Friday, August 24th

After spraying my ass with hand sanitizer, I walked out of the restroom and back into the food court to find my son Reece. The chicken didn't look very appetizing through the glass and I was so close to skipping over it, but I said yes please to the barely fresh or grilled when the nice man pointed excitedly to it. We had just hiked several blocks to find a place to eat and would have to hike the same distance back plus some, so I knew my body needed something that resembled the likes of a protein.

  Eating the first few bites of my fast deli food salad I realized I had no carb, so I walked back over to the counter and bought two small bags of potato chips, highly hoping he wouldn't want one. I have to say, it felt really good to sneak in a "bad for you" kind of food once in a while—especially when unforeseen circumstances allowed for it.

Loudly, I whispered, "Do you want any cookies?" to my son who was already sitting at the table enjoying his massive hoagie. Cookies are one of the treats I have no hesitation giving in to for my kids. That and brownies. Well, come to think of it—cake too. Surprisingly, he said no thank you and later told me that he stopped adding sugar to his coffee. Wow. I guess all that guilt I poured into him about paying a few thousand dollars out of my pocket for his dental work was really paying off.

Satisfied with my simulated salad I was ready to burn off my little bag and a half of chips and we walked over to admissions together to meet my husband. It was a slight change in the original plan, which was to meet him at one of the train stations in Boston. But we missed ours and had to make the drive into the city.

I was not particularly fond of the train idea to begin with, and caught myself saying quite a few times in the weeks leading up to the college tour date, "Oh, and if we miss the train…" So, when we raced into the parking lot and heard the horn sound as the train started to pull away—I wasn't surprised. It's funny how my subconscious mind was the one steering us. Driving into the city must have been plan A all along.

They were taking the train home together to practice though just in case it was the college he chose. So when the tour was almost over, I said goodbye. As I was pulling up to the first light I said a quick traffic-less prayer to myself and noticed at least 15-20 homeless men and women gathered on the sidewalk. The tired drooping fence—their built-in couch.

Luckily, it wasn't raining. Some of them were sleeping on the ground and some were clustered in seemingly intent conversations. I assumed the one man slightly bent over while walking toward a huddled few was discreetly getting his fix—hidden in plain sight.

Many emotions came over me as I let go of my silly little highway prayer. Strong emotions like fear, guilt, compassion, pity, gratitude, and even shame. They looked dazed and confused, struggling with each and every aching moment. I wasn't struggling nearly to that degree but over the years my problems had accumulated to something a little more than mediocre. My challenges were of a different scale, *and they got me to thinking—what was my drug?* Sugar? Carbs? Wine? Or maybe even worse—*Victimization.*

Back at home, before dropping my son off at a restaurant to put in an application, I said goodbye and then I love you. He returned the sentiments by saying I love you back and wrapped his words inside a gift by saying it louder than expected—openly in plain sight.

Day 326: Saturday, August 25th

My guided meditation by Deepak-Oprah was all about the power of unbounded awareness. It was brilliant and unleashed an even broader understanding for me.

Scooting out to the dealership, I was on a mission this time. My car was long overdue for a trade and I made a conscious decision to find a lemon-less one. Seeing that I practically live in my car as an entrepreneur, I wanted to invest in something that would increase my energy this time—along with my desire to keep it.

Practicing what I preach and letting go of my ego, I was ready to look for a car with colors that were right for me. Colors that were actually in alignment with my personality and boosted my unique energy. My current car was perfect for someone else—like my daughter. She loves white.

My car had a flat stark white exterior and a tolerable charcoal interior. It was not me. I don't even wear white. If I were to swing over to the side of gratitude though, the previous car I was driving depleted me inside and out with layers upon layers of light-grey sucking energy. So at least I wasn't driving that.

I was on the hunt for something very specific. An off-white, sparkly diamond coated SUV with a soft camel or sweet caramel interior. I thought it was a great goal. "But you're looking for a needle in a haystack," my husband said to me very "un-secretly." His self-imposed limiting belief was not mine though and I knew I could manifest what I wanted. I found that other needle and it was only two state-stacks away in Maine—waiting for me.

The manifestation was physically possible. Just like the cranberry jumpsuit outfit in my closet that was waiting for me too. The thrift store find is one of the visuals that I hold up often and dream of wearing in my everyday eight-hour four-inch, toddler-less heels and I couldn't wait for that day when it would almost be too big. A fall day perhaps, to a brunch or lunch. I could adorn my oversized outfit with some really cute stockings, ankle boots, and a mildly warm scarf that almost didn't match in that wicked cool European way.

When I told my husband about manifesting my body into that short jumper ensemble, he said, "Yeah, you used to wear some really hot outfits." I wanted to smack him upside his head, but instead—I said, "Yeah, and you used to have a head full of Gregg Brady hair." Checkmate.

As it turned out, that needle in the Maine haystack didn't fit my numbers at all. So, I opened up my mind to needle number two. Perhaps the real deal was the second one that still sparkled in the sun. The beautiful cranberry one. It was in a much closer haystack too, only 30 minutes away. And it was more beautiful up close and personal than it was online. It had a multi-colored tan and brown interior that made the metal shine like gold. And it was just shy of three-years-old.

This time when I dropped my son Logan off for his interview, I returned the gift by saying I love you to him, louder and prouder.

Day 327: Sunday, August 26th

Staycations are something I would love to have more of and over the weekend I was literally smelling my own roses.

Perhaps if we owned a pool, we would see our backyard more clearly as the oasis that it is. But a pool is merely a conduit to pour more love and attention into myself and my family. And that was something I could do, *and have*, any time I wanted. It's still a great thing to have on my bucket list though, along with wearing that barely-there, age-appropriate one-piece—without the unnecessary body-shaming of course.

It takes practice though, to master living mindfully in the present moment. And I was making the effort to live in that beautiful space of unbounded awareness. But I am still learning the art. And it appears the paintbrush doesn't ever truly get put down.

Nicole Perry

Day 328: Monday, August 27th

It was coming down to the wire with only 37 days left of my love diet journaling experiment. And I felt like I was slipping away from optimism to pessimism. Sure, revealing the many ups and downs that I've experienced throughout my journey was part of this process, but we all know—the proof as they say—is in the pudding. And in my case, there was still too much of it.

In my opinion, detoxing still resembles the likeness of another outward drive-thru fix and can be just as seductive as a diet. Engaging in a detox wasn't in my original plan nor was it anywhere on my radar. But desperation was rearing its ugly head again and in the eleventh hour, I was looking for an easier button. Engaging in a detox felt like the swing vote or the last-minute hanging chad. In that moment of weakness, on Day 328, I was resorting to the idea of a foxy detox.

Bringing my mind to a higher state of consciousness while reaping the rewards of an inner body cleanse felt like a reasonable intention and of course it was sincere. But I was rationalizing. Because in my mind, any effort to detox also came with a higher expectation of receiving an incidental bonus of slimming down and losing weight.

It's probably safe to say that most women have opted into some type of detox at least once in their life. And a typical detox suggests participating in many things—all at once. Like drinking a lot more water than we usually do, eliminating processed and refined foods, steering clear of carbs or anything white, going gluten-free and/or dairy-free, removing alcohol and sugar, letting go of caffeine, and getting more active. That's a whole lot of shit. And already, I was doing most of it.

Slowly, I was eliminating what wasn't good for me—and introducing better and kinder foods filled with more love. Some could even go so far as to say that my love diet is in fact, a one-year-long detoxing journey. But there was one thing I hadn't considered removing yet—and it wasn't caffeine.

For what it's worth when my love diet began, I never had any intentions of letting go of my friend Chardonnay from Monterey. And believe you me, I am just as surprised as anyone that I was even considering it. But like many other women, mothers, and really, people, it was the crowning vice for me that ruled over all other vices. And the fact that I was taking a moment to look a little closer into my personal consumption of the adult-beverage called wine—was actually love in disguise.

Cleaning my body up from many other toxins was organically happening anyway. And as much as I liked living like a refugee at the end of a long hard day, I thought why not give it a let-go. I had no real plan other than to make the simple decision to eliminate wine from my diet for a few days. Alcohol could actually be playing a part in why the weight wasn't coming off as quickly as I thought. *And I was curious to see how my body would react, and how I would feel without a perpetual medicinal mask.*

Day 329: Tuesday, August 28th

The tables had turned. I wasn't quite sure what to expect because this time I was the guest. But I embodied a sense of humility because I was grateful for the invitation and excited for whatever the experience would bring.

Once I had arrived, the stress of the drive was over. But the oppressive heat wave grabbed hold of my face as I got out of the car and took the less than one-minute walk into the building. I did my very best impression of a person trying to perspire as little as possible and as I made my way inside, immediately I looked for a place to powder my pits. My face had practically fallen off too and I wondered if it was all worth it. As I walked up the stairs, I hoped that anyone I met would kindly forgive the ginormous pit stains on my satin blouse right along with me.

Settling into the air conditioning I placed my focus back on my story and my business. Marketing is all about energy and I brought it to the broadcasting table and to the microphone when it was time to turn it on. Overall, it was a good experience and helped me to see podcasting through a new set of eyes.

A variety of turkey and veggie burgers along with chicken sausage were on our family menu for dinner and I gave the eclectic proteins uniformity by popping a tray of homemade french fries into the oven with olive oil and sea salt. I used to make fries the exact same way so begrudgingly as a teen.

We hated having to lift a finger when we were kids and loved everything that came from a frozen bag. Individually-quick-frozen, aka IQF, is the term I learned in my twenties when I was a sales rep and worked for Kraft. For the restauranteur, IQF was ideal but it was ideal for any kid growing up in the '70s too and it continues to be what most people reach for today. Now that I'm an adult on a better path to a healthier body—making my own baked french fries is one of the easiest go-to vegetable sides.

I was doing everything I could to love myself more and it was all indeed my own choice. But I was allowing myself a little extra sugar in the form of ketchup on my plate since I wasn't having any wine. Sugar is by far the most talked-about food topic in our home, so of course, they knew they were preaching to the choir when they tossed in their relentless two cents. And from their peanut gallery view, the opportunity was too good to let go of. They couldn't help but poke a little fun at my perfectless meal and pile on with their opinions. And it was only wineless day two throwing my panties in a bunch.

On a constant ongoing daily basis, I was making the effort to love myself more and I was making huge strides. I was on such a good path toward finding more balance and I may detox my body and mind more often along with reducing sugar.

Ketchup was one of those things that I was eating less of but suddenly had tripled in size on my plate. I couldn't let their musings instigate a sense of panic in my psyche though. So, very openly with a hint of sarcasm, I gave myself the verbal compassion they weren't giving to me.

I could still use a little more fine-tuning how I react to other people's comments about the choices that I make. I know. But I had to remind myself that I was doing my best through this little detoxing experiment and I was only conducting a test. Had I not felt a sense of urgency coming to the end of my journaling journey, I wouldn't have thought twice about their broadcasted opinions—or let them into my system.

Day 330: Wednesday, August 29th

The only thing I knew about analyzing sleep came from watching a Laverne and Shirley guinea pig episode. It was really just a sleep deprivation study though in the form of a comedy as well as a major fasting followed by a formal gathering looking for Mr. Right. *I* was just an ordinary woman looking for ways to love myself more.

In any case, whether physically or mentally, the lack thereof or plenty of will eventually show up. And anyone can venture to guess what one would have to remove in order to improve one's sleep.

The shortlist is probably in alignment with a simple detox. And at the top of that list is absolutely caffeine. But the one or two restaurant-style cups I drink each day was hardly worth the consideration to remove. And since I was already removing the majority of sugar from my diet, realistically, alcohol was next on my agenda to reduce.

One of my favorite red wine accomplices is chocolate. And chocolate is one of those fabulous foods that contain caffeine and sugar. Seventy percent or higher is what I always try to buy and to only eat a few squares after lunch. Nice and early so the caffeine wears off. It was only during those start and stop dieting years that I would stop and start eating chocolate. And when I removed the good chocolate there were plenty of other less healthy sugar substitutes that would work their way in.

We all know what happens when we remove something we love from our diet. And even though I couldn't remember the last time I had chocolate; now was the perfect time to bring it back because I was removing wine. The bottom line—simply testing out the wineless waters was the least I could do to feed myself more love. And bringing back dark chocolate was a good idea, especially in the form of a dove.

Day 331: Thursday, August 30th

Working from home helps make the end of summer taste so sweet. And like most women entrepreneurs with kids, the end of

I AM ON A LOVE DIET

August is one of the best times of the year to come out from the woodwork to network.

Free lunches hinged to seminars had replaced the days of door-to-door selling a long time ago. And the meeting I was invited to was about a variety of relevant topics to me. It wasn't just about a free lunch. I wanted to attend. I had turned 50 and one of my four kids was in college. Organically, planning for my future in smarter ways was what I was already getting more curious about.

The meeting was thought provoking and got the wheels in my head turning on every dime. I was drinking their Kool-Aid and wanted to sign up for everything under their sun. But like most people in a similar situation, I already had too much on my plate.

Putting my desires on the back burner where I knew they would begin to collect dust didn't feel good to me. But it was only temporary. I still wanted to put a better plan in place for myself and the seed had been planted. My mind was slowly growing toward the direction of how to love my money by making it more futuristic.

This time my mother-in-law served pork for dinner. I was grateful that it wasn't redrum raw and I was lucky that she usually serves green vegetables and potatoes with her meals. But when it came time for dessert, I knew she had no idea how much sugar she was about to serve her loved ones.

From the dining table, I could see her in the open kitchen cutting the double chocolate layer cake giving every plate a giant slice. A large heaping scoop of ice cream was placed on each side and she topped off every dish with even more whipped cream and chocolate sauce. In my mind I counted up the sugars easily.

And each plate was in the range of 40 grams at least—maybe upwards of 60.

My mother-in-law grew up in the '40s and '50s and raised her husband and family in the '60s. So of course, serving dessert to her family with a lovely meal is the love she knew. I imagine those were the days you were expected to make an exception for dessert, which was practically a daily thing. And she served her two to three course meals with love.

I wondered just how many meals she had to skip throughout the years to accommodate and still be able to tie her apron in a bow. Serving foods that are filled with additives bad for the body and basically addictive is not easy to stop doing—or even to see. But it was clear to me. From where I sat, those plates of sugar were the opposite of love. No matter how home baked it was.

I didn't want to eat it and my body was not equipped with a 1950's foundation of fewer chemicals in it either. I sat there watching and wishing I had learned about the dangers of sugar a long time ago and had been able to share that knowledge with her. I wished someone had taught her that sugar is the root cause of cancer. Or maybe it's that cancer feeds off sugar. Either way, if she knew how bad sugar was, she may have thought twice about feeding it to the people she loved.

Feeding our loved ones is love. And eating the food we are kindly served is also love. But I said no thank you to that 40 gram or more chocolate cake dessert and poured myself another glass of wine with the built-in modest two grams of sugar instead. I had already loved myself by going three days without.

It was not my intention to insult or reject, but I was on a better path of eating more cleanly and I only wanted to enjoy the evening by consuming as little sugar as possible. At the table though, I took every judgmental dart to the heart and did my best to stand strong in my decision to not eat something at the risk of my own demise, just to make everyone feel more comfortable.

Day 332: Friday, August 31st

Sometimes the families that eat together—cheat together. And our extended families can play a significant role in our lives, whatever dietary path we are on. The question is, how do I help my family understand gracefully—that I no longer wish to cheat on love?

My decisions have everything to do with my health and nothing to do with anyone else's choices or cooking. It shouldn't matter what I do, when I do it, or for how long, because if I am loving myself in a new way, nothing else should matter. Even if the decisions I make are fleeting, so be it. At least I'm on a better path toward a healthier body. But where does the protocol fall? And what is the dietary refresh etiquette? How do we move on with our families without placing unrealistic demands on any given host without abandoning our own principles or employ compromises to our guests without diminishing theirs?

What I'm doing is simply changing a part of my life by what I choose to put in my body. And in doing so, some of my beliefs had shifted. What was good for the goose was no longer good for this gander. Still, it remained a challenge for me to continually explain why I was choosing not to eat steak, pork or dessert. My intention was not to insult anyone else's choices or cooking and I certainly wasn't dessert or meat-shaming, but I tell you what; I sure did feel wine and veggie-shamed.

I couldn't even imagine if I became a real vegetarian. Or worse, a vegan. But my main focus remained the same, which was getting my cholesterol under control, through tweaking my diet, instead of taking a pill. The proteins and sugars that I used to eat had in fact, become toxic for my body. And that's all that should have mattered.

We all know that some things are easier said than done. And we have to be considerate and not cross that very fine line that lies between our immediate and extended families in this reality game of life. All I wanted was to be mindful about my diet during our family visit, and not give up on myself so easily, just to be polite. *I had done enough of that already.*

Remaining cautious was all I really had done by not eating anything that was not in alignment with my plan. I had no desire to eat what they were eating anyway, but I couldn't help but to ask myself; Was I missing out? Would eating those foods carry me safely into my future? And were their choices truly the luxury they claimed them to be? Or was the proclaimed luxury just a way to free the guilty?

Our family visit was what it was because we are who we are. And the only person I can control is me. It wasn't easy to change to new ways. and change alone can easily introduce stress and anxiety. Which is why I was doing everything I could to introduce and eliminate each new concept or idea slowly and carefully. My diet simply had changed. And through the eyes of an outsider it could have been considered unnecessary or even complicated.

The evening with our family did provoke many questions for me. Like was it disrespectful to serve food knowing that your guests can't eat it? Or was it disrespectful not to take a "no thank you" helping? I think it's all up for debate. But even if there are people in my life who continue to serve the very food that I can't eat, well, that's not on me. I think my love diet is easy. And my mission is stronger than ever; to continue this path of feeding my body cleaner love.

Day 333: Saturday, September 1st

My husband and I had a light sushi dinner and I hardly needed to eat any of it. Seriously, this love diet had to be working.

Day 334: 194 lbs. Sunday, September 2nd

It was already well into the morning. I had two cups of coffee and a light breakfast. Still, the temptation to check my weight was strong. She was almost done shaving her legs in the sink when I jokingly said to my daughter, "How about if I blindfold myself and you can check the number for me?" But as I was getting ready to hop in the shower, I realized how silly that sounded. And if I were to be somewhat clothed, I was still torn—between getting back to my old habit, and apprehensive to see the mysterious number.

My energy had shifted, and I could feel a tinge of depression setting in. It was the perfect opportunity to spend the day snuggling up with a blanket and watching movies. So, I decided to do just that. Tuck myself away from family and even from work or writing and deposit myself into a few chick flicks. I wanted to collect my thoughts and emotions around why I was letting outside energy dictate how I felt.

Giving myself permission to dial it back and take a mental health day in the comfort of my own home—was pure love. But as soon as my in-laws picked up the kids for a late breakfast, I did it. I stepped on my scale for the first time since we left for our vacation. And it was not the mind-blowing reveal that I was hoping it would be.

Day 335: Monday, September 3rd

My plan was to drive my son Logan to his new dorm room in my new-to-me SUV and then head back home to spend the day with the rest of my family.

My energy wavered with every inch of pavement under my tires between dropping my son off blahs and back over to recycled car bliss. I sincerely wanted to keep my car this time, beyond the two or three years I typically did, and I arrived back home to chicken being cooked on the grill while we all admired our latest family decision.

Day 336: 192.5 lbs. Tuesday, September 4th

On July 3rd I had weighed in at 199 pounds so the new number of 192.5 pounds must be the real shift that was happening. My body had taken eight months to recover from the copper and could finally be off the recovery road and crossing into newly reclaimed territory.

I must be back on track. I had been dancing since late July, almost six weeks of daily consecutive dancing and sometimes I did it twice. It was only a few pounds but surely I would be looking back at this moment as a pivotal and major one inside my love diet.

His lily-livered words stung as they clung to my awareness. It was a short video I happened upon by Dr. Oz. and I got sucked in when he said, "If your liver is not happy, then losing weight will not be easy." Was my liver indeed the next organ in need of a cleanse?

Day 337: Wednesday, September 5th

Everyone was back to school and at the office, so I spent a few minutes sitting at the island after they all left.

I poked around on social media falling immediately down one giant rabbit holding hole after another and started to watch something extremely interesting. Dr. Gundry was explaining the thing called lectin and how it was not good for the gut at all and that one of the top four foods that are in fact, high in lectin, tomatoes ranked number one. Evidently they can also cause issues in the skin.

Rosacea is something I had lived with for well over two decades and was just about to give up some spices next to help reduce the inflammation in my face, so this new information was quite revolutionary to me. We had just cooked ourselves a tomato sauce-based meal the night before and ironically, when I woke up my acne was flaring up again.

The video I watched continued to intrigue me because evidently foods that are higher in lectin can wreak havoc on the stomach. Looking down from my computer screen to my plate of scrambled eggs I was eating, the three grape tomatoes on my plate were staring back at me. And the other items on the shortlist higher in lectins were eggplant and peppers. So far, all of those vegetable foods were staples in my diet.

Another item the doctor mentioned that was high in lectin were beans. Which I thought was worth investigating further since most vegetarians and vegans appear to be healthy and beans are a staple in their diets. Cashews were also on his list, and were in fact, not a nut, but a bean. How did I not know this? There is so much I don't know. And the final item he mentioned was whole grains.

Particularly brown bread and whole grain are significantly higher in lectin. Which brought me to my next thought; Was my body actually feeling better because I had been cutting out grains in the form of gluten, that were actually lectins?

Day 338: Thursday, September 6th

The newest addition to my love diet. Try to live mindfully and as much as I can—lectin-free, before officially adding it to my love diet list.

Our meeting was held at a restaurant and the chef brought out a slow-baked pear drizzled in local honey and infused with gorgonzola and pecans. It was delicious but it was not on my low animal fat or low sugar plan. And to top it off, it wasn't lectin-free either.

Not giving myself room to breathe was not living a life filled with love either. Sometimes rules are meant to be broken. It's only when the broken rule becomes the new rule. *That's where the danger lies.* It's a good plan to allow for the unexpected, as long as I am still respecting.

We made chicken and broccoli stir-fry for dinner and I found a good enough recipe to follow and only had to replace the soy.

Day 339: Friday, September 7th

On a phone call with my mom I did my best to explain my newest lectin-free discovery and she warned me that we do need some bacteria in our bodies. I get that. But, it's another big butt, sometimes the acne that I have actually hurts and feels more like an infection. So, if choosing to eat a "mostly" lectin-free diet may help my skin get more consistent, and be less painful, well, what can I say?

Choosing to let go of tomato-based foods was a huge decision for me. It wasn't easy but it was a good one. I was light years ahead of where I was eleven months ago. I had come farther than I ever could have imagined and acquired more information about the human body and diet than I ever thought I would. And yet, there is still so much more to learn.

I love tomatoes. And pizza, salsa, hot sauce, ketchup, etc. but it just might be the red foods causing the red rosacea on my face. Deciding to eat a diet filled with mostly greens was not a bad idea at all. And like everything else I have tried; I was just going to give this a try.

Trying one thing at a time and seeing how it goes is such a good idea. One change at a time. And for me, eliminating something 100 percent hardly ever stays at 100 percent. For me, all I want to do is try to love myself in new ways.

Day 340: Saturday, September 8th

I am shrinking. My clothes are fitting better, and I can wear two pairs of slacks that I haven't worn in about two years including the skinny grey size 12 slacks that I felt so good in.

At our farm-to-table dinner date night, ordering dinner was getting a little trickier. There were more foods I needed to eliminate that were high in Lectin. Talking with my husband I told him that I wouldn't be able to eat the crunchy almond nut butter I had just purchased either, because it had cashews in it. He just sighed.

I read almost every single label from every single product I look at, but why didn't I turn this label around to see what was in it? Was it because I assumed almond peanut butter was made purely from almonds?

Parmesan cheese was the next thing to discover that was not lectin-free and I was devastated. No Romano either. Starting a list of lectin-free exceptions was looking pretty good right now. And even if I did eliminate most of them and allow a few, I was loving my body better.

Day 341: Sunday, September 9th

I have one word for this day. Football. So, I took my glass of sparkling water over to reality television and snuggled up to Big Brother.

Day 342: Monday, September 10th

Monday. It was a hard day for some reason. The energy of the universe was not aligned with me. Or vice versa. I felt like I couldn't make a single decision and I am such an action person! Typically, I am the queen of decision making—most of the time both personally and professionally. I love to hit the send button! But something in me was off.

Day 343 Tuesday, September 11th

In a pinch I had to work around what they offered during the lunch-and-learn because I completely forgot to bring my brown bag. I made the best of the situation, but it was still frustrating.

While I was focusing on eating better and consuming only the healthiest nutrition for my body, I had to work with what was in front of me. And the invitation to eat white bread deli sandwiches, soda and bags of chips for sides held very little to be desired. It had taken me over eleven months to get to the positive mindset and place I was at around food, but why did it feel like I was the only one who was trying.

The lunch looked lovely and very typical, but there wasn't anything remotely healthy. I think people have a theory that if it's not fried food then it must be healthy. It felt like I was the only fish swimming against the current.

Along my journey to eating more cleanly, I wished and prayed that more people would want to work on their nutrition like I was. I wished I didn't have to work around the rest of the world and the world was divinely working with me. I was grateful though for the egg salad option and scooped out the innards from the gluten-filled bun onto my plate. And I started to eat the popcorn from the bag and realized it was drenched in fake white cheddar.

Day 344: Wednesday, September 12th

My peanut butter breakfast toast had come a long way from what I used to make. The first transition began with letting go of the kids' white bread and switching back to wheat. Then I moved on to gluten-free, to lectin-free, and now also using my new soy-free butter. And the crunchy almond nut butter that I was just finishing up, that may or may not stay.

The point really is that I was still enjoying some of the same things that I had been for years, but everything just looked a little different now. A little more sophisticated and grown up. My taste buds were adjusting pretty darn fast too and I was sure they would continue. The human diet is such an ever-changing process.

When I got home from my board meeting, I enjoyed some beet chips with artichoke dip while watching a little TV with my daughter.

Chapter 17
The Calm Before the New Norm

"Had I done nothing different over this last year, or worse, signed up for a bunch of trendy diets, I wouldn't have learned nearly as much as I did or likely changed anything at all."

Day 345: Thursday, September 13th

His meal looked fantastic. It was a gourmet pizza and a fairly healthy one. Not one of those greasy large pizzas with a crust stuffed with God only knows what. It was a flatbread that was topped with ricotta, sausage, and leafy basil pesto. His cholesterol was not perfect, but his healthy HDL was through the roof. He didn't have a single issue with his weight aside from getting older—so he was eating what he loved.

Honestly, I wasn't jealous at all. My husband was enjoying something I no longer had any desire to eat and I was happy for him. But to coin myself as "happy" was not quite the correct term. I was feeling more content than anything else. My mind was completely focused on eating my meal—which was a salad, and I was immersed in our conversation—which was lovely. No matter how gourmet his pizza was, I didn't wish I could eat what he was eating. I had absolutely no signs of animosity toward him or anyone else for that matter. And I didn't even wish it was gluten-free.

I used to think pizza was sort of healthy and I ate it routinely, automatically, and even mindlessly. But it really is one of the worst foods we consume as Americans. The crust is processed, not typically gluten-free, the sauce is full of sugar and the cheese is definitely not good for anyone cholesterol challenged. Pizza was not love. And at that very moment, I realized *pizza* no longer held any power over me. With a family full of people who all love it, it wasn't easy to even think about letting it go. But as it turned out, it was possible—and I was free.

Throughout these past several months, I noticed a few people making a snarky comment or two about my healthier choices or smaller portions and each time I just laughed it off, chiming in here and there pretending I didn't care. But like sticks and stones that can break my bones, their words no longer diverted me. I don't feel deprived when people are eating the foods I no longer choose to eat, because like Janet Jackson—I was in control.

Maybe floating their thoughts into the air are just little tests to see if I can easily be swayed or pulled back in. In the beginning, I let that happen a few times with bacon. But living in a sea of uncertainty wasn't healthy. *And removing pizza from my diet or any other food similar thereof—wasn't a punishment*

I was inflicting upon myself—it was a lifesaver I handed to myself. A life-line that arrived in divine timing.

Day 346: Friday, September 14th

Before picking my son Logan up at his dorm room, I stopped to get myself a small salad with chicken and avocado and ate just a little very carefully in my awesome new energy-infused SUV.

While waiting, I thought about all of the journaling I had done in the last year and how quickly it flew by. Everything I did from the start was out of pure necessity. *And I had to hear every piece of news, the way I heard it, in order to see it the way I needed to see it. Then and only then, was I able to change my diet the way I needed to change it.*

Reducing my sodium to begin the process of healing my heart was the beginning. And that first discovery paled in comparison to the everyday challenge of working at lowering my cholesterol. Then came making the decision to cut out gluten, which came with so many benefits. And even though it was scary finding out about the Copper IUD—I was so grateful that I did. I can only imagine what I would look and feel like had I not started those wellness visits in the first place.

Everything I have learned has led me to so much accumulated progress, and it was all equally significant. Each simple step I took revealed even more hope. I was a good student and had taught myself well. But above all, the most meaningful discovery was the amount of sugar that I was taking in—that most people take in. That most manufacturers put in.

My eyes had been opened to the simple notion that putting my body into motion could actually be whatever I wanted it to be—and I finally found what worked for me. If I wanted to, I could have even more dancing diversity. I was only down about six pounds and my ego hurt, but the truth is curt—my mind was what needed to change first.

All of the changes I made led me to create my own personalized diet and exercise plan that has been the most elementary, realistic, and adaptable plan that I could have ever imagined. It was something I had practically searched for my entire life. And all I had to do was respect myself with a little more love.

When we got back home from my son's dorm, I ate the rest of my salad and blocked out several hours in the afternoon to get some work done. The turkey burgers I made for dinner came out a little dry, so we came up with a great idea to add some of my homemade breadcrumbs to them the next time. It's easy to whip together in the Cuisinart and I make it with only a few ingredients: gluten-free rice bread, olive oil, onion powder, garlic, parsley, salt, and pepper. We wouldn't add as much to the burgers as one typically would to a meatloaf, but just enough to make our burgers juicier again.

Day 347: Saturday, September 15th

Stopping only briefly to make myself a quick egg-over-easy with a slice of gluten-free toast I added a little goat cheddar in between the two layers. I squeezed in a small sweet potato with butter, salt and pepper and a handful of walnuts later for a snack. Saturday mornings are practically pressure-less, and I was getting quite a bit accomplished.

Switching gears my husband and I decided to do the family grocery shopping together. It was something we rarely did and for the first time in ages, it was actually kind of fun. We were in sync with each other and shared tips and tricks about where to find certain healthier items. Whizzing through each aisle we made the most of our time while still keeping our recipes in mind.

It was very different from how we used to shop together. Which is why we usually tackled the task separately. When the kids were little, I was the one who used to do most of the shopping of course. And as the kids grew older, I got a reprieve once in a while if I needed some help and asked. A few of those helpful shops turned into many and inevitably, my husband took over the grocery shopping chore completely. He liked it. But little did I know how happy he was about "chipping in."

He loves buying the food and would come home excited to show me the great things he found, but what was interesting in his mind was altogether different than mine. I was the one who had to cook our dinners with what he bought. And stranger things started to make their way into our home—pulling me far out of my comfort zone. Weird things like octopus, monkfish, and smelly cheeses.

When I caught wind of what he was doing I got smarter sending a kid or two with him to "help." And that's when the real junk food purchases started to work their way in. I found myself running in circles of gratitude when he left, hoping when we unpacked, followed by frustration until the next time. The one consistent positive—the food bill was significantly smaller because the "interesting" and "junk" foods were always cheaper.

Since I took the reins back over, the paradigm shifted. There are far fewer junk or weird items to work with and my husband was grateful not to have to go. He was also glad that I was bringing home some things that were less than boring and passed the entire family taste buds test. The kids were grateful too because I wasn't eliminating their junk food 100 percent.

Overall, our little shop together was not so horrible. I had a little pep in my step each aisle we walked down, and I danced a little in my seat on the car ride home. Life is good indeed, living with love.

Day 348: Sunday, September 16th

Whether it's funk, disco, or hip-hop, if it's got a great beat and you can dance to it—I'll probably love it. Even slower songs will work to get me going and in the mood of moving my body. And boy did I move around my bedroom like I was giving the best 30-minute performance of my life. Someday I'll tape it.

Dancing has struck a chord with me. And even though I did plenty of dancing in clubs when I was younger and then a fair amount at the occasional wedding as I aged, the simple concept that dancing could be my workout was revolutionary. I love to dance! And now that I am in tune with dancing actually being my exercise of choice, the memories of the moves from the workout machines made their way into my mind and my muscles were falling back into line.

Real exercise was working its way back into my life and introducing dance revealed layers of benefits. I was slimming down. I was more agile, which would help tremendously as I age. But it was also helping my brain and played a huge role in diminishing the feelings of depression that seeped in every now and again. I can't even listen to music without having the desire to get up and dance. Similar to yoga, I was feeling strong, flexible and practically limitless.

My workout was fantastic. I was beyond proud of myself and couldn't wait to dive headfirst into my day, letting the positive energy I exuded spill out into the world. My mental health was heightened and jumping into the shower, I was elated to every degree, high on life and simplicity. Then I reached for the shampoo and there was none.

Day 349: Monday, September 17th

The new school year had barely begun and already my son was sick and had to stay home. It isn't easy being a mother and I didn't sign up for it thinking it would be. But I have to admit—it is easier to be a mother—who happens to be an entrepreneur.

Being there for our kids was what made sense to us. So, my husband and I made the decision early on with our firstborn son that I would be their caregiver and I gratefully adapted to the term stay-at-home mom. But I needed more than binky fairy lessons and I wanted more than discussions on why an egg won't become a baby chick living in your sock drawer—no matter how many times you try or how many days you leave it in there. So, I embraced becoming a homemaker.

When I stopped hoarding the dramatic energy inside of me and started to pour it into decorating my home and cooking for my family, I owned it. When other families were going on Disney vacations and weekend trips to Six Flags—I was buying furniture and cooking up Today show recipes after watching my stories. Overall, becoming a parent has been the most challenging role I have ever had the pleasure of knowing.

Deciding to be the caregiver to our children was easy for me. It wasn't until I made the decision to share a dark part of my history with my kids as they got older that was hard. A few years back I came out to my kids about being a suicide attempt survivor. With the subject of suicide coming up a few times on the news and having to explain it at the dinner table—sharing my story felt like the right thing to do. It was important to me—for them to hear it from me. I wanted them to understand that my attempt all those years ago was simply a part of my past that has led me to who I am today. Everyone has a past. And I had embraced mine. It felt good to tell them that I love myself, that I want to live, and that I want them to want to live too—for a very long time.

It also felt really good to point out the obvious—that we all make mistakes. And that this particular mistake from my past was a huge one. I wanted them to know from me that without question—it was an erroneous decision and it wasn't the answer. And finally, I wanted them to know that the one single event from my past did not define me as a person, who happens to be their mother, but it did let them know that I am human.

Day 350: Tuesday, September 18th

The days were getting shorter, so I sat outside soaking it in and focused on being in the present moment. I let go of my past, but as the end of my journaling journey got closer, I was getting tangled up in my future. I couldn't help myself.

My legacy was something that I was thinking about more and more. I had spent my twenties finding myself and my thirties raising a family. When I reached my forties the desire to circle back to having a career was strong. Now that I'm in my fifties—my legacy and embracing my life purpose were both taking the stage.

The old pictures on our walls of generations before us told me many stories without even knowing most of my ancestors. But what were their portrait eyes saying? And what stories would be told to the generations to come through my eyes behind the looking glass? Had I done my part in placing my little stamp on our planet? What would my grandchildren and their children know about me by looking at my photos through their frames? And how could I ensure that I would be a positive influence in their lives long after I'm gone?

Luckily, I had more than pictures to leave behind. But still, I kept asking myself, was I doing enough? Or had I spent more time worrying about when to have my floors redone than being fully present about what I was doing while walking on them.

Day 351: Wednesday, September 19th

My intuition is generally spot-on, and I've easily let it guide me as I age. I want to listen to my own instincts and it usually takes me in the best direction. Even when it doesn't, I know it's still the best direction I was meant to go in. But on occasion, my inner guide can lead me down a storytelling road.

There's such a fine line that can get crossed—when the intuition I receive leads me to the story I believe in my head. Sometimes I can't help it. It's humanly natural to want to fill in the blanks. But filling in the blanks about why people do what they do and did what they did are just that. Stories. And sometimes, like the portraits on my walls, it's just easier to jump past my intuition—and finish the untold story. Closure feels good.

Day 352: Thursday, September 20th

It wasn't an ideal breakfast, but it was better than eating nothing. I needed something fast so just before running out the door I grabbed what I had; a frozen, gluten-free, coconut ice cream sandwich. *Yum.*

I enjoyed a lighter and more practical lunch with some egg salad lettuce wraps and a side of radishes while searching the top ten foods to avoid if you have rosacea. The list was long but similar to when I first perused the world wide web on the subject about 25 years ago when the net was in its terrible twos. From what I remembered nothing really changed. Coffee and hot tea beverages were ridiculously high on the list and practically unrealistic for any adult to avoid. Of course, spicy foods were on the list along with citrus, chocolate, and cinnamon. Everything was listed as "rosacea aggravators" and one item on the list that I had been fully aware of was red wine.

I was already at risk for developing rosacea just by being a woman with somewhat fair skin. But looking at the list made me feel like I was faced with having to remove several staples from my diet in order to change what was happening to my skin. And removing all the items didn't feel realistic. Come on, cinnamon?

Some of the aggravators went beyond food and included everyday stuff like being exposed to sunlight and wind, extreme temperature changes, and of course my favorite—emotions. I had already resigned to living with flush and saving a few bucks on blush. But the cute little pinkish cheeks that began when I was in my mid-twenties after a brisk sun-filled day skiing had evolved. And I wondered what was considered a real aggravation for me and my body. Aside from being aggravated by the suggestion to remove a ton of stuff I loved.

My husband is a huge advocate of vitamins and we talk about the benefits of vitamin D a lot in our home. Our kids all take it when they see any signs of acne flaring up and I thought it would be next on my list to bring back. But here's the thing.

I AM ON A LOVE DIET

Taking anything on a daily basis hasn't really worked for me. I've tried every pill-popping, plastic convenient Monday through Friday tray there was. Which is why I was changing my diet to begin with—by treating my body with the food I put in it.

For the first time in years, I noticed something else that was different. It may seem insignificant to the average person but for me it was very interesting. My elbows felt smooth and silky. They used to be cracked like I had dermatitis or something. And what I noticed may be another sign that what I was already doing was, in fact, working. A subtle sign but possibly a huge one.

I was so grateful that I noticed how healthy and almost buttery soft they felt. It was a little strange to think that just because my elbows were a little dry and scratchy that it might be an underlying sign that something else was going on. But it's true. And it is quite remarkable to be able to see the little signs that our bodies show us that give us the clues to what's really going on. So, if I did have dermatitis, it was yet another auto-immune issue.

When my dermatologist checked my elbows, he agreed that they looked good. And then I told him that my face was looking much better too—and there was probably no need to do anything.

The makeup coverup job I was used to putting on each day was like that of a pro and I knew I should have removed my makeup to show him what my face *really* looked like. But I was too embarrassed to let anyone see my skin in its most-rare form. Scared and ashamed.

If he saw my face naked, reddish-purple and raw—there's no doubt in my mind that he would have prescribed medication. Likely with a sense of urgency too. But whether it's over the counter or not, I was still refusing to believe that a topical Band-Aid cream was the final solution for me. And I was willing to temporarily cover-up and conceal—than to surrender to a mask of medication.

Day 353: 191.5 lbs. Friday, September 21st

Holding the towel rack ever so slightly before stepping onto it— I placed my right foot first. Only letting go after gently placing my left foot. It was a very delicate daily dance. And I used to do it several times until I got my final number to keep in check with my progress.

I was smack back into my old habit and asked myself; How many times would stepping on and off a scale would be considered obsessive-compulsive? Maybe the better question to ask myself would be whether the routine was helping me or in fact, holding me back—which led me to my next question. Was sharing all of my personal thoughts about my scale and my routine of weighing in actually helpful to the reader. It's not like I had come up with a solution.

When I arrived at the networking lunch, I wasn't even hungry. I had a late breakfast, so I chose to listen to my body and hold off eating until I felt hungry again. Feed my body only when I actually need to. What a concept. Magically, my old skinny grey slacks that arrived from the dry cleaners fit like a glove.

Day 354: 191 lbs. Saturday, September 22nd

I was so organized I actually had a little extra time on my hands, so I baked some gluten-free muffins. They were, of course, lectin-free, but I still wasn't sure if sticking with the new theory of eating a lectin-free diet was the right thing for me. It was however, worth it to keep going a little while longer if only for the benefit of my skin.

My life was starting to fall into place. The kids were getting settled back into school and I was getting organized. I was nesting too and getting caught up on work. I felt like I could breathe easy and relax a little. I was back to my work-at-home mode and it felt good. My clothes were starting to fit better and get looser. Weighing in at 191 pounds—I was finally starting to see the light.

Day 355: 190 lbs. Sunday, September 23rd

Weighing myself several times before getting an acceptable pre-coffee reading was taking the term obsessive-compulsive to an entirely new level of disorder. Each day my routine involved a pre- and post-elimination check. Stripping off every ounce of clothing and jewelry and before standing buck naked on my scale, I was really hoping to make it to 189, but I didn't reach the inspirational number, which would have been more outside proof that represented progress achieved.

Eating less of the nightshade vegetables was the latest food diet fad going around and I bought into it. Day 365 was fast approaching, as well as a fair amount of fear and anxiety about where I was going and where this was all taking me. I was resorting back to finding an easy button to get slimmer in less than ten days. It's amazing how I was openly looking for it and how I gravitated right to it.

Resorting back to the old limiting belief that the stuff "out there" was going to fix my "in here" was not good. Even after almost an entire year of creating my own mind-and-body customized diet that was helping me to transform. Convincing myself that foods higher in lectin were the reason for the rosacea was a reasonable rationalization—and getting skinnier was the incidental bonus.

Getting the skinny on the lectins wasn't the easiest thing to figure out either, but what I did understand was that we have both good and bad bacteria in our gut. And eating foods that are higher in lectins can "eat away" at the good bacteria, which is the one we want to increase, not reduce. I also read that different lectin foods can do different things, which made learning about the pros and cons even trickier.

When I stripped the lectin stuff down to the bare basics, it was the seeds and skin found in the nightshade vegetables like tomatoes, peppers, eggplant, and potatoes that can-do damage to our gut. And still, on my path to higher self-love, I have to take everything with a grain of salt.

It just isn't my life purpose to become a scientist or professional chef and I didn't have the time or energy to change my career path again. So, *until I learned otherwise*, the best thing I can do on my journey to better health and having a sound mind, body, and soul, is to run with what I know.

The fact of the matter is—removing tomatoes, peppers, eggplant or potatoes from my diet—is hardly life-threatening. And I decided I was okay with continuing to test the lectin-free waters. The only question that I kept asking myself was would I truly find happiness becoming lectin-free, or was it just another thing to trick me on my journey?

Day 356: 190 lbs. Monday, September 24th

Not being able to sit outside was bringing my spirits down a little and my inflamed rosacea wasn't helping. To help lift my mood I treated myself to a couple of gluten-free muffins to start my day. I was fully aware of how sometimes depression can hit me when I least expect it so very early on in the day, I thought it would be a good decision to abstain from having any wine with dinner.

I didn't want to feed my depression, so I thought it was a perfect time to abstain and once again, see how my body would feel through the lesson. Obviously, alcohol is a stimulant, but only when consumed in the way of moderation. And when it isn't, it can easily transition and become a depressant.

Day 357: 191.5 lbs. Tuesday, September 25th

After dropping my kids off at the bus stop, I looked up into the rearview mirror on my way back home and saw the word "Hi" drawn into the dust on my window. Which let a long-overdue smile come through. Then, after parking the car in the garage, and walking toward the back of my car to wipe it off I saw "suck dick" directly below it. *Lovely.*

Combing through the last day or so I realized I wasn't in the best of spirits. And I may have said or done something to one of my kids that frustrated them enough to lash out passive-aggressively. I felt bad about not being able to control my own emotional descent and I was even hoping that it wasn't one of my kids who did it. But then another thought occurred to me. Maybe it was a sign.

Within vulnerability there is freedom. I believe that. And the old mindset that I have carried with me for years was almost gone. I was embracing a new healthier one and it had taken quite a lot of time and effort to get myself unstuck from the old ways of thinking. And they may never be completely gone. It's all still a journey. And like many, loving myself 100 percent didn't come naturally to me, because I have been chained to a variety of limiting beliefs. But I was getting so close to being free. And I knew that freedom was somewhere in here waiting for me.

The immaculate conception marked the beginning of my journey and carried me through to that sugar challenge—all the way to this day. I learned about what I can let go of by teaching myself how to live with love by eating healthier. And to feel better about my body by giving myself all that I can give. In doing so—the real journey organically began.

Public humiliation was never an ideal driving force for me. It didn't help me want to do better or work harder; it was merely an incentive to hide. No matter how much desire was with me at the start—the embarrassment of it all toyed with my heart. In my mind it was easier to recline. And it was a blessing in disguise to find a fresh new perspective around exercise.

The dance workout I found was real and changed my view about how I could be moving my body. Every day I was stepping into my new starring role and gave it my all. Of course, there were a few times that I didn't feel like doing the workout at all. And it wasn't easy to ignore the old voice taunting me to quit. And how going back to doing nothing was far more appropriate. Especially when an unflattering image of my fat would fill up the mirror as I passed. It wasn't easy to stop judging myself, but I kept the music turned up on high. My unchoreographed workouts got easier and I started to remember some of the movements from a typical workout machine and organically worked them into my clumsy routine.

Looking at my body with love in my eyes I began to care about the workout clothes I wore and did my best to embrace my thick core. In many subtle ways, I was inspiring my own positive mental health strategy. And the changes I started to see were slowly working their way into my psyche. I was beginning to see the light and it was getting brighter. I persevered through the mess and exercised my heart with finesse. On the other side, I found forgiveness.

After almost twelve months of many major moments of self-discovery, my personal puzzle was still not complete. I wish I could say that I love my whole self; 100 percent. I want to. I really do. But there's no point in lying to myself. I am getting there. And I love many pieces of me. But I know that before I can love myself whole-heartedly, I have to embrace yet even more vulnerability. This has been by far the most eye-opening experience for me. To make this journey to the center of my worth, while I still have plenty of time left here on earth.

Sautéing some frozen turkey meat without hormones or antibiotics into a pan with plenty of olive oil, I added some salt and cracked black pepper. Then I sprinkled in only a little parsley. Since eliminating a lot of foods higher in lectin, it appeared that I had to avoid mostly red foods and spices. And I was happy to eat mostly green foods to help my skin turn olive again.

Everyone was fine about adding in their own taco seasoning because I was avoiding cayenne and paprika. I layered my lettuce first into the small bowl, then added some ground turkey, a few black olives, guacamole with fresh basil, leftover rice and our new substitute for sour cream—plain yogurt. My taco salad was delicious, and everyone enjoyed theirs with taco shells. The meal has always been a big hit for everyone in my home, and I was falling in love with taco night again.

Day 358: 190.5 lbs. Wednesday, September 26th

Our taco night spilled into brunch. I had a networking thing and had to leave early in the afternoon, so I brought some easy almonds with me for a snack. I brought walnuts too because they were of course lectin-free. So I brought them back into my diet. Nuts are not the best thing for a woman getting long in the tooth, but I was no stranger to flossing and driving.

Day 359: Thursday, September 27th

Literally, there was not a single thing I could eat at the breakfast meeting that I paid for. It was a hotel, so it was sort of continental. And their breakfast had nothing conducive to my new love diet.

But I had to eat food. I had to feed my body love. Starving myself was not an option. I stuck as tightly to my own rules as I could. *It's my diet and I can apply when I want to.* I don't have to box myself into such a tight corner that there's no wiggle room at all. That's not loving either. I gave myself the chemical egg omelette with the yellow fake cheese, two small pieces of potato and one slice of bacon. It was what it was. And I had to do what I had to do.

What I didn't do though, was seize it as an opportunity to swing the complete opposite of the pendulum, quit and dive into the well-known territories. And I didn't feel the least bit of guilt either. It was out of my control. I just hoped that someday, hotels would start serving more food with love and less sugary chemicals. Hotels are usually for vacations, which are for relaxing, not backtracking and weight gaining.

Treating myself to some baked haddock at lunch to balance out my breakfast, I thought I would have some asparagus with it and rice. A nice hot and healthy fish meal. The rice pilaf was a no-no though since it had orzo and I didn't see any other substitute on the menu. I was about to go without, but at the last second, I asked the waitress for some kalamata olives on the side to be sure I had plenty of healthy fats.

The weird look I received from the ladies was complimented by the whiplash from our server. I quickly explained the need for healthy fat and moved on. It wasn't ideal, but what was even more ridiculous than my weird olive choice was the fact that chefs can be so creative, but at the same time so fearful of people with allergens that they spice our foods with next to nothing—deducing me to using table salt.

We ordered a pizza delivery for the kids for dinner along with a side of onion rings, curly fries, and two cupcakes. For me, I opted for the Greek salad, with the very appropriate kalamata olives.

Day 360: 188.5 lbs. Friday, September 28th

Crystal took me by surprise. I stepped on and off several times before I could believe it. What I was doing WAS working! It took time for my body to adjust to the new ways of eating and eliminating the foods that were no longer serving me. *What it took was time.* And on day 360 I had come down a total of 14.5 pounds. Wow.

It felt really good. To reap the rewards of pouring all of that hard work and effort into myself. I took my own body and health into my own hands and I cleaned up my own act. On my own—with a little help. More importantly, I lived most of this journey without any outside quick fad diet fixes.

For lunch, I had my leftover Greek salad and realized that the pepperoni peppers I love so much were indeed a pepper, which meant they had seeds and skin and were high in lectin. I had to let them go—for the time being. Just like I let go of watermelon and walnuts. Every small change was just a test.

Even the detox was temporary. And the lectin-free, who knows. What I do know is that I have always known that I was on the right path, even when there weren't any obvious signs for me to grab hold of.

For dinner, we made delicious chicken tenders with basil, avocado, and sweet potato sides.

Day 361: 188 lbs. Saturday, September 29th

They were secretly hoping I would go away and leave them to their gaming, but I needed to brag. I was finally hitting a stride and down 15 pounds. When they mustered up a little too much enthusiasm, I caught their clue and moved on. They were happy for me though—but more that their mother was getting healthier and not sicker.

On the first day I was at a weight that I never thought I would be at without being pregnant. And then climbing up over 203 was so devastating to me. It was my personal rock bottom.

The weather was beautiful all weekend and I had my son's indoor senior portraits to shoot. I had a light hard-boiled egg and half of a sweet potato for breakfast. When we got back, I had two radishes and two celery stalks with my homemade guacamole dip. So, was what I was eating sustainable? The somewhat plain and limited eating style was bound to get boring quick. And healthy food can be fun and delicious. All I had to do was get a little creative.

Day 362: Sunday, September 30th

Caught between embarrassment and wit, I said good morning quickly to my husband and shared that I had diarrhea and was heading up to weigh myself. It's a gift and a curse all at once that OCD of mine. But I was coming to the end of my 365-day journey and my scale was still a crutch.

I needed it though, because I was filled with such joy and gratitude when I was beginning to see my body change in a new way. And beyond the number on my scale, I could almost see my vagina without lifting my stomach out of the way. It was the beginning of a glorious day.

Day 363: 189 lbs. Monday, October 1st

Day 365 was only two days away and I was flip-flopping back and forth from knowing I was on the right path, to again wondering if everything I was doing was worth it. Would it all eventually pay off to more than 13 to 15 pounds of lost weight? Why wasn't I prouder of myself? Why couldn't I feed myself more positive encouragement?

Because of the many years of self-sabotage that's why. And the recent self-criticism that was kicking me, was speaking louder to me that I still needed more time. I wondered what it would truly take for my thoughts to catch up with my body. And for my body to catch up with my thoughts again. I wondered how long I would have to go through these cycles before my mind and body would equalize? Thirty more pounds and another year or two? The fact that this wasn't really over was a little disheartening.

My process had been self-guinea-pigging. And I really needed to step it up for myself and be the best friend I needed to be for me. I had spent the better part of the entire year working on cleaning up my body from the inside out and had shed an amazing fourteen pounds. But yet, I was swinging back and forth from half full to half empty—more than I wanted to admit. And I was certain that there are plenty of women and even some men that were faced with the same amount of frustration.

Day 364: 189 lbs. Tuesday, October 2nd

After having some simple rice toast with an egg-over-easy for breakfast, I thought about what I would say to my board at our meeting. I was two months away from fulfilling the two-year term.

Stepping down from the role of President of the women's group was not an easy decision to make. Fulfilling the term didn't matter, in my heart I wanted to continue. But I knew it was time to stop pouring myself into everyone else and start pouring all of my energy into me.

So, I gave my final notice that at years' end I would be moving on. It was bitter-sweet, but it was time. I had poured my heart and soul into the group and every ounce of my time that I could give. And it was time to pour my attention and intention back toward me—wholeheartedly and into my personal journey. It was a tearful beginning of a two-month goodbye.

My energy and dedication had originally stemmed from believing in the longevity of the local group and all of the women who came before me. As I touched on how so many women came to appreciate the energy that I brought to the table, I knew it was time to go.

Day 365: 188.5 lbs. Wednesday, October 3rd

I did it. I journaled my way through 365 consecutive days, of feeding myself love. My first thought—thank God it's over! But here's the thing. It isn't over.

This is my love diet. A forever diet that I've created. And it will continue to shift and change and evolve. Everything I have chosen to put on my list organically filtered its way into my brain—and therefore has been easy for me to want to keep doing it and easy to remember.

Some of the things I had forgotten about like the 80 percent rule and the not eating carbs after 12 or 2 pm. But that's the shifting of it. It continues to shift until the important things that I really need to be mindful of, stick. The only thing that is really over is the daily journaling to discover the emotional attachment to the food I was eating, notating what I had been eating, and connecting the dots. And—my love diet continues.

Had I done nothing different over this last year, or worse, signed up for a bunch of trendy diets, I wouldn't have learned nearly as much as I did or likely changed anything at all. In fact, I'm certain I would have landed even higher than 203 pounds, and on my way to medication, or worse, diabetes, stroke, or a heart attack.

Shedding fourteen and a half pounds was not too shabby. I was grateful and thanked my lucky stars that I weighed in at a respectable weight less than 198. I had climbed down and then up a few times in the beginning and finally started to see the weight really let go around ten months in. In fact, all of the changes I had made took about ten months just to settle in. And my mindset has still not come full circle yet.

I don't know how much more time it will take for me to reach 100 percent of optimal self-love, and maybe that's the point. I love myself more than I ever have before. I am in control and I am living in a state of mindful awareness.

There's no going back to the way I was living before. There's no way I want to go back to ignoring salt, animal fat or sugar. At this moment in time, I know that I wouldn't dream of putting deli meat inside my body or even bacon. I have let go of the foods that no longer serve me for good because I want to. Because my body is becoming a sacred place of love.

Almost every meal on my plate, in my bowl and in my cup is filled with love. Binge eating is almost non-existent and if I do, I am fully present and aware. Turning the binging into smaller and more moderate binges have transformed and are even considered snacking. The journey of journaling the first 365 days is complete, but more journaling will continue. And the 365 days that I spent feeding myself love was just the beginning.

I spent the last 365th day doing the usual. I had an interview on the schedule, this time with a local actress. I was excited about it and during the interview one of my questions led me from asking if she would be willing to do anything—like play the lead role in my book—even if that meant putting on a fat suit.

Sitting alone at a local sandwich shop getting some work done afterward, I watched a barely 2-year-old little girl toddling around and wondered if someday she would be holding my book.

Nicole Perry

<u>*My Love Diet*</u>:

1) Feed Myself Love
    a. Is Love on My Plate, In My Bowl, In My Cup?
2) Minimize Sodium
    a. Remove High Sodium Caesar Salad
    b. Remove or Reduce Soups, Dressings, Sauces, Gravies and Dips.
3) Reduce Animal Fats
    a. Red Meat, Pork, Shrimp, Yogurt and Soft Cheeses
4) Be Mindful of Carbs
    a. Remove or Reduce to Size of Fist
5) Let go of Pizza
6) Remove Deli Meat
    a. Including Bacon, Sausage, Linguica, etc.
7) Live Gluten-Free
8) Exercise Any Amount—Three Times a Week
9) LOVE My Body as It Is Today
10) Eat Slower. Listen for the 80 Percent Tinge
11) Prioritize Meditation Daily
12) Reduce Sugar to Less Than 20 Grams Per Day.

I LOVE my diet!

Chapter 18
I Love My Diet!

"It feels good, now that my choices come without hesitation—and it feels even better to get a true taste of unconditional self-love."

From the beginning, I knew that creating my own diet was going to be a defining moment in my life. Slimming down, was of course, the original intention that held my attention. And during the process I wanted to quit several times, but each time I wanted to give in and give up, I picked myself up. And I am so grateful that I knew better and am extremely proud of myself for persevering.

My blatant honesty and putting myself out there was the blessing in disguise, because as soon as I discovered that my body was in fact, desperately in need of love and attention—in my mind—that's when my real love diet began.

Nicole Perry

THE SEED WAS PLANTED

Walking down to the mailbox with my two-year-old, first-born son Logan, I explained to him that the binky fairy was coming. We were expecting our second child and we had to pull that plug cold-turkey. I happened to be on the phone with my mom during that short walk and mentioned what we were doing. She said, "Wow, you should write a book."

I laughed, but I smiled just a little too at the thought of my being a writer. But what would I, Nicole Perry, write a book about? I've always done a fair amount of journaling, but beyond a little binky fairy insight, what did I have to say? I was just an at-home-mom all those years ago who had some semi-career success prior to becoming a mother.

Fast-forward to the year of 2017 in early October, that two-year-old boy was at his first year of college and I was writing my debut book.

It has hardly been easy, over these last several years of my adult life, shocking my body and removing the foods that inspire guilt and deprivation. And to quit almost every single diet I had ever started because I wasn't seeing the weight coming off fast enough, or at all. And through the first ten months of my love diet, it was no different.

Feeding my body with food that was not serving me was not love. And ignoring the signs my body was giving me by hiding behind makeup and clothes or even disappearing into glasses of wine was not love either. It wasn't even an illusion of love, but merely shielding myself with blame. Ultimately, I am the only one who can clean up my body and I had to do it from the inside out. The power within me finally started to come through—and now I feed that power—instead of the helpless emotional binging monster.

Never had I considered myself a victim of anything until I realized a few years ago that blaming and complaining was keeping me stuck in the victim mode. I had always thought my experiences in my life were just life lessons. But ignorance is bliss. And now that I can see that I was a victim of some circumstances, I wanted to transition out of victim mode and into a better title. Survivor was another term I never coined for myself and I really didn't want to hold a title that heavy either. Love-inspirer sounds much better.

It is all about finding an equilibrium between ease and struggle, frustration and delight, and of course comfort and vulnerability. And it's the in between that I have been looking for and where I am finally finding my own sense of balance.

BEYOND 365 DAYS

Getting curious and taking action was how I spent an entire solid year. And during that time I climbed over the original weight I revealed somewhere mid-stream. I was beyond embarrassed and didn't even want to admit it. But I continued on and completed the year-long commitment I ultimately had made to myself.

Many times throughout I circled back to tired habits and old ways, but each time I picked myself up, I dusted myself off and got my butt back on the better track—through love.

That 365th day came and went and what I felt was a sense of relief that the pressure had been lifted. Not in the sense that it was a relief that I didn't have to work so hard at loving myself anymore, but really that I could focus on continuing my journey toward achieving more love in a way that was only for me, rather than recording it for the book-world to see.

Many times throughout this journey, huge doses of doubt washed over me. And I wondered; What the heck was I doing? Why wasn't I loving myself enough? Why was it taking so long? And would I ever get there?

Sure enough, the intention to love myself transitioned into holding myself accountable through self-care. Whether or not the book would ever come to fruition was a whole other story.

On October 27th I was officially down 19 pounds. It was only a few short weeks after my experiment had come to an end. Was love the answer? Would being mindfully aware of whether or not I am feeding myself more love actually be the secret to weight loss, a healthy body and state of mind?

Putting on my jewelry I took a sneak peek into two books on my nightstand; Oprah's "What I Know for Sure" and "The Best of Erma Bombeck." I was saving them for when I finished writing my own book, because I couldn't bring myself to pick up anyone else's words while I was crafting my own.

I didn't want to risk getting derailed or having my own style and voice get crushed by inferiority or doubt. I already had all that I could handle, and I didn't dare send myself into stage fright. So I was saving them. But I took a sneak peek. And the two sentences I read from each book gave me the dose of confidence I needed to keep going.

It was January 23rd when I finally discovered that tomato puree was lectin-free because the tomatoes were actually skinned and seeded before they were canned. Green food is delicious, like homemade guacamole and basil pesto, and it was where my focus

I AM ON A LOVE DIET

was on, but I was in love with my red sauce again!

My husband told me that our bodies have a short-term memory. And maybe he's right, but it feels like my body is accepting that what I am doing is long-term and permanent. It feels like my body is following my lead.

By February 4th I was back up to being down 18 pounds. I didn't give in to the helpless emotional binging monster though. It still lives and breathes inside me and it tugged on my heart strings. In a moment of frustration, exhaustion, and feelings of emptiness—it was begging to be fed. But I didn't do it. I didn't feed the helpless voice that wasn't coming from the real me. And it became weak.

I know now, that in those moments, it's even more vital for me to hold the key to my own control center. Because when I give in, I never win. Whether it's sugar, carbs, wine or some kind of junk food that still sits on the high horse; whatever that binging monster wants, I have to be the one who decides and learn to hear the helpless emotional cries. I can't ignore it and I have to answer the calls, in healthier ways so my soul stays alive.

March 6th was day 1 of 40, and I was back up to being down 17 pounds. When I wrote about trying to give up something I love for Lent during my journey it was an honest-to-goodness effort. And I only got a few days of tasting what sacrificing something I love would feel like. This time I made a conscious decision to give it a solid try. This time I gave up potato chips, pizza, white and red wine.

I was ready to embrace the humility. And I saw this second chance as a time in my life solely as an opportunity to crush the other experience. Engaging in the Lent experience wasn't a punishment, but an experimental gift that I wanted to give to myself. To know what it would feel like to completely let go. I was curious to see how I would feel on that 40th day after ridding my body from the fatty, medicinal, greasy and salty.

When I went to bed I wasn't thinking about wine, chips or pizza. All I could think about was how my clean body would feel through 40 days and 40 nights. Even when my husband poured himself a second glass of wine at dinner, I could care less. What I cared more about was my new mission to love myself yet even more.

Lying in bed I decided to give in to one of my books that was staring back at me. The "Seat of the Soul" by Gary Zukov. And while I was learning about my own soul, I felt myself opening up to the universe just a little more.

On March 7th my blood pressure was 115 over 70. It was the first time I had checked it in a while and it was proof that what I was doing was in fact, worth it. I had been so curious if changing my diet was really working and it turned out that salt was indeed the slut of all seasonings. Inside the doctor's office results—my state of health was solidified—with a little peace of truth.

When my husband walked in the door his energy wavered a little. We were having our date night and he wasn't sure if I was going to be okay with him having wine at the restaurant. But I was totally fine with it. *What I was doing was for me.* At our table for two I had sparkling water with lemon and our conversation was good. It didn't bother me in the least to have a full view of other people celebrating at the bar either.

It was day 24 of 40 on March 29th when I was sitting in the patient room at the express clinic. Four days previously I had gotten up out of bed in the morning and my body threw myself across the room.

It was like nothing I had ever felt before and I had been paying close attention to my every move for four days, but I knew I had to be seen. They ruled out an ear infection and of course, pregnancy, and even though I passed the neurological exam, they wouldn't treat me for vertigo. Not unless I went to the emergency room first.

Driving myself there and on the phone with my insurance company, they told me that my co-pay was in fact, $700 and I hadn't met my $2,000 deductible yet. Needless to say, there was no way I was going to pay $2,700 for anyone to tell me they had great news—that the brain tumor results came back negative. So I made an appointment with my doctor and chiropractor instead. And picked up some Dramamine on my way home.

On April 16th I was officially down exactly 25 pounds on day 42 of Lent. You would think I would be excited, but I had lingered at the same weight loss for about five days and my heart wanted to see the next number. The fact that my body was following suit with every choice I was making was still not good enough to feed my spirit.

I felt like I was falling out of love. *I was still conditioned to be unsatisfied with slower progress and I wanted to shrink faster than my body was capable of.* So I gave in to crinkle cut potato chips! They are one of my favorite binges and I ate bite after delicious bite. It's so interesting how I can easily be swayed and pulled back under—by my own impatient thoughts.

April 18th had arrived, and I completed 44 days of Lent. I kept it going even through the four Sundays of reprieve too. And even though I gave in two days early to the potato chips, in my eyes this Lent experience, was a huge success. I had sacrificed things that I loved. And I did it because I wanted to.

But of course, I was ready to bring back the adult-beverage called wine and for the first time in 44 days, I ordered a glass of chardonnay. It was the house brand at a chain restaurant, and it tasted awful. But I drank it anyway because I knew my taste buds would readjust.

On April 27th I was down 26 pounds. It felt like my body was finally listening to me. It had been *18 months* since my love diet began and I prayed that my body would continue to let go of even more fat.

While having lunch, a couple of friends told me I looked great and really didn't need to lose any more weight. Which I thought was supportive, but also very interesting. The funny thing was, at this stage I wasn't trying to *lose* anything. I was just sticking to my love diet plan.

It was May 3rd when I was searching for information about fiber and what foods have good amounts of it. What came up on most lists were beans, broccoli, berries, avocado, popcorn, whole grains, apples, and dried fruits. I was avoiding fruits of course because of their sugar content, and I was confused as to how I would know if I were consistently getting the proper amount of fiber each day, without taking a supplement.

I didn't have any issues with irregularity unless I ate too many almonds or almond crackers. But my cholesterol was still not where it needed to be. I was planning to go back and get it

I AM ON A LOVE DIET

checked again when I had a solid three months under my belt without the fatty pizza. And in addition to removing pizza, I wanted to add fiber into my diet because adding fiber is known to reduce cholesterol.

<u>By May 16th I was down 27 pounds.</u> Almost immediately after seeing the number—I ate chips. It sort of made sense. To treat myself right away with something I loved and then, get back to my love diet plan. My love diet was far from perfect. And to compensate, I chose to remove carbs at dinner for three days.

I made another decision: to completely let go of red meat. And another; to remove palm oil from our home and our diets. All variations of it which included palm, stear, laur, and glyc.

My son had to watch a documentary for school and asked us to watch it with him. It was with Leonardo DiCaprio and it's called "Before the Flood." From watching the simple documentary, it made the decision for me to remove red meat and palm oil easy.

Reducing animal fats was what I was already doing anyway to lower my cholesterol. But having a healthy body will do me no good if there's no planet for me to live on. The damage we do to Mother Earth might not come full circle in my lifetime, but it could in my kids' and for several generations of my family that follow. I was just one person, but I was more than willing to do my part.

On a bigger scale, letting go of red meat and palm oil were two of the smallest things I could do to help the planet that would indeed help me to love my body. Palm is found in most packaged junk foods anyway. They were two simple things that I could easily live without. And by living without, I was in fact, helping the planet. The decision to me came effortlessly. *It feels good, now that my choices come without hesitation—and it feels even better to get a true taste of unconditional self-love.*

<u>On May 22nd</u> my restaurant owner friend said, "Do you really believe that you can make a difference? You're just one person." I said, "Yes, I totally believe that I can make a difference*!* One person can make a huge difference. I'm starting with removing palm from my home and not eating red meat. And I'm sharing that with everyone I know. If we all don't do our part to support the planet, there will be no planet to live on." He just smiled like he wished he could do the same.

I want to live to be 108 years old or older. So I need to do my share. None of us can comprehend the weight of the world on our shoulders alone. But if we all try not to eat beef and remove palm oil wherever and whenever we can, we will all be helping make that positive and sustainable change happen.

<u>At dinner on May 25th</u> the couple sitting next to me declined the dessert offer from our barkeep. I overheard her say that she was dieting, and her husband wasn't allowed to eat any sweets in front of her. I couldn't help but smile while waiting for my husband.

Reaching for my business card I shared with her that I'm creating my own diet and writing a book about it. And we both jumped right into many conversations about diet and food, stealing the stage and barely letting her husband take a seat. And she was very determined and proud that she was sticking with her new diet.

The diet she was following didn't allow for any sugar at all, or carbs or dairy. No beer or wine either. She said she would love to read my book, but she wanted to stick with her new diet for now. Then I asked her, "Do you think you can live this way for the rest of your life? I think we need some sugar and carbs in our bodies." I went on to tell her that I still eat carbs, sugar, dairy and still enjoy wine and I've lost 27 pounds since July. And I had kept it off for about ten months. She said, "Well, maybe I'll be doing your love diet next."

My hope is that my love diet will become a household name. Just like BubbaGump Shrimp.

When <u>August 29th</u> arrived I was down 29 pounds. When we got home after our date night dinner with pizza for the kids, I sat at my island and watched all of my kids pacing while eating their pizza. The energy was high. My husband was eating a slice too and enjoying another glass of wine. The energy was palpable, and it wasn't easy to shield myself from it.

Still, I had no desire to eat the pizza they were all oohing and ahhing over. I did want to have a glass of wine though just a little, but I was choosing not to and trying to abstain until my book was complete. I wanted to keep my head clear.

Looking around the room and watching my loved ones consume food and beverages that I no longer chose to have was interesting. A little sad too. Only because I had no food in front of me. Just a glass of sparkling water. Reaching for the popcorn in the pantry I realized we were out, so I stood in the kitchen absorbing their energy while making popcorn for myself the old-fashioned way—on the stove.

<u>By August 31st</u> my diet was becoming so easy for me to live with, even on vacation. It's not so strict that I can't enjoy eating out with family and friends. And I even bent my own rules

with a little extra sugar, cheese and glasses of wine. It's so great though because when I return, it only takes a day or two to shrink back down from the three pounds I climbed up.

I had been toying with a variety of titles for this chapter and after we came home from our weekend getaway on Martha's Vineyard, almost two years after the start of my diet, it came to me. I said to my husband, "*I love my diet!*"

FROM "OUT THERE" TO "IN HERE"

When I think about what I used to look like before my love diet began, I still wonder how I could have ever let myself get that far off track. I was practically oblivious to everything that was going on inside my body. But maybe I'm no different than anyone else. And placing so much padding around my heart was an unhealthy way to exist. It's not easy—to not judge the old me.

Just like smoking was not a healthy way to exist. Luckily, I was able to quit. Twice. The second time was when I was trying to conceive my first child and I quit cold turkey. Ironically, what helped me get through it was to count the days I accomplished and accumulate my successes. In turn the days of successfully living smoke-free became more powerful than the desire to take a drag. And I got myself to a point where there was no way I was willing to start all over again on Day 1. My mind made the shift from wanting a cigarette to wanting to increase my smoke-free power.

The first time I successfully quit was when I was around 18 and a friend said he would hand me $100 cash if I quit smoking for an entire year. Additionally, he mentioned that he made that bet with several people and none of them lasted the total 365 days. Selfishly, I did it to be the first. I did it to win.

Two and a half years after the start of my journey I have kept off 24 to 29 pounds. I am listening to my body more than I ever have in my life and I can only imagine what I will look like in another two or three years of living this way. I don't even exercise vigorously or in high quantities. I just dance on occasion and practice yoga daily. Whether it's for eight minutes or eighteen doesn't matter. As long as I move my body.

Reducing my sodium was the best place to start for me. But I had to go deeper than counting milligrams. I had to remove or significantly reduce many things whenever possible like soups, sauces, spreads, gravies, dips and dressings. I knew that doing this one simple thing would indeed help lower my blood pressure within a few weeks. And it did.

Animal fats got a little trickier for me. The concept was easy to swallow, but it took a little more time to avoid the fatty foods that I had been accustomed to eating throughout my life. It did get easier to let go of some of those foods that clung to me, because I knew they were clogging me. Deli meat was one of the easiest things to let go of first. Then it took a little more work to say goodbye to most cheese, bacon, pepperoni, and red meat. But I got there. In my heart, I knew it was what I needed to do to love myself up a notch—and my mind came around in time.

Becoming gluten-free-sensitive helped pave the way to one of the biggest challenges of all—removing most sugar. The tiniest morsel had made the biggest impact because it's practically in everything. So, learning about it meant a lot of trial and error in the beginning. I still get stuck at things like fruit, because my mind tries to tell me it's a good thing to eat. But even the dumb caveman only ate fruit in the warmer months. Sugar was hiding in the food I was eating, and it wasn't easy to let go of one of the biggest team players. Sugar was the star.

The suggested pyramid has been upside down on my cereal box for years. And now my pyramid starts with vegetables with just about every meal and healthy fats of course. Then I think about rice, potato, gluten-free pasta or bread. The low hanging fruit now sits upside-down with the point at the bottom of my pyramid.

Who knows how much further my love diet will take me, but my future is much clearer now than it ever was. I am choosing foods that help me thrive and will keep me alive and strong for many years to come. It isn't always easy to keep it up, but most of the time it is easy, even when other people are enjoying the types of food I no longer eat.

I know that everything I do today will help me achieve healthier days in my future. And I have said often and openly that I want to build my business slowly, so that it's achievable and also sustainable. Building a healthy foundation for my body is the same. It's in complete alignment with my overall mission. *What's important is being consciously aware of my choices and making smarter decisions because I care about myself.*

What I have done is open up my arms to love and it's what I've needed the most of. Not a fad diet. But true love. It made more sense for me to slow down and stop looking everywhere else but "in here." I wasn't broken, but I am malleable. And I began by paying attention to whether or not I was in fact feeding my body love. Most of the time I wasn't. I was feeding into the old and regurgitating the pain.

Stopping for a moment to watch a short video with Dr. Wayne Dyer, I took a moment to be guided by his soul. He talked about when he was a professor at St. Johns' University in Queens,

I AM ON A LOVE DIET

New York where my son was currently attending. It was the year his first book was about to come out and what he said stuck with me. He thought really hard about whether or not he wanted to live for 90 years—or spend 90 years living the same year over and over again.

Like him, I wanted to live. And it turns out it's possible to create positive and sustainable change. It's also easy to fall back into old ways or through the process, become impatient. And bringing my thoughts back into focus takes practice. Eventually I saw a clear path and began carving it out for myself.

Educating myself and my kids through this process is part of what it took. And I am beyond proud of myself for being their thought leader, and my own love-inspirer that I have become. I am over the moon excited to continue learning and sharing what I discovered with everyone on the same path to better health and world-wide wellness.

I imagine I will be spending more of my time in the years ahead enjoying my loved ones and my life, rather than struggling or fighting with myself—within it. And now that I am fearlessly speaking my truth through love, my relationship with myself will evolve and expand even more gloriously.

On Day 223 I had italicized *"I was a binger"* and when I was editing that day, I saw the words for the first time—in the past tense. And it was simply because I could hardly call myself a binger anymore. I still do it, but it's very different. I am fully aware, and I know myself better. I love myself through each challenge.

None of us have a crystal ball. And what I have done is choose to pencil in my future by taking one small step at a time. Day by day and week by week, which has now transitioned into month by month and year by year. As much as I'd love to see the number on my crystal scale shrink even smaller, I don't have a goal weight. It's more like a range. I let go of my original idea of fitting into a size eight plan too. In my mind, I am not at my final number—even though I don't have a number in mind.

Before I had my first child I was about 160 pounds and after my second child—I had slimmed down to 148. Searching the "ideal" body weight for a woman my height and age was anywhere from 118 to 148 pounds. But trying to reach either of those numbers or any of the ones in between feels heavy, drastic and even unhealthy. Maybe if I were 20, but at my age, I just want to keep loving myself. I still look to crystal to follow my progress, and through each day my body is getting smarter. Organically, I will land where I land.

My energy is different now and it's because I am different. I wasn't really living when I was hiding behind conversations about all the wrong that was going on "out there" in the food industry, dieting world, or even in the past. And I didn't want to hide behind rationalization any longer. I wanted to break free from being told how to eat or live. Free from righteous theory after theory. I love my diet now. And what I've created is easy to tweak as I continue to learn better ways to feed my body love.

It took over two years of living this journaling experiment to be able to see my own patterns. And I fell back into old ways many times throughout. I saw myself blaming and complaining again in December. And I caught myself saying things like "I've put a few pounds back on because it's the stress of the holidays, and I'm drinking a little more wine than usual, and the wedding, and transitioning to vegan." The list goes on. But chaining those excuses together was not love. And it was making it easier to not care about myself by rationalizing. So I took back ownership and

I AM ON A LOVE DIET

made the decision to stop blaming and get back to taking action.

There is no rewind button and it's important for me to pay attention to where I need improvement. On December 12th I held myself accountable again and decided to do yoga for the twelve days until Christmas. And those twelve days grew into almost five months.

I don't want to be somebody I'm not. It's uncomfortable and it throws me off. I just want to be me. I want to set organic intentions for myself that are achievable. I like slowing down now instead of living in that go-go-go mode. I like continuously striving to live in the present moment. What I know is that it took me a long time, longer than one year to arrive at a place of inner peace. And I'm still not there 100 percent.

What I had to do was the dirty work. I'm almost there, and it's as though the floodgates have been opened and the abundance of love is finally rushing through me organically and gracefully. It feels really good to make better decisions about my overall health and my future. *And I'm so glad that my kids have front row seats to watch me love myself more.* I'm so grateful for all that I have achieved and through healing my own body it shows exponentially in my heart, my nails, my skin and even on my scale. Every choice I have made can't help but to show up on the outside. And I'm so blessed to have the creative insight to share my thoughts and actions that may inspire someone else to pour more self-care and love into their own body and life.

It still makes me sad to see the people I love continue to eat the foods that are filled with negative energy because I am living proof that we can heal our own bodies. And it had to start with my mind before my body could adapt.

My relationship with myself is a more loving intimate one. Every day I work on my desire to give only the best to myself.

When doubt steps in the way, I crush it with the positive reality that I am literally doing this. Each tiny thing I do is accumulating and getting me closer to where I want to be. Every day I turn my beliefs into actions. I am finally able to keep some thoughts out of my meditation and journal them instead because I care more about the benefits of quieting my mind. I'm beginning to crave the clear and clean. I am open to exercising my body and I'm cooking healthy meals that are beautiful and delicious. I am taking better care of myself through love.

Sustainable love is what I strive for. Because I want the loving relationship I'm having with myself to continue to spill over to the ones I love and even the world of people that I don't. And that comes from focusing on me, being with me, and doing things for me. Not from looking for other things "out there" to fix or complete me.

My book is just a small piece of my story though. It's raw and real, but it's more about asking the why's, what if's, and who says and how about I try it my way. I made the decision to spend an entire year of my time journaling my thoughts around my struggle with dieting, the challenge with junk foods, the reality of binging, and the practically non-existent nutrition inside my body. I turned many of those provocative thoughts and questions into some statements and answers.

My hope is my intention. That sharing my story can and will make a positive difference in the world when it comes to our diets and how we think about the human diet. Because what I needed was to strip down everything I knew and thought to be true about health and wellness, back to the simple basics of loving myself and my body more. I know I still have a ways to go, but I will be able to let go of more weight over time. Because it takes time.

Now, I can't imagine living my life without giving myself the extra care and love that I needed and still need. As I sit here writing this final chapter, approximately two and a half years from that first day, I am amazed at how much I have discovered and shifted. But more astounded at how much love for myself that I have organically acquired. I was a diamond in the rough as they say, and I still have so much more polishing to do—to reveal even more brilliance from within.

What I've created is sticking. I still get stuck. Like eating a muffin with my butter dish handy for reapplying. It's just smaller now, gluten-free, and homemade. And most of the time it's just toast. Each decision I have made has accumulated and brought me to a better place of health and wellness. And through it all, what I was actually doing was working on my mental health too. In a little over two years, I've gotten better at knowing what living a healthy life really feels like.

The love I have for myself has come through and I was finally able to see clearly that I did have what it takes to turn my own life around. Even when the emotions of depression settle in, love is stronger. Depression is just an emotion and it's the one that gets stripped away just before love breaks through.

Love has not always been easy for me to turn to. Even when I tattooed the word onto my wrist to see it each day it eventually faded into the every day. Loving myself 100 percent all day, and every day is still not what I have done, but I keep on keeping on. I keep striving to love myself more. I keep staying curious and asking myself the harder questions that I really never wanted to ask. I keep on trying and doing. And eventually it clicked. Love has become my magical trick.

I'm almost 100 percent vegan now. And that came after two years of working at eating cleaner, struggling with my own cholesterol, and learning about the environment. Ironically, it wasn't deep seeded emotional compassion for other living creatures that led me to becoming vegan, but mostly compassion for myself—and the next several generations of my family that will live long after me that made me reintroduce a vegetarian life. And within two weeks I quickly and effortlessly transitioned to vegan.

When I asked my vegan friend what he ate for protein his response reflected a bit of accumulative irritation. "Protein is in everything!" he said. Instinctively I said, "Oh like mushrooms?" He stood even stronger in his statement. Again he said, "It's in everything!"

The meals I make for myself and my family now are far more creative, and taste better than one would expect. And eating tasteless food or a salad twice a day is boring. It feels like a punishment. Someday my goal is to eat almost entirely whole food, plant-based or WFPB, which isn't easy. And trying out just a few recipes takes a lot more effort than hamburger helper and so far, it's so much easier to be a healthy or even a lazy vegan.

When I watched "Forks Over Knives" for the first time and learned that the body doesn't need as much protein as we thought we did, it was huge to me. Additionally that consuming twenty percent of animal proteins with each meal can in fact, "turn on" cancer while decreasing our proteins to five percent can turn it off. Well, what can I say? The theory made perfect sense to me.

Perhaps the cure for cancer was right in front of us the whole time in the form of greens. And that theory sent me quickly and effortlessly from only two weeks of becoming a legit vegetarian to going full vegan. Watching "Forks Over Knives" was an education and it was eye-opening to learn that filling my

I AM ON A LOVE DIET

body up with turkey burgers was not necessarily "filling my stomach" because, in fact, it is the vegetables that are what fill our stomachs up, more than any other food. Excitedly, I brought back whole corn and popcorn without skipping a beat.

I don't know why I was so surprised that the two gentlemen at my local grocer, one 30 years younger than me and one about 15 years older, were not on the same page as I was about our health and the world we all benefit from. It was so strange but interesting that I was the one teaching both of them. And they both thanked me.

They thanked me. First came the vegan millennial at check out. He brought me the vegan butter he uses, but I kindly told him that it didn't pass my *free from palm oil* test. I told him I'd rather keep eating real butter because it was better for the planet. He didn't know that just because something was labeled vegan, that not all vegans will eat it. And the product he handed me had one of the worst hidden ingredient terms there is, "vegetable oil." Unless the nutrition label states clearly what vegetable oils are, in fact, in the product, it's their way of hiding palm oil—in the product. I wasn't willing to support the continued destruction of palm trees and said I was continuing on my quest.

Then there was the 65-year-old politician dude trying to get signatures outside. I wanted to get something in return for my signature, so I asked him kindly what his thoughts were about the environment and the planet. He immediately went right into a speech about water with a seemingly go-to responsive tone. I let him know that his campaign would benefit from watching the Leonardo documentary and handed him my business card. I thanked him in advance for being open to learning and when I wished him luck I said if he promised to watch it he'd have my vote.

Now that I am eating even more cleanly because of my passion for the environment and the earth that I will leave behind for my children and their children and their children, I feel physically and mentally elated, educated and empowered. The world is ours. And together we all need to respect it. The frustration I felt was equivalent to the elation I had in the new driving force behind my mission to heal, support, and motivate. *Love IS in the palm of our own hands.*

Just because something can be recycled or we are told it can be, doesn't mean it's a good idea to keep buying it too. Is it really recyclable? Do we need it? How will this impact the planet where my children will continue to live and my grandchildren and my greats? Not everything is recyclable. Not all numbers one through seven are recyclable. Only the one's, two's and five's, can in fact, be transformed. Most recycled products will still find their way into landfills.

Plastic worries me. And I pay close attention to every product that comes into my home. And I want to do whatever I can to reduce and reuse. Recycling just isn't what it's supposed to be. Everything I purchase now is questionable. Is it worth it? Is it a single-use product or can I reuse it multiple times? I question because I care.

The expectation of practicing what I preach and my desire and willingness to actually love myself wholeheartedly is going to take more time. And I have come such a long way to revert back to how I used to eat and live and how I wasn't really caring for myself.

It's such a cliché but it's true. From love, through love, with love, for love, in love, and about love. When everything I do

I AM ON A LOVE DIET

stems from love, most worry, fear, anxiety and depression can disappear. I found a good place, but really what I found is a lot more peace. And the love inside of me that has always been there didn't come through by losing a lot of weight, but by working diligently to loving myself more and more each day.

When I think about it, the two and a half years I have spent living this way is really not that much time at all. And the one year of true discovery was my quick fix and what it took to kick-start myself into a healthier direction. The eighteen months that followed by continuing gave me a taste of a newer life and what was still to come.

My eyes have been opened and have shown me that slowing down and really taking a strong hard look at all of my habits and behaviors was a positive thing. And it helped me to see that *proactive doctor visits* is love and I need to keep those appointments ongoing for the love of my future.

My love diet has helped me to take it slowly and only do things and make changes when I was ready. And I realized that I did in fact have an eating disorder that my mind wanted to hide. Through my love diet I have been able to shift an old and tired mindset into a stronger healthier one that will continue to evolve.

Embracing my love diet has helped me to take a stand and take control of my own body. Through my love diet I have transformed. I am a completely different person than I was two and a half years ago. And I have kept off 24 to 29 pounds. An average of 27 pounds of lost weight isn't a lot to some people for 30 months of effort and time invested, but it's not just about the weight. Through my love diet I have changed my body on the inside.

I am cleaner because I eat cleaner and my relationship with food is healthier. I look at everything differently now. Food,

Nicole Perry

body image, wine consumption and the planet too. My love diet has helped me to see sugar for what it is and to really pay close attention to where the sugar lies. My love diet was in fact, not too good to be true. It was simply a door that I decided to walk through. And it led me to a place where there was more love.

I AM ON A LOVE DIET

Made in the USA
Middletown, DE
14 September 2020